DATE			

OMNI'S
FUTURE MEDICAL
ALMANAC

OTHER BOOKS BY DICK TERESI

The Three-Pound Universe (1986)

Laser (1982)

Omni's Continuum:
Dramatic Phenomena from the
New Frontiers of Science (1982)

OMNI'S FUTURE MEDICAL ALMANAC

edited by
Dick Teresi and Patrice G. Adcroft

An OMNI Book

McGRAW-HILL BOOK COMPANY

New York   St. Louis   San Francisco   Toronto   Hamburg   Mexico

This book is not intended to replace the services of a physician. Any application of the recommendations set forth in the following pages is at the reader's discretion and sole risk.

1 2 3 4 5 6 7 8 9 DOC DOC 8 7 6

ISBN 0-07-063505-6

Library of Congress Cataloging-in-Publication Data

Omni's future medical almanac.

  Includes bibliographies.
    1. Medical innovations.   2. Medical innovations—
Forecasting.   3. Twenty-first century—Forecasts.
I. Teresi, Dick.   II. Adcroft, Patrice.   III. Omni
(New York, N.Y.)   [DNLM: 1. Forecasting—popular works.
2. Medicine—trends—popular works.   3. Research—
popular works.   WB 130 055]
RA418.5.M4056   1987   610   86-21314
ISBN 0-07-063505-6

Book design by Sharen DuGoff Egana
Editing Supervisor: Margery Luhrs

Contributors

Chief of Research: Catherine Spencer

    Writers:

Healing Currents: Ellen Kunes

Redesigning the Brain: Judith Hooper

Super Tests: Mary Ellin Barrett

The Real Bionic Man: David Masello

Childbirth 2000: Linda Marsa

The Biochemistry of Desire: Peter Tyson

An End to Pain: Peter Tyson

Off the Disabled List: Jane Bosveld

The Healing Ray: Jeff Hecht

The Heredity Factor: Linda Marsa

War on Fat: Randy Steele

Super Foods, Megavitamins: Kevin McKinney

Immortality Made Easy: Susan Ellis

The Last Whole Body Catalog: compiled by Murray Cox

Contents

---

14. The Last Whole Body Catalog   336

Breathing Easier. Bucktoothed Kids. Knifeless Face-Lifts. Pollen Cure.
Pain Free, Naturally. Short-Circuiting Migraines. Dry Mouth. Innovative
Hearing. Sweet Treatment. Anti-inflammatory Drug. Male Infertility.
Allergy Consult. Healing Bubbles. Titanium Teeth. Heart Patches. Bioptic
Lenses. Healing Toxin. Blood-Clotting Aid.

Introduction
Taking Advantage of Medical Breakthroughs

We were among the first nonscientists in the world to hold the Jarvik-7 in our hands.

Long before the polyurethane, titanium, and dacron heart was beating away inside Barney Clark, we were disassembling it in the lab. "Go ahead, pull the two ventricles apart," urged one of the scientists. We pulled, and the artificial heart split in two, making that satisfying ripping sound that only Velcro can make. The researcher laughed at our surprise. So, it's as simple as that, we thought. Someday a man will owe his life to a plastic pump that's stuck together with Velcro.

The year was 1978, and we had traveled to Salt Lake City to cover a story that was to become the most frequently reprinted article in *Omni* magazine's history. Called "The Real Bionic Man," the article told of the bioengineering exploits of medical researchers at the University of Utah, scientists who were building artificial vision systems, synthetic ears, artificial kidneys, blood vessels, and various other organs, and even a computerized arm controlled by human thoughts.

But the Utah group was proudest of the Jarvik-7, designed by the now famous Robert Jarvik, head of its heart program. At the time, the Jarvik-7 was only being used to power the circulatory system of Theodore, a frisky veal calf in Utah's artificial heart lab. But the Jarvik-7 was man-sized, and clearly the Utah crowd had its sights set on bigger game.

As soon as the article hit the newsstands, the criticism began to roll in. We were accused of writing "science fiction disguised as science fact." An artificial heart to be implanted in human beings? Harumph! Not only scientists, but other science journalists as well, thought we had gone one toke over the line in publishing such nonsense. The implication: Either the scientists we interviewed were crackpots or we had made it all up.

Of course, as everybody who hasn't been vacationing under the South Pole now knows, the Jarvik-7 was implanted in Barney Clark only 4 years after the article appeared. Despite problems, the bionic heart has kept other patients alive for a full year or longer. And, of course, the same critics who had derided the Jarvik-7 as science fiction a few years earlier have now hailed it as the medical advance of the decade.

Which all goes to prove that, when it comes to medicine, the future often gets here faster than one expects. The book you're about to read is dedicated to that position. What we are attempting here is to report not only on the most advanced therapies now available to the public, but also on those pills, devices, and operations that are still in the research or experimental stage. We are treading that line where the present meets the future. And in each case, we will help those who wish to step over that line, by providing what we hope will be useful information on where to go next.

How to Read This Book

We have divided the future of medicine into fourteen different categories—electrohealing, tests, childbirth, pain control, sports medicine, etc.—and sent a team of reporters to ferret out the latest innovations in each field. Each chapter presents medical science's cutting edge, but we also take a hard look at what the future will bring. We are looking at the current basic research and ongoing clinical trials, along with the fantasies of medicine's brightest minds, dreams that will change the face of health care in the 1990s and beyond. Included in each chapter is a Timeline, an informed estimate of when we can expect such breakthroughs as home medical robots, artificial eyes, and effective aphrodisiacs, to name a few.

More important, though, is a special feature we've included for the *present*. At *Omni* we have learned that any story on a medical advance, no matter how futuristic, brings an influx of mail and phone calls for more information. After our "Real Bionic Man" article, for example, we (and the University of Utah) were deluged with letters from amputees who wanted bionic limbs. We heard from the families of blind persons who wanted to know more about artificial sight. From dialysis patients who wanted portable kidney machines. It seems that the most adventurous people in medical science today are the patients.

So, at the end of every chapter, you'll find an Access Guide with suggested names, addresses, and sometimes phone numbers of practitioners, clinics, and institutions to be contacted for more information. For example, if you're interested in any of the pain-relieving techniques described in Chapter 7, you'll find a list of pain clinics in the Access Guide. Be forewarned that many of the therapies described in this book are futuristic or experimental. But the Access Guides will allow you to track down those treatments that lie in the twilight zone between common use and basic research, where the future seeps quietly into the present. How many times have you asked your family doctor about some medical breakthrough you read about in a newspaper or magazine, only to find that he or she had never heard of it? Obviously, the average general practitioner cannot keep up with the rapid advances of medical science. The Access Guides are your chance to take matters into your own hands—at least in terms of gathering information and helping you to find more informed medical help.

A Word of Caution

Finally, we should stress that we are not physicians, and that this book is not meant as an endorsement for any of the practitioners, clinics, institutions, drugs, or devices mentioned. We are journalists who have set out to report on what is state of the art in medicine and what are its frontiers. We hope the following serves as a guide to the future and as a sourcebook for the present.

1

Healing Currents: Electric Cures for the Mind and Body

It happened the night of her high school graduation in June, 1978. Nan Davis and a few friends were returning home from the graduation ceremonies when the boy driving the tiny Volkswagen lost control of the wheel. The car flipped over and rolled into a nearby ditch. Nan, who had played on her high school's track, basketball, and gymnastics teams, who had waterskiied since the age of 4, had broken her back and her neck. She would never walk again.

Or so doctors thought at the time. But with the aid of an electrical stimulation device hooked up to a microprocessor, Nan *was* able to walk again. At a much publicized news conference in 1982, Nan took her first difficult steps, and a year later she slowly walked up to the podium at Wright State University to collect her college degree.

Thousands of people today are overcoming paralysis, pain, bone fractures, bedsores, drug abuse, and a host of other disorders with the healing powers of electrical current. More and more, doctors are beginning to do as poet Walt Whitman professed he did—that is to "sing the body electric."

"Electricity will become as ubiquitous in medical practice as surgery or drugs; in many instances, it will supplant them," predicts Dr. Andrew Bassett of Columbia Presbyterian Hospital. Bassett and scores of other researchers have blazed trails in electrical healing, a struggling branch of medicine with ancient roots. Doctors have known of electricity's therapeutic powers as far back as the time of the Roman Empire, when they treated headaches by pressing electric eels to the temples of the stricken.

In more recent times, though, with charlatans including "elec-

trical cure-alls" in their little black bags, acceptance of electricity's
healing powers has been slow. In the early twentieth century, Dr.
Hercules Sanche promoted the Oxydonor, an electrical device which
he claimed would make people thirst for oxygen—and breathing
in more oxygen, he said, would cure them of a number of diseases.
Perhaps the most notorious example of electrical healing quackery
was San Francisco physician Albert Abram's Oscilloclast, an im-
pressive-looking electrical box which he claimed would diagnose
and treat such serious ills as tuberculosis, syphilis, bacterial infections, and cancer.

But what doctors around the world are now beginning to recognize as fact is that we do have a "body electric"; our internal
communication network transmits messages in a language that is,
by and large, made up of electrical signals. Each special signal
determines whether our cells will grow, proliferate, repair
themselves—or if they will die. By tapping into this internal communications system with external currents, some so weak that they
wouldn't light up an electric bulb, scientists are finding that they
can alter the messages to the cells. It may one day be possible to
regenerate severed spinal cords and weakened heart muscle, to
regrow the limbs of the amputee, or even to stop the runaway
growth of cancer cells.

The progress researchers have made toward these goals in the
past 35 years is startling. The catalyst for much of the heightened
interest in the field has been Dr. Robert O. Becker, who began his
career as an orthopedic surgeon in 1956 at the Veteran's Administration Hospital in Syracuse, New York. "The concept that human
beings respond to magnetic fields, is, I think, going to revolutionize
biology. It will revolutionize medicine."

At the rate research is going, the revolution Becker speaks of
may soon touch each and every one of us. Electrical currents are
now being used to heal stubborn fractures that refuse to mend on
their own. Doctors believe electricity may also cure other afflictions
of the bones, including osteoporosis, the brittle-bones disease which
is responsible for 1.3 million fractures yearly in American women
over 45. Exciting advances are being made in the area of spinal
cord regeneration: Researchers around the world are reporting success in stimulating the regrowth of severed peripheral nerves—

those found in the limbs—and many believe that ability to regrow the damaged spinal cord, thereby restoring movement to the paralyzed, may not be far off.

Drug addicts, alcoholics, and smokers are also benefitting from advances in electrohealing. A little black box developed by Scottish surgeon Margaret Patterson tunes into the electrical frequency of an addict's brain and alters the signals in a way that alleviates the painful symptoms of withdrawal.

Victims of spasticity disorders, such as cerebral palsy, are being aided by a spinal cord tuner. Electrodes imbedded into the spinal column and controlled by what looks like a Walkman unscramble the garbled signals being sent to the spastic limbs of cerebral palsy and multiple sclerosis victims, allowing them to function more normally. And some electrical treatments stimulate growth of bone, nerves, and soft tissue.

"Electricity is a tremendously powerful tool," says Andrew Bassett. Another pioneering electrician named Benjamin Franklin would have agreed. After being jolted by a few stray currents during one of his own experiments, Franklin was said to have muttered, ". . .if no other use is discovered for electricity, it will always serve to make a vain man humble."

The Spine Tuner

Today, Carmen Scozzari, 31, is able to move with ease. She walks without a limp, speaks clearly, writes smoothly—she can even play the guitar. Carmen appears so normal that it's hard to believe that a few short years ago she was confined to a wheelchair, her entire body locked into braces to straighten her twisted torso and limbs.

The victim of a rare, disabling disease called dystonia musculorum deformans, which garbles the messages the brain sends to the muscles, Carmen was unable to control the movements of most of her body and limbs. Her legs would go into painful spasms for hours at a time. It was difficult for her to swallow or speak, and she needed a mouthplate to keep her jaws from clenching. She experienced double vision and had lost control of her bladder.

But with the aid of a new spinal cord stimulation system, Carmen is able to move her body and limbs normally—with much less pain—and she's regained control of her bladder. Electrical spinal cord stimulators were first implanted in patients in the late 1960s to relieve chronic pain. But in 1973 it was observed that a patient with multiple sclerosis in whom a spinal cord stimulator had been implanted to lessen pain also experienced a marked decrease in spastic movement and great improvement in motor control.

As a result, Dr. Joseph Waltz, a neurosurgeon at St. Barnabas Hospital in New York City, began implanting stimulators in patients suffering from a number of other disorders characterized by uncontrollable spastic movements. These afflictions included cerebral palsy, spinal cord injuries, and post-stroke disorders, as well as multiple sclerosis and dystonia, the disease from which Carmen suffers. Dr. Waltz has treated 735 patients with electrical stimulation. He claims that 70 to 85 percent of them have experienced a moderate to marked improvement in motor control and function, with virtually no side effects.

In essence, muscles normally behave like finely tuned instruments: When given the correct messages from the central nervous system, they act in symphony with each other, and a nice, smooth movement results. But when the information they're given is distorted, this smooth balance is lost; there's no harmony between the muscles, and a spastic, uncontrolled movement results.

"What we do with electrical stimulation is essentially speak to the central nervous system on the only terms it understands," Waltz explains. "We try to alter the abnormal coded impulses and bring about a more normal system." To accomplish this, the patient has four electrodes, each the size of an eyelash, implanted into the upper area of the spine via a thin, hollow needle. Once they're threaded into place, the electrodes are hooked up to a radio frequency receiver, which is implanted just beneath the skin in the patient's lower side. Finally, a flat, round "antenna" taped to the patient's skin is hooked up to a battery powered transmitter the size of a small transistor radio (generally worn on the patient's belt). This transmitter sends signals to the receiver, which converts them into electrical impulses that speak to the brain, clearing away the wrong messages and sending out the right ones.

Each patient must have his or her stimulation system programmed specially. It generally takes from 6 to 8 weeks to hit on the electrode combination and frequency that gives the correct coded message to the muscles. "There's just no set frequency for each different disorder," Waltz explains.

The spinal cord stimulator cannot help most victims of paralysis, although Waltz contends that if a patient has spinal sections that are still intact, it may be possible to restore some function. Patients interested in the stimulator are carefully screened. "You don't want to perform a surgical technique unless the person has tried all the medications available—without success," Waltz adds. Currently, the spinal cord stimulator is being implanted at 24 institutions across the country—including UCLA, the University of Texas, Johns Hopkins, and Baylor University—on a clinical basis, and FDA approval is expected in 1986. A totally implantable system is now being readied for clinical testing.

The Brain Tuner

Of all the electrical devices developed to cure human ills in recent years, perhaps the most controversial is a little black box that is said to help drug addicts, alcoholics—even cigarette smokers—free themselves from their destructive habits. Technically known as *NeuroElectric Therapy (NET)*, this Walkman-like device was invented by Scottish surgeon Margaret Patterson and has been used by scores of British addicts of one kind or another to help them break their dependence on chemicals.

Just as Waltz's spinal cord device is able to "tune in" to the frequencies of the nerve impulses in the spine, Dr. Patterson's black box literally tunes in to her patients' brain waves: The NET box transmits a tiny electrical signal that seems to harmonize with natural brain rhythms. In doing so, it stimulates production of the body's natural painkillers, thus reducing craving, anxiety, and other symptoms of withdrawal from drugs and alcohol.

It sounds a little like black magic, but the black box seems to work. Patterson claims that in 1981, after a decade's worth of detoxifying patients with the aid of the box, a startling 98 percent of the 186 patients were drug-free at the end of the detoxification process. "I can take anyone off a drug of abuse, no matter how severe his or her addiction, with only minimal discomfort," Patterson says. Of course, Patterson points out, not all who successfully finish the NET treatment remain free of drugs—the therapy seems most effective when combined with counseling and strong support at home. Even so, the treatment does seem to be long-lasting. While in most drug programs, an average of 90 percent of addicts are unable to kick their habit for good, less than 20 percent of drug addicts who've completed Patterson's NeuroElectric Therapy have returned to their old habits.

Peter Townshend, the songwriter and lead guitarist who helped propel the English rock group The Who to stardom, turned to the NET box when he became addicted to alcohol and a variety of drugs in the early 1980s. Beset with marital and financial difficulties, Townshend began drinking heavily, then got hooked on cocaine, sleeping pills, and finally heroin. But after 10 days of tuning into the NET box, and receiving psychological counseling, he was drug-free—without having experienced the severe withdrawal symptoms that prevent most addicts from breaking their habits. "NET reeducates the brain to produce its own drugs, and in the process, you learn something about your human potential," Townshend said in an Omni interview. "You come to realize that somewhere within you is the power to deal with crises, tensions, and frustrations. So the treatment reaffirms one's faith in the self-healing process."

Patterson first stumbled over the idea for NET in 1972 when she was head of surgery at Tung Wah Hospital in Hong Kong. A colleague there, Dr. H. L. Wen, had recently returned from China, armed with knowledge of a technique known as electroacupuncture. He found that these electrical needles did more than curb pain; they also seemed to lessen the withdrawal symptoms some of his drug addicted patients were experiencing. The runny nose and stomach aches, and the anxiety that's symptomatic of withdrawal, seemed to disappear quickly after the needles had been inserted. A study done by Dr. Wen showed that of 40 opiate addicts treated with the needles, 39 left the hospital drug-free 2 weeks later—a remarkable achievement.

Patterson returned to England to try Dr. Wen's treatment there, but found that English addicts were far more wary of needles than the Chinese were. Believing it was the electricity generated by the needles that somehow helped curb withdrawal symptoms, Patterson set about developing an electrical device that did not use needles. She experimented first with surface electrodes, varying the type of current, the voltage, and the placement of the electrodes. After exploring all the variables, she found that the most important seemed to be that of electrical frequency. Apparently, a special frequency was required to eliminate withdrawal symptoms for each type of chemical an addict could ingest. For instance, cocaine and amphetamine addicts responded best to frequencies set as high as 2000 hertz, while those addicted to sedatives were helped by frequencies between 75 and 300 hertz.

By 1976, Patterson had developed her NET tuning box; it could be clipped onto one's belt, and two wires leading from it were attached behind the ears, allowing patients both mobility during the day and comfort at night. Although the 10-day treatment has been administered on an outpatient basis, it appears to be most successful when patients spend the entire period in a clinic.

The success of the box is hard to refute. In an evaluation made by Patterson of her former patients, from the years 1973–1980, 80 percent of drug addicts, 78 percent of the alcoholics, and 44 percent of the smokers who wished to achieve total abstinence said that they had done so. (Patterson admits those figures may be too favorable because those patients who'd returned to their former habits may have been less likely to respond to her evaluation questionnaire.

According to one national survey, 60 percent of all addicts who have ditched narcotics take up heavy drinking instead. But Patterson also found that NET users were far less likely to exchange one habit for another.

But exactly how does the little black box perform its magic? Dr. Robert Becker believes that the stimulator causes a "profound alteration of the central nervous system." Patterson theorizes it may work by affecting the production of endorphins, the natural brain chemicals which seem to spark euphoria. Apparently, opium, heroin, morphine, and other drugs have a molecular structure that resembles that of the natural endorphins. Thus, when these artificial endorphins are ingested, they produce sensations that are similiar to those caused by the natural brain hormone. To redress the chemical overload, the brain cuts back on its own production of endorphins, and a condition known as tolerance develops. The addict must increase the dosage, and the brain reacts by virtually shutting down endorphin production. No natural hormone is being produced then, so if the artificial drug supply is cut off, painful withdrawal symptoms are unleashed.

Dr. Patterson believes that NET acts as a catalyst to the natural endorphin system and, in effect, gets the "juices" flowing again. In an experiment performed at the Marie Curie Memorial Foundation in Surrey, England, Patterson and collaborator Dr. Ifor Capel examined the blood of rats treated with NET and found that the low-frequency currents increased endorphin levels in the rats by as much as threefold. Furthermore, they discovered that at the 10-hertz frequency, the production and turnover rate of serotonin, a neurotransmitter that acts as a central nervous system stimulator, was hastened.

But couldn't the black box itself become addictive? Isn't NET just an electronic fix? Patterson claims that no one has ever become addicted to the black box. "Drugs, for the very reason they are foreign, upset the brain's chemistry," she explains. "NET, on the other hand, simply coaxes the brain to restore it's own chemical balance. The body heals itself."

What's the future of Patterson's brain tuner? Currently, a number of doctors in England are using it—but general acceptance of the device is not at hand. The seventh model has recently been developed, which Patterson feels is easier to use than past models. With this one, she says, the doctor would simply prescribe the box and, using the booklet that's provided, the patient would find the correct tuning combination for the chemical he or she is addicted to and then program the box accordingly for the 10-day treatment. Patterson expects the new tuner to be available in England in 1986, and she intends to come to the United States to conduct clinical trials for FDA approval. Patterson is also researching the use of NET for several other conditions. These include mental disorders such as severe depression or anxiety, chronic pain, arthritis, and multiple sclerosis.

Controlling the Bladder

Incontinence is generally thought of as a childhood problem. But for several million Americans, bladder dysfunction is a grownup trouble which is not only socially embarrassing but sometimes life-threatening. Most paraplegics and quadriplegics have impaired function of the urinary bladder, and the difficulties they suffer as a result include a predisposition to urinary infections and to kidney stones and other kidney ailments. Many people suffer from incontinence as a result of diseases such as multiple sclerosis, Parkinson's disease, diabetes, tumors of the spine or central nervous system, and strokes. And more than 1.5 million victims develop urinary difficulties for reasons doctors cannot explain.

In essence, the bladder has two functions: to store urine and then to empty itself when a person wills it. But these functions can go awry when the coordination between the bladder and the activity of the urethral sphincter is thrown out of whack due to a spinal injury or a disease of the nervous system. The sphincter is a ring of muscle located at the neck of the bladder, and it controls the timing of urine release. When the sphincter is tightened, the bladder is relaxed and is able to store urine. Conversely, when the sphincter is relaxed, the bladder is tensed and will rid itself of urine. If the messages to the sacral nerves in the vertebral column, which help control the bladder and sphincter, are somehow distorted—as they would be if one had suffered spinal cord damage—all control of the bladder is lost and incontinence results.

Until recently, there was little doctors could do to treat this condition. In some cases, drugs were used to relax a spastic bladder or to improve bladder contractions. But drugs did little to help urethral sphincter troubles, so surgery—often to implant an artificial sphincter—was tried, but with little success. Now, researchers are developing an electrical alternative; a sort of bladder pacemaker, which helps the bladder and sphincter to get their movements in synch and thus improve the patient's control. FDA approval of the *neuroprosthesis pacemaker* to control bladder function seems just around the corner.

The bladder pacemaker has three essential components, the first being a set of electrodes implanted in the sacral nerves. Each sacral nerve has thousands of small fibers that carry information both to and from the bladder and sphincter. When the sacral nerves are stimulated, the sphincter contracts, allowing the bladder to store urine. The second component of the pacemaker is a receiver, which is implanted in the abdomen. When the patient places the antenna from an external transmitter (the third component) over the spot where the receiver is implanted, the receiver tenses the bladder (through the sacral nerves) while relaxing the sphincter muscle, allowing the patient to eliminate urine.

The most advanced work in this area is being done by Dr. Richard Schmidt at the University of California at San Francisco. He is currently conducting clinical trials on an implant system that aids a greater variety of incontinency problems than other devices have.

In addition to treating those with spinal cord injuries, prostate disorders, and diabetes, he is helping those patients whose incontinence stems from no discernible organic problem. So far, he can claim a 75 to 80 percent success rate (as defined by a 50 percent or better improvement in function) in the 60 implants he has performed since 1981. "We're able to make people much better," he says. "I mean, if you can cut leakage by half, well, that's a big improvement. The rule is that the milder the problem, the easier it is to correct it." If the implant is to be successful, it's also vital that patients with spinal injuries still have their sacral nerves intact and that the bladder not be too deformed.

Breathing Easier

It's just one of many life-threatening conditions that people with spinal cord injuries must deal with. If damage to their spinal cords has occurred above the origin of the phrenic nerves in the neck (which help to ennervate the diaphragm), the diaphragm and the other muscles that enhance breathing are paralyzed; people with this type of damage cannot breathe on their own.

In the past, such a patient would have been hooked up to a mechanical ventilator—for life. And it wasn't a life that lasted very long. The mechanical respirator, which is the modern version of the iron lung used by many polio victims, could only extend life by about 1 to 2 years. But an electrically stimulated diaphragm pacer is extending the lives of quadriplegics, as well as those who suffer from other chronic pulmonary problems such as lung disease. Dr. William Glenn at Yale University was the first to construct a pacemaker similar to the heart device to stimulate the phrenic nerve, pacing the diaphragm of patients who couldn't breathe without aid.

When a healthy person breathes, complicated chemical sensors detect the carbon dioxide and oxygen levels in the body and stimulate breathing. The phrenic nerve stimulator, which consists of a radio frequency transmitter, an external antenna, a receiver, and one or two phrenic nerve electrodes, bypasses most of these sensors. The external transmitter sends special coded signals through the antenna to a receiver that's implanted just under the skin in the chest. The repetitive pulsations governed by that signal are then conducted through stainless steel wires to electrodes implanted around the phrenic nerve. According to Glenn, the benefits of this treatment are obvious: "We have patients who have been pacing since 1970—and if you turned it off, they'd die. That's unequivocal proof that this is an important technique." Glenn believes that getting patients away from their mechanical tethers is vital. "You've got to keep the spirits of these people up. Pacing helps them live a more normal life. We've got one woman who graduated from college and law school while using a pacer, and now she's practicing law. Several others using the system have also gone to college, graduated, and are now involved in careers."

In order for the diaphragm pacer to be effective, the phrenic nerves of the patient must be intact and the lungs and diaphragm must be in good shape. There may be some drawbacks to the system: Patients must have a permanent tracheostomy (a hole made in the tracheal tube in the neck) and there's apparently some danger that the implanted electrodes may damage the area surrounding the phrenic nerves. Still, the life-saving benefits of the pacer, most doctors agree, outweigh the potential drawbacks. Researchers are now working to correct these problems and to develop a totally implantable system.

And the Lame Shall Walk

In 1791, Luigi Galvani, an anatomy professor in the medical school at the University of Bologna, discovered that electricity, when applied to the main nerve surrounding the muscle of a frog's leg, would make that muscle contract. While medical science has known since then that electricity can move muscles, what wasn't known was how to synchronize this movement in any useful way. With the advent of the Computer Age, however, researchers are using microprocessors to mimic cerebral impulses that fail to reach the arms and legs due to spinal cord injury. As a result, those with paralyzed limbs may soon regain the ability to use their hands— and perhaps even to walk—with the aid of *functional electrical neuromuscular stimulation.*

"We discovered that the computer could do most of the book-keeping," says Dr. Terry Hambrecht, the director of the neural prosthesis program at the National Institute of Neurological and Communicative Disorders and Stroke, a federal agency. "It could decide how much to stimulate which muscles and in what order, thereby coordinating the intricate patterns of muscular contraction that underlie even the simplest of movements." The computer acts as a sort of general, issuing orders in the form of pulses to move the muscles. Both the duration and the frequency of those pulses determine the size of each muscle contraction.

Several achievements have taken place in recent years in the area of neuromuscular stimulation. Though similar work is going on at about a dozen research centers here and abroad, probably the best publicized work has been that of Dr. Jerrold Petrofsky, executive director of the National Center for Rehabilitation Engineering at Wright State University in Dayton, Ohio. After 13 years of research in the area of neuromuscular stimulation, he and his team of 30 researchers were able to put paraplegic Nan Davis back on her feet—if only temporarily—in 1982. Then again, in June of 1983, Nan—with the aid of Petrofsky and his colleague Chandler Phillips—took some halting steps from her chair to the podium during her college graduation ceremony at Wright State. She's even ridden a special bicycle designed for paraplegics across the Wright State campus.

Getting the paralyzed to walk is no easy trick. What makes it possible is that legs paralyzed from spinal injuries and strokes are usually left with muscles and nerves intact. The legs don't move on their own because the brain, which normally sends nerve impulses through the nervous system, can no longer communicate with the muscles of the limbs. The link has, in effect, been broken. While a computer can't reconnect that link, it can be programmed to imitate the brain's function. And when it's connected to the proper nerves in the muscles, the microprocessor can feed electrical signals to the paralyzed limbs, thereby making them move.

To use the system, Nan Davis must don what looks like a pair of ballet tights which have a number of surface electrodes sewn into them. These electrode sensors cover the three major muscle groups in each leg. Nan also wears a lightweight external leg brace which helps the researchers position the sensors correctly. These electrodes are connected by wires to the computer stimulation system, which is 6 inches by 4 inches by 2 inches—the size of a small tote bag. It uses four 9-volt batteries and is generally worn on the patient's belt. Finally, Nan is equipped with either a walker, Laufstrand canes (two canes often used by the elderly) or crutches, all of which have push button switches on them to activate the system.

Each time Nan wants to move, she must hit the button—either for her left or right leg—and the computer, noting the position of the leg and the movement it has already undergone, generates an electrical current of from 40 to 80 milliamperes. This moves through the electrodes to the muscles in the correct sequence to get a smooth movement. Because this is what's called a "closed-loop" system, the sensors on the legs monitor both leg position and movement, giving the computer the feedback it needs for the next move. The system also helps protect against muscle fatigue and stress on the bones, and if the patient loses her balance, the system can help to stabilize the muscles and activate the appropriate ones to get her back on her feet.

Both Nan and another paraplegic at Wright State have walked over a mile using the system (the feat was accomplished in the halls of the research lab) and Nan asserts that she could have kept on walking if she hadn't developed a blister on her toe. Says Chandler Phillips, professor of engineering at Wright State, "We see the system as very safe, very reliable and yes, very practical. Our ultimate hope is that it will benefit anywhere from 200,000 to 500,000 spinal-cord-injured people."

Phillips believes the system could be available at the end of 1987, though the research team is still seeking a manufacturer and FDA approval. A totally implantable system is also being researched, but Phillips speculates it may not be ready for testing for another decade.

Unfortunately, not all spinal-cord-injured people will be helped by the system. "They can't have any major deformities of the knees and hips," says Phillips, "and they need to move easily. It also won't be available to those who have been paralyzed for more than 15 years and probably suffer from severe bone demineralization as a result. Trying to stand on limbs that haven't been used in such a long time could lead to fractures."

To get patients like Nan ready to walk, Wright State researchers developed computer-controlled exercise equipment, which they claim increases the muscle mass of paralyzed limbs. The exercise system includes a leg-lift machine on which a patient's paralyzed muscles are stimulated to pedal against a weight. Studies conducted at the University of Miami by Dr. Barth Green and by researchers at Wright State indicate that the exercise system can reverse the muscle atrophy that occurs in the limbs of the paralyzed, while increasing muscular strength and endurance.

Hands-On Stimulation

In the summer of 1983, Robert Morris, a 26-year-old ceramics engineer, had his spine severed in a tragic car crash. The accident left him totally paralyzed from the shoulders down. He could no longer work, feed himself, or care for himself in any way. And his doctors told him not to expect to ever regain the use of his limbs.

But today, thanks to a team of researchers led by Dr. P. Hunter Peckham at Case Western University, Morris, though still "paralyzed" is able to move his hands. He is just one of 20 quadriplegics who are helping Dr. Peckham to test a neuromuscular stimulation system that enables them to feed themselves, comb their hair, shave, brush their teeth; simple tasks for the healthy, but nothing short of miracles for the paralyzed.

Using a hypodermic needle, researchers implant into the muscles of the patient's arms tiny multistranded stainless steel wire electrodes bent into the shape of springs. Part of the electrode remains outside the skin, and these bits of wire are hooked up to a stimulator which is controlled by a microprocessor. This is contained in a box the size of a small portable radio, which is clipped onto the back of the patient's wheelchair. To activate the system, a patient must move his or her shoulders up or down, forward or backward. (Only quadriplegics injured below the fifth cervical vertebra in the neck can manage this.) This moves a joystick of sorts, taped to the chest, which will in turn set off the computer-controlled pulses that coordinate muscle movement in the hands and arms.

Right now, the microprocessor can produce two different hand grips, each of which requires the stimulation of four or five muscles. These are the "pinch grasp," with the thumb held down against the side of the index finger, and the "three-jaw-chuck," which involves the three-fingered action needed to grasp a pencil. "The system, says Robert Morris, is a real help." It makes me a lot more independent. I can go out to dinner and hold a sandwich, drink with a cup. Most quadriplegics depend on other people to feed them. I can even write a little with the system." Peckham is hoping to ready an implantable system, in which all the electrode wires and the stimulator would be placed beneath the skin, by 1987. He's not so certain, though, that the technology will ever be widely available to quadriplegics. "It may be used in a few major rehabilitative centers in a few years," he says. "But it's hard to say how many doctors will have the interest and the expertise to put these things in correctly."

Wright State researchers are working on a hand stimulation system of their own. Unlike Case Western's semi-implantable system, Wright State uses a glove with surface electrodes sewn into the fabric; the electrodes are hooked up to a tiny microprocessor. When patients move their shoulders up or down, forward or backward, the computer is cued to send out electrical impulses to the appropriate muscles of the hand. Currently, four patients are using this system and Wright State researchers are hopeful that it will be more widely available in 2 years.

Another exciting innovation that Case Western researchers are developing is a sensory feedback system. Because the paralyzed have no sensation in their fingertips, it's difficult for them to know if they're grasping an object too tightly when using the hand stimulation device. With the system being developed by Dr. Michael Newman, a pressure switch is mounted on the fingertips of the patient. If he or she grasps a cup too tightly, for instance, a signal fed through the computer electrically stimulates the skin in an area where the patient can feel—generally in the upper arm or back. Very brief pulse whips, giving a buzzing sensation, let the patient know that the grip should be loosened. Testing on this equipment began at Case Western in late 1985.

Straightening Spines

Scoliosis (a curvature of the spine) is a crippling disease which afflicts somewhere between 4 and 14 percent of all school-age children. In most cases, the problem is a mild one. Until recent years, though, a child suffering from progressive scoliosis—in which the curve of the spine becomes increasingly marked as the youngster matures—was subjected either to years of wearing a confining neck-to-hip brace 22 hours a day, or to major corrective surgery. But now electrical stimulation applied to the back muscles is being used to stop the progress of scoliosis.

The idea was first conceived in 1969 by Walter P. Bobechko, now chief of orthopedic surgery at The Hospital for Sick Children in Toronto, Canada. Dr. Bobechko noted that children with cerebral palsy often had a muscular imbalance in their backs that seemed to curve their spines. He theorized that if a muscle imbalance could cause scoliosis, building up the muscles on the convex side of the curve might act to straighten the spine. Unfortunately, an ordinary exercise regimen designed to strengthen back muscles will not stop the progress of a curvature; in order to build up enough muscle to influence a curvature the muscles in the back must be stimulated constantly. In addition, it is difficult to increase the muscle mass on one side of the back through exercise without augmenting the other side, too. But in studies with rabbits and pigs, Bobechko and his associates discovered that they could produce and then correct spinal curves by stimulating the muscles in the animals' backs, using an implanted "pacemaker" which produced 6-volt pulses that made muscles contract 70 times each minute. In clinical studies with children, the researchers found that a muscle twitch induced every 10 seconds would build up the muscle being stimulated and, by strengthening it, keep a child's curvature from becoming worse.

Now, a child with a spinal curve of less than 40 degrees can have an electrical stimulation system implanted during a simple operation performed under general anesthesia. In some cases, the system will actually straighten the spine—in others, it will prevent the curve from becoming worse.

The child has a small radio frequency receiver implanted just beneath the skin in his or her back. Before going to bed each night, the child tapes a tiny antenna over the area where the receiver was implanted and then connects it to an external transmitter that runs on a 9-volt battery. In the morning, the child switches the transmitter off, removes the antenna and can then go to school, play ball, etc. The receiver is removed surgically when the child has reached puberty—the age when the bones will have stopped growing. The electrical stimulation device has been shown to be about 75 percent successful in stopping the progression of the spinal curvature, and, in some 30 percent of cases, it even helped to reduce the amount of curve.

According to Dr. Morley Herbert, who worked with Dr. Bobechko in Toronto to develop the implantable system, this success rate is comparable to that attained with a brace.

"No current treatment—not even surgery—will leave those with scoliosis perfectly straight," he says. But he believes that electrical stimulation is preferable to the use of a brace because so many children simply refuse to wear one.

Indeed, studies show that about 40 percent of children saddled with a brace won't wear it regularly—which can't help but reduce its effectiveness. One 16-year-old boy (a patient of Dr. Herbert's) who played on his high school football team, had a curve that had progressed from 22 degrees to 30 degrees in a year's time. He refused to wear a brace, which would have prevented him from playing football, and yet his ever progressing curve would have required surgery if it had continued to worsen at such a rapid rate. Dr. Herbert implanted a stimulator in the muscles near the boy's spine and within 18 months—when his bones had matured, thereby "locking" in the amount of curve—the curve had been reduced to 25 degrees.

Another electrical stimulation device, one which works externally to correct scoliosis, is proving more popular than the implantable system. Developed by a research team at Rancho Los Amigos Rehabilitation Engineering Center in Downey, California, the device consists of two electrode disks connected to a small, battery operated stimulator. The disks are placed on the skin, over the convex area of the child's curve and, like the implantable system, are activated when the child goes to bed, and then removed upon waking. The system seems to be just as effective in stopping the progress of scoliosis as the implantable stimulator, although about 25 percent of the children using the external stimulator develop a skin irritation from the gel that's used with the disks. Some of the children also complain of the buzzing sensation they experience when the stimulator is on. Even so, says Howard Schulman of the Scoliosis Association, most U.S. doctors prefer to treat children with the surface method, rather than perform surgery—however simple the procedure. Both methods are being used by more than 250 orthopedic doctors throughout North America.

Straightening Teeth

Orthodontia is probably one of the biggest growing pains many teenagers ever encounter. It's not just the discomfort of the wires being tightened to straighten crooked teeth that's hard to bear; it's also the length of time one is required to wear the socially unacceptable braces—from 2 to 3 years. In recent years, adults who didn't have their gaps closed or their overbites corrected during adolescence have also been getting braces. In fact, an estimated 20 percent of the 4.4 million people wearing braces today are adults.

All sorts of innovations have been taking place in the orthodontics field to make patients feel less like social lepers while getting their teeth fixed. Now there are braces made of clear plastic, which makes the appliance somewhat more difficult to see. Researchers have also developed what they call "invisible" or "lingual" braces. These are attached to the back of the teeth so that there are no telltale metal bonds in front to mar one's smile.

The newest innovation, though, is *electrically stimulated braces*, which doctors claim may cut the time you would normally have to wear braces by almost half. The electrical device includes a tiny battery pack encased in a capsule which is attached to special brackets mounted on conventional braces. When turned on, the 10 to 20 microamperes of direct current stimulate the tooth's surrounding tissue, doubling the rate of movement.

The original device was developed at the University of Pennsylvania in 1979. Test subjects' teeth moved at the rate of 2 or more millimeters a month (the normal rate for conventionally braced teeth is 1 millimeter or slightly less a month). But the electrical stimulation seemed to irritate the gums of the patients and the trial was discontinued. At nearby Drexel University, Dr. Richard Beard, professor of biomedical engineering, developed a new electrode system that used a gel instead of metal electrodes to conduct the electricity. Successful animal studies have just been completed with this new technique, and human clinical trials are expected to begin shortly. Penn Med, the company set to market the electrical braces, is hoping to obtain FDA approval and get the device to orthodontists in about 2 years.

While the electric braces, which would be turned on from 4 to 8 hours a day (perhaps while patients sleep), may make the tooth-straightening experience a shorter one, there's no word yet on whether it will also cut the cost of orthodontia by half. Nathaniel Lieb, chairman of Penn Med, says, however, that the cost doesn't matter much. "Adults, in particular, want to spend the least possible amount of time with braces on. This will speed up a normally tedious process."

The Bone Menders

One night back in May of 1977 Skip Lambertson was driving his motorcycle to his job as a firefighter in Greenwich, Connecticut, when a car swerved into his path, knocking him from his cycle. When the surgeons got a look at his mangled left leg, with the bones shattered in three places, they decided they would have to amputate. But Lambertson's wife insisted they set the bones and hope for the best. They let him keep his leg, and for the next year and a half, Lambertson lived inside a cast that came up to his chest—but still the fractures refused to knit. When the doctors began to feel that amputation was the only answer, Lambertson read about the then experimental use of electricity to heal bones and he told his doctor, "Let's try this electric stuff." He was fitted with the pulsed electromagnetic coils devised by New York's Columbia-Presbyterian Hospital's Bassett, and about 6 months later, Lambertson's leg had begun to heal. Today, the 51-year-old Lambertson is able to run—though he prefers to walk.

The use of electricity to heal bones that stubbornly refuse to mend is the most widely accepted of all the electrical practices being used in medicine today. Presently, there are three FDA-approved methods of healing nonunion fractures. In the late 1950s, Bassett and Robert Becker discovered that bone becomes electrically polarized when bent or broken. This finding was made at about the same time by two Japanese doctors, Iwao Yasuda and Eiichi Fukada. Furthermore, Becker found that the electric voltages bone produced seemed to guide the cellular repair mechanisms when the bone was fractured. Sometimes, though, for reasons scientists can't explain, the normal healing process just doesn't take place. Some theorize that there may not be enough blastema cells (a cluster of embryonic cells that mark the beginning of the regeneration process) at the scene in the crucial hours after the break occurs. In any event, the bones refuse to mend and a nonunion develops.

Researchers reasoned that electricity applied at the fracture site might stimulate growth—and animal studies backed the theory up. Interestingly, the three FDA-approved methods of healing nonunions with electrical currents, though different in approach, heal bone equally well; they're all about 80 to 85 percent successful. Dr. Carl Brighton of the University of Pennsylvania Medical School uses a semi-invasive method which employs four electrodes inserted around the break. These are connected to a power pack anchored in the patient's cast. The batteries emit a steady current of 20 microamperes to the electrodes, and the break generally heals in 3 months. Another method, developed by Australian researchers, requires both electrodes and battery pack to be surgically implanted, and so two operations are necessary, one to implant and a second to remove the device.

The third method, the one created by Bassett (with the help of electrochemist Arthur Pilla, of Mount Sinai Hospital in New York City), consists of a pair of electromagnetic coils covered in soft plastic pads. These are connected to a small generator that plugs into an electrical outlet. The pads are applied to the cast at the site of the break for up to 12 hours a day. Though no one knows exactly why, the *pulsed electromagnetic fields* (*PEMFs*) generated by the coils also heal nonunions effectively. Healing generally takes from a few months to a year with the Bassett method, which is the most popular method because no surgery is needed.

Bassett's PEMF coils are also being used to combat avascular necrosis, which could be described as a heart attack of the hip. The bone at the hip joint dies because the blood supply to it has been nipped off. It's a disease that strikes between 25,000 to 30,000 people a year and it commonly afflicts young adults—the average age of those who suffer from avascular necrosis is about 30. In the past, the hip would self-destruct in the course of a few years, and a total artificial hip replacement would be necessary. And since hip replacements can't take much wear and tear—50 percent of those people who receive them need to be operated on again within 5 years—doctors hesitate to implant artificial hips in younger, more active patients.

Diane Resciniti was 8 months pregnant when her legs began to ache and walking became difficult. After she had her baby in August, 1984, the pain became worse and she went from cane to crutches to wheelchair in a few months. A hip replacement seemed out of the question: Diane was too young. So she placed the PEMF coils on her hips for about 12 hours each night. Three weeks after the beginning of therapy, she could walk again and nine months later her hips were 90 percent healed. Since 1979, over a thousand others have used the PEMF coils nationwide, on a clinical basis, to cure avascular necrosis, and FDA approval is expected in 1986. Although, once again, Bassett cannot be certain how the coils work to cure the disease, he believes that the special pulsed signal they impart may improve the blood supply to the hip.

Pulsed electromagnetic coils may also be used soon to slow the progress of osteoporosis, the debilitating disease that weakens bone. Bassett's preliminary studies show that when PEMFs are tuned to the appropriate pulse, they stop bone loss and even put some bone back, preventing the loss of height, the dowager's hump and the porous, brittle bones that mark the disease. He believes the treatment will be used widely in 3 to 4 years. "We'll either get a very large coil covered with a pad which we'll put over the spine, the pelvis, and the hips, or patients will sleep in the PEMFs bed."

In fact, such a bed may be used by NASA astronuats to prevent what's known as astroosteoporosis. When in space, the astronaut's bones become thin and brittle due to a loss of calcium. If the space flight is prolonged, the condition can become so severe that the astronaut can't walk when he or she returns to Earth. Bassett has been working with NASA since 1977 to develop a PEMFs coil bed that would, as he puts it, "help them grow bones while they sleep." He expects that such a bed may be ready to board the space shuttle in 5 years.

Healing Wounds

Electricity may not only promote the healing of bone: A number of researchers are investigating the possibility that it may also enhance the healing of soft tissue, such as skin wounds, ligament and tendon aches, and bedsores (which afflict 20 to 30 percent of all bedridden patients).

Virtually all types of soft tissue normally heal in the same way: a complex process in which the injured tissue is replaced with a scar. For this to take place, the blood at the wound site must first clot. Then the area becomes inflamed so as to get rid of the damaged cells, and new cells grow to replace these. Finally, "remodeling" takes place; this is the body's way of recreating the structure of the tissue as closely as it can. These stages normally take hours, weeks, months, and years, respectively. But complete healing can be prevented if the process is interrupted by infection, an inadequate blood supply to the wound, repeated opening of the wound—even by poor nutrition.

Using low-intensity direct currents with a negative copper mesh electrode placed over the skin ulcer, Lester Wolcott and a team of researchers at the University of Missouri Medical School were able to "clean" chronic sores. Then, by reversing the electrode current to positive, they stimulated the growth of tissue in 151 patients with 175 previously resistant skin ulcers. Forty-five to fifty-nine percent of these ulcers were healed completely when stimulated. Using pulsed electromagnetic fields on the skin's surface also seemed to significantly increase the number of fibroblasts (the predominant cell type in wound healing) and the amount of collagen in the healing wound. And a recent study showed that pulsed electromagnetic fields could relieve the symptoms of patients suffering from chronic painful tendinitis. In the study conducted at Addenbrookes Hospital in Cambridge, England, 85 percent of the patients outfitted with electromagnetic coils got well after only 4 weeks of treatment. And these were people who had already tried every other available treatment, including steroids and ultrasound.

It isn't clear yet why electricity seems to heal soft tissue. Scientists doubt that the electricity is actually penetrating the cells. Instead, they theorize, it may somehow affect the cell membrane, which in turn affects the cell itself. It's also been hypothesized that electricity enhances blood flow to the wound area or increases the amount of energy across the cell membrane triggering the internal repair system. Much more investigation is needed, says Andrew Szeto of San Diego State University, before electricity can be used widely to heal soft tissue. "Currents do have the potential to heal," he says, "but we must show it's also cheaper and faster than other techniques are, and we're not yet at that point."

Killing Cancer Cells

What are the chances that electricity, which enhances the growth of bone and soft tissue, could slow that of a cancerous tumor? According to a few studies, the chances may be quite good. Electrochemist Arthur Pilla asserts that he and other researchers have found that certain pulses kill lymphoma cells grown in culture. The team of researchers, led by Pilla and William Riegelson of the Medical School of Virginia, injected mice with deadly melanoma cells and found that those left untreated lived an average of 27 days and those given chemotherapy lived 36 days. But the mice treated with both chemotherapy and low-energy pulsed electromagnetic fields (PEMF coils were placed around the cages) lived an average of 43 days. Observes Pilla: "Although the electrical currents didn't get rid of the tumor, they did increase survival time."

A second study, conducted by Dr. Larry Norton at Mt. Sinai Medical Center in New York, also showed that when chemotherapy was combined with PEMFs, better than 90 percent of the tumor growth in rats was inhibited. "When used separately," says Dr. Riegelson, "neither treatment was as effective. When combined, chemotherapy and electricity seemed to have a synergistic effect. Together, they made the most effective treatment."

Some researchers believe, however, that electrical currents will cause cancer instead of cure it. Becker is a vocal opponent of the freewheeling use of electrical currents for this reason. "We just don't know how all the currents and the magnetic fields will affect us yet," he explains. A study he conducted in 1981 showed that when the same type of current and voltage used to promote bone growth was applied to a human fibrosarcoma (cancerous fibroblasts), the growth rate of the tumor cells in the culture increased by more than 300 percent in 24 hours. Magnetic fields may have the same effect on cancer cells. A study done by Dr. Jerry L. Phillips, Director of Biochemical Research at the Cancer Therapy and Research Center in San Antonio, Texas, showed that a flow of 60-cycle current increased the amount of growth of cancerous cells 200 to 2400 percent. Says Becker: "Everyone seems to believe that you can influence bone without influencing everything else; that you can turn on bone growth without turning on the growth of other tissue. But that's extremely simplistic thinking."

Until more is known about *how* electrical currents produce the effects that they do in the body, the possibility of their use as a cancer treatment seems limited. Dr. Pilla estimates that it may take another 10 years before electricity can be used to combat cancer. But, adds Dr. Riegelson, "there is tremendous potential for pulsed electromagnetic fields in helping to halt the growth of tumors. Like chemotherapy and radiation, I think it will one day become a standard method for treating cancer."

A Total Eclipse of Heart Trouble?

With heart disease still the nation's number one killer, finding a way to heal the body's pumping machine is a number one priority for scientists. Valve replacements, pacemakers, transplanted hearts, mechanical hearts—all of these treatments help to artificially restore heart function and maintain life. But could electrical currents help the heart to heal itself?

Scientists predict that electromagnetic fields will someday be used to heal damaged heart tissue—perhaps even to regenerate it. Right now, Chicago heart surgeon Robert Gordon is attempting to treat atherosclerosis—a disease common in the elderly—with electrically charged particles. Atherosclerosis is caused by the buildup, over the years, of fat within the artery walls, where it restricts the flow of blood to the heart. Commonly called hardening of the arteries, the disease is irreversible; at present, the only way to treat it is by rerouting the blood flow through healthy blood vessels with bypass surgery. But Dr. Gordon is developing a nonsurgical electromagnetic technique that could melt the fatty deposits in the blood vessels.

In his experiments, Gordon has been injecting a solution of tiny magnetic particles into the bloodstreams of rats and rabbits. These collect in the atherosclerotic lesions, which are more permeable than healthy blood vessel walls. The animals are then subjected to an alternating electromagnetic field low enough in current to excite only the particles, not the rest of the tissue. The magnetic field interacts with the magnetic particles, generating heat—and the heat melts the life-threatening fatty plaque, while leaving the surrounding healthy tissue undisturbed.

Gordon is excited about his new technique because it may cure a killer disease. Even more significant, it may help to prevent it from occurring in the first place. "It looks like the plaque can be treated at a very early stage," he says. "So theoretically, people could get this treatment done periodically to prevent large buildups of plaque," Gordon claims, though, that he's still about 2 years away from testing his technique on human subjects.

Electromagnetic fields are also being used to regulate hearts that beat irregularly. Tecnic Research Laboratories in San Leandro, California, is developing the first wireless cardiac pacemaker worn outside the body. According to William Van Bise, Tecnic's chief of biomedical research, the tiny transmitter will generate magnetic fields that stabilize the firing pattern of the cells that keep the heart beating. Elizabeth Rauscher, inventor of the external pacemaker and president of Tecnic, says the device could be worn as a necklace or implanted just beneath the skin.

Bassett believes the use of PEMFs could help victims of severe angina, who experience pain due to a diminished blood supply to the heart. Recent animal studies conducted by Bassett show that PEMFs can make blood vessels grow, allowing an increased supply of blood to reach the heart. There's no solid evidence yet that PEMFs could stimulate enough vessel growth to eliminate the need for bypass surgery. But patients with intractable angina who aren't candidates for surgery or the new "kissing balloon" technique (in which a small, deflated balloon is placed in blocked arteries and then blown up to stretch the artery, increasing blood flow) might be helped.

At the farthest end of the spectrum of heart-healing possibilities is this one: That surgeons could induce the heart to heal itself with a little help from electrical currents, rather than seeking outside aid from transplanted or mechanical hearts. Heart disease, in which heart muscle dies as a result of a blockage to the coronary artery, could be overcome by literally cutting away the dead tissue and regenerating healthy new tissue. A surgeon, Becker theorizes, would cut away the scar tissue that had formed as a result of a coronary blockage, and would then apply ready-made preblastema cells (perhaps taken from the patient's bone marrow) to fill the defect. The correct doses of current would take the heart wound through the regenerative process, replacing damaged tissue with normal cardiac tissue.

Becker is confident that the human heart can be made to mend itself. "The benefits far outweigh the risks," he says. The difficulty lies in convincing the medical community that the healing potential is there, he explains, prerequisite for obtaining the funds for necessary research. "If we could get the funding," he says, "we could develop clinically relevant heart-healing techniques in 5 years."

Healing the Spinal Cord

In the whole human catalog of destructive diseases and catastrophic injuries, there are few that rival the total devastation that damage to the spinal cord engenders. Everything from breathing difficulties and incontinence to bedsores can make life miserable for the paralyzed. Not long ago, many people who suffered spinal cord injuries died, not from the accident itself, but from infections and complications resulting from their paralysis. There are researchers, though, who seem hopeful that one day soon they'll be able to regrow a severed or damaged spinal cord, thus restoring the use of limbs, respiratory muscles, excretory and sexual organs—even the sense of touch—to millions of paraplegics and quadriplegics around the world.

"I think that with pulsed electromagnetic fields," says Bassett, "it would be possible to impart different healing messages. One might actually be able to regenerate parts of the spinal cord— particularly if the treatment were combined with appropriate surgical approaches." Although scientists are not yet attempting to regenerate severed spinal cords, there has been remarkable progress in stimulating regrowth of peripheral nerves (the peripheral nerves are all the nerves located outside the skull and spinal column). A number of animal studies now show that the use of electricity can double—sometimes even triple—the growth rate of peripheral nerves. Bassett, along with Dr. Hiromoto Ito of the Nippon Medical School in Tokyo, has demonstrated that his electromagnetic coils stimulate peripheral nerves in rats to grow back at twice the normal rate, restoring function to the damaged limbs in half the normal time.

Dr. Davis H. Wilson of the Leeds General Infirmary in England successfully used a *Diapulse* machine (a radio wave generator employed in Canada and in the United Kingdom to mend bone fractures) to stimulate peripheral nerve growth. "Peripheral nerves usually regrow at the rate of 1 millimeter a day," he says. "Using the Diapulse machine, though, growth is speeded up to 3 to 4 millimeters a day." In one experiment, 40 cats paralyzed by spinal cord injuries were hooked up to the machine; after treatment, 38 of them could walk again. Wilson has also grafted peripheral nerves into the spinal cords of cats that had theirs severed and then turned on the Diapulse machine. Although the animals didn't recover the use of their limbs, the nerves in the spinal cords did grow back.

Another soon to be published study shows that low-level direct electrical current can enhance and guide peripheral nerve regeneration. Dr. Gustav Roman, assistant professor of neurology at the Texas Tech University Health Science Center, cut the sciatic nerves of rats, placed the severed nerves inside a vinyl tube, and then applied the electric current. As a result, the two nerve ends rejoined—although nerve function itself didn't return.

While peripheral nerves can reconnect naturally if the space between the severed ends is less than a centimeter long, human spinal cord nerves do not possess this ability. There are some species whose spinal cord nerves do regenerate. Salamanders and goldfish can regrow severed spinal cord nerves (although their ability to do so declines as the animals age). But why can't higher species perform this feat? Becker theorizes that there's a critical period during which regrowth must be completed or it will fail. All animals, he says, who suffer a spinal cord injury endure a period of spinal shock, in which even the simplest reflexes disappear. When the shock wears off, the nerves below the injury become hyperactive, and this can lead to spastic paralysis of the muscles.

In goldfish and young salamanders, the shock seems to last only a few minutes, while in mammals it can go on for as long as 6 months. According to measurements Becker took with salamanders, the electrical current during spinal shock is highly positive.

In the salamander, this current soon becomes negative—the type of current known to stimulate regeneration. But when Becker manipulated the current—keeping it from becoming negative—for 5 or more days, the salamander's regenerative abilities were stymied and the animal became paraplegic.

Becker believes that if scientists could cancel out the positive current at the injury site of a human spinal cord and replace it with a growth-stimulating negative one early on in the process, spinal regeneration in humans might occur. Although Becker doesn't predict that paralysis victims will be able to walk normally anytime soon, he does feel the potential for healing damaged spinal cords is there, and Bassett agrees. "I don't think we'll ever regenerate the spine to the point that there's no evidence that anything was ever wrong, but I do think that down the road, we will be able to improve function."

Electrical Limb Regeneration

A man working at a construction site falls off a beam two stories up and lands on his left arm, crushing it. The doctors have no choice: They have to amputate. But instead of fitting the man with a prosthesis and sending him home to disability checks, they apply carefully mapped out electrical currents to the wound. Two months later, the man leaves the hospital with a healthy left arm, identical in every way to his right arm. He returns to work.

That's the future of limb regeneration—and it may only be a few decades away. While some researchers have doubts that humans will ever be able to regrow limbs, others believe that human beings once possessed this ability, and that, with the use of electrical currents, it may be restored to us.

Perhaps the strongest believer is Becker. "If we can identify the mechanisms that stimulate and control regeneration in the salamander," he says, "I see no reason why man cannot be stimulated to do the same thing."

In 1960, Robert Becker decided to investigate whether nerves in animals provide an electrical signal, which he believed was vital to triggering the regenerative process. He reported the differences in the "current of injury" after he amputated limbs of the regenerating salamander and the frog, which is a nonregenerative animal. While both animals' wounds emitted a positive current at the site of the wound right after amputation the salamander's current switched its polarity to negative within 10 days. The frog's wound never really shifted polarity, but instead crept back to its original value. From this, Becker hypothesized that the negative current brought forth the all important blastema, and that perhaps by manipulating the frog's current to negative with electrodes, regeneration could be induced.

Then in 1974, Stephen D. Smith of the University of Kentucky achieved full regrowth of a frog's limb by implanting an electrode that migrated down the limb as the tissue grew back. Becker, also using an implanted electrode, stimulated a rat to regenerate an amputated leg all the way to the elbow joint.

The work of these researchers—and others—opened up the possibility that electrical stimulation could also induce limb regrowth in humans. But their speculation came close to certainty when one English physician made an amazing discovery in the early 1970s: Young children possess the ability to regenerate their fingertips. Usually, when a young child's fingertip is cut off in an accident, standard treatment is to stitch the wound closed or to try reattaching the section by microsurgery. But due to a mixup in the emergency room at Sheffield Children's Hospital in England, one child whose fingertip had been accidentally amputated, didn't receive either of these treatments. When the error was detected several days later, Dr. Cynthia Illingworth saw that the child's fingertip was regrowing all on it's own; the skin, the fat, the bone—even the fingernail— were regenerating perfectly. After treating several hundred more children with such "neglect," Illingworth was able to report in 1974 that in children aged 11 or younger, fingertips sheared off above the uppermost joint will invariably grow back in approximately 3 months time. Like limb regeneration in salamanders, this regrowth will only occur if the wound isn't stitched closed.

This proved that humans *do* possess the capacity to regenerate multi-tissue structures in limited amounts. But why do children have this ability—while adults do not? Says Becker: "The younger the animal, the better the regeneration. You need plenty of marrow in the bones in order to get regrowth, and kids have more marrow than adults do."

Although artificial limb regrowth has not yet been attempted on human beings, the top researchers in the electrohealing field are confident that regeneration through electrical currents will soon be achieved. "All of this right now is just a gleam in the father's eye," Bassett says. "And it may take more time than *I* have. But knowing what we know now, we might do it before the end of this century."

=Timeline=

1987 to 1990
- *Totally implantable spinal cord stimulator alleviates symptoms of cerebral palsy and multiple sclerosis.*
- *Electrical tuner that helps break cigarette, drug, and alcohol addictions now sold by prescription.*
- *Electrical braces cut orthodontia straightening time in half.*
- *Heart pacemaker available that can be worn on a necklace.*

1991 to 2000
- *Electronic bikes for paraplegics sold in sporting goods stores.*
- *Electronic implant allows quadriplegics to move their hands and "feel."*
- *Electric coil beds sold in every department store to keep bones healthy.*
- *Broken legs take only a few weeks to heal.*

2001 to 2010
- *Every paraplegic is able to walk with muscular stimulation system.*
- *Over-the-counter device heals skin ulcers and tendinitis.*
- *Tumors can be "zapped" with electric current.*
- *Atherosclerosis (hardening of the arteries) can now be cured—even prevented—using electric particles.*

2011 to 2030
- *Spinal cords regenerated, restoring life to paralyzed limbs.*
- *Cancer eradicated through use of electric coils.*
- *Amputated limbs can be regenerated.*
- *Transplant organs no longer needed from donors. All vital organs can be regrown with use of electrodes.*

Access Guide

The Spine Tuner

For information, consultation, and/or referral to another institution for surgery, write to:

Dr. Joseph M. Waltz
Department of Neurological Surgery
St. Barnabas Hospital
4422 Third Avenue
New York, NY 10457
(212) 960-9476

Waltz requests that he be contacted first so he can refer patients to the proper medical institution for treatment. Although the program is still in clinical process, it's open to new patients. It requires a week's hospital stay for implant procedure and daily outpatient care for 6 to 8 weeks. Cost is approximately $8,500 for hospital and doctor's fee. Cost of surgical implant and other equipment is $6,235. Consultation and preliminary studies fee is $300.

The Brain Tuner

Dr. Patterson expects U.S. clinical trials to take place next year, possibly at the University of Texas and the University of Oregon. Right now, the cost of the NeuroElectric box is £500 or approximately $750. Patterson hopes treatment will soon be totally on an outpatient basis. At present, it may require a 10-day hospital stay. To learn which doctors presently are using the box in the United States and Canada, or to find out more about the upcoming FDA trials, write to:

Dr. Margaret Patterson
32 Chambers Lane
London, England NW10, 2 RJ

Bladder Pacemaker

At present, implanted devices to control the bladder are available only at the University of California at San Francisco. Some types of therapy are available on an outpatient basis. Patients with spastic bladder or who are incontinent can become outpatients. The cost of evaluation, doctor's fees, equipment and hospital stay is about $15,000. Dr. Schmidt says surgery will be available in about ten university medical centers across the country within the next year. For more information, write to:

Dr. Richard Schmidt
University of California School of Medicine at San Francisco
400 Parnassus A610
Urology Faculty Practice
San Francisco, CA 94143

Or contact the urology or urodynamics department of the nearest university medical center or rehabilitation center.

Diaphragm Pacer

Implantation of a diaphragm pacer is available at most major medical centers (though it isn't a routine procedure and some centers have much more experience in the surgery than others).

The centers with the most experience in performing this surgery are Yale University School of Medicine (the institution where Dr. William Glenn developed the device) and Case Western Reserve University. The surgery may require a lengthy hospital stay.

While nonquadriplegics may only need hospitalization for 6 weeks, quadriplegics could require a 6-month stay. The pacer itself costs between $12,000 and $18,000; surgery ranges from $2,000 to $3,000. Hospital costs are usually covered by insurance. For more information about the procedure and referrals to medical centers experienced in the procedure in your area contact:

Dr. William Glenn
Yale University School of Medicine
Dept. of Surgery
333 Cedar Street, Box 3333
New Haven, CT 06510
(203) 785-2703

Dr. Michael Nochomitz
Biomedical Engineering
 Department
Case Western Reserve University
Cleveland, OH, 44106
(216) 368-4093

Neuromuscular Stimulation System

About a dozen research centers are working on systems for helping paralysis victims use their arms and legs. The National Center for Rehabilitation Engineering at Wright State University is currently conducting clinical studies for their system. Treatment for clinical patients is free. If interested in becoming a clinical patient there, write to:

Dr. Jerrold Petrofsky or Chandler Phillips
National Center for Rehabilitation and Engineering
Wright State University
Dayton, OH 45435
(513) 873-3248

Ohio State University is working on a walking system similar to that of Wright State. If interested in becoming a clinical patient there, contact:

Herman Weed
Director, Biomedical Engineering Center
Ohio State University
Columbus, OH 43212
(614) 422-6018

Wright State's exerciser for the paralyzed is presently available at hospitals and rehabilitation clinics across the country. Its use is covered by insurance. It should be used by patients two to three times a week. In addition to quadriplegics and paraplegics, stroke victims may benefit from the system. The home system was introduced in January, 1986, and costs between $7,500 and $8,000. It is sold by physician's prescription. For more information, and/or a list of hospitals and clinics with TTI systems, and how to buy the home version, write to:

Therapeutic Technologies, Inc.
2200 West Commercial Boulevard
Fort Lauderdale, FL 33309

Related Information for Spinal-Cord-Injured Patients

For the latest information on what research is being done in the area of muscular stimulation, diaphragm pacing, bladder pacing, soft tissue healing, spinal cord regeneration, and other areas of importance to those suffering from spinal cord injuries, contact:

American Paralysis Association
2655 Old Springhouse Road, Suite 104
McLean, VA 22102
(703) 556-7782

For information on electrical treatment you may also wish to contact the National Spinal Cord Injury Association. This organization puts out a directory that includes information on where research is being done and refers readers to other important information sources, including those that give information on how to get financial assistance for various treatments. The book is called *National Resource Directory: Information Guide for Persons with Spinal Cord Injury and Other Physical Disabilities*. For spinal-cord-injured people, the cost is $4.50; for others it's $20. Write or call the Association for the book:

National Spinal Cord Injury Association
149 California Street
Newton, MA 02158
(617) 964-0521

Scoliosis Treatment

Both the external and implantable devices are available at most major medical centers in North America. The implantable device requires two surgical procedures, with two short hospital stays; the external device is used strictly on an outpatient basis.

While the cost of the electrical implant is about $2,700, the surface device costs between $1,100 and $1,200—a price comparable to that of a brace. These prices do not include doctor's fees, which vary widely, according to Dr. Herbert. All devices are covered by most insurance companies. For more information on where to find an orthopedic doctor in your area who uses either or both the external or electrical implant device, write to:

The Scoliosis Association
Department O
1 Penn Plaza
New York, NY 10119

The two companies that manufacture the external electrical equipment also have toll-free numbers to call for information on orthopedic doctors who use their device.

They are: Medtronic (800) 328-0810 and EBI Medical Systems (800) 526-2579.

Electric Braces

With clinical studies set to begin soon, those interested in becoming electric orthodontics patients may do so by contacting:

The University of Pennsylvania Dental School, Orthodontics Department
4001 Spruce Street
Philadelphia, PA 19104
(215) 898-8982

Bone Healing

The electrical devices described in this chapter are available at most major medical centers (though some centers favor one method over the others). The cost of treatment varies depending on the type of device used. The implantable devices require surgery and a 3- to-4 day hospital stay. Including the cost of the device, doctor's fee, hospital, etc., the fee usually runs between $4,500 and $6,000. The external device, pulsed electromagnetic field coils, don't require a hospital stay and the cost of using the device combined with doctor's fee is $2,600 to $2,950, depending on where the fracture is. Patients cannot keep the device: It must be returned at the end of treatment. All methods are covered by insurance. For more information, contact the orthopedics, rehabilitation medicine, or sports medicine department of the nearest medical center.

Avascular Necrosis

Patients are being accepted into the 30 to 35 clinical testing centers using the PEMFs device across the country. The device itself costs about $3,000. With doctor's fee, the cost may run to $5,000. The cost is about one-third that of a hip replacement, which—with doctor's fee, hospital, cost of artificial hip—is about $14,000 to $15,000. The PEMFs device is covered by some insurance companies. For more information on orthopedists using the device and clinical testing centers in your area, contact: the PEMFs manufacturer, Electro-Biology or the office of Dr. Andrew Bassett.

Electro-Biology
300 Fairfield Road
Fairfield, NJ 07006
(800) 526-2579

Andrew Bassett, M.D.
Columbia Presbyterian Medical Center
722 West 168th Street
New York, NY, 10032
(212) 305-3432

Soft-Tissue Healing

Soft tissue electrohealing is still very much in the experimental stages:
most testing is still being performed on animals. For more information on
progress of research, contact the American Paralysis Association (listed on
page 35), the National Center for Rehabilitation and Engineering (also
listed on page 35), or:

Dr. Norman Schacher
Calgary General Hospital
841 Center Avenue
East Calgary, Alberta
Canada T2 EOA1

2

Redesigning the Brain

At Brookhaven National Laboratory in Suffolk County, New York, two schizophrenic men were led into the Positron Emission Tomography (PET) room. Both were in communication with otherworldly voices.

"One heard voices telling him he was God, and the other guy thought he was the devil," recalls Alfred P. Wolf, chairman of Brookhaven's department of chemistry. "We had them here on the same day and they kept arguing with each other." The PET scans showed that God and the Prince of Darkness had something in common. On the color-coded display the patients' frontal lobes (at the front of the brain, behind the eyebrows) glowed bluish green. That meant abnormally sluggish activity in a part of the brain thought to govern insight, foresight, and empathy. "It was very exciting," says Wolf, "because it was the first demonstration of a clear abnormality in a schizophrenic brain."

For most of human history the human brain was a terra incognita all but inaccessible to scientists' probes. In the late 1800s a young Viennese neurologist named Sigmund Freud, who had done some creditable research on the nerves of lampreys and crayfish, despaired of ever deciphering the complex wiring and decided to explore the brain with words instead. For the better part of this century the behaviorist psychologists, following their mentor B. F. Skinner, focused on input (stimuli) and output (behavior) and ignored all the murky territory in between.

Today, for the first time, there are windows on the organ of thought. One of them is *Positron Emission Tomography*, or *PET*, an imaging technique invented in 1973 at Washington University in St. Louis by Michael E. Phelps. The patient is injected with a radioactive form of glucose, a sugar used in brain metabolism, which "lights up" the brain cells that absorb it. The result is a vivid picture of the brain's *activity*, not just solid structures.

Thanks to PET, scientists can now "open the hood" of a living, thinking brain and see hallucinations, epileptic seizures, the spreading dementia of Alzheimer's disease, or the seesawing moods of a "rapidly-cycling" manic depressive. They can watch how the brain reacts to music or Sherlock Holmes stories, how a memory decays in time, which parts of the brain are involved in panic attacks and in the strange attacks of coprolalia—uncontrollable bursts of foul language, tics, and grunting—that plague people with Tourette's syndrome.

But high tech imaging techniques such as PET and Nuclear Magnetic Resonance (NMR) aren't the only new windows on the human brain. Remarkable breakthroughs in our knowledge of brain chemistry made in the last decade are making it possible to decipher the subtle chemical messages that cause depression, pain, hallucinations, serenity, sleep, panic, or food binges. Today, as more and more "mental" illnesses turn out to be biological, scientists are searching for the secrets of schizophrenia and depression in spinal fluid samples, not in psychological excavations of the patient's childhood.

What scientists look for in these bodily fluids are abnormal levels of neurochemicals, hormones, brain enzymes, and metabolites (breakdown products) that may explain something about the biology of mental disease. Schizophrenics are known to have abnormal levels of dopamine, a neurochemical, and all the drugs used to treat the disease (such as Thorazine and Haldol) work by suppressing dopamine in the brain. (Unfortunately, these drugs don't actually *cure* schizophrenia—they merely suppress the most florid symptoms. A number of neurochemicals appear to be unbalanced in the brains of depressives and manic depressives. Chemical abnormalities have shown up in people suffering from panic attacks, certain phobias, obsessive compulsive disorder, anxiety neurosis, anorexia nervosa, and many other ills. Just as an internist can tell if a person has diabetes from a simple urinalysis, a psychiatrist in 1998 will probably need only a vial of blood and urine to detect anorexia, melancholia, obsessions, double identity, and suicidal tendencies.

Designer Drugs

A curious experiment was in progress at Stanford University's Hormone Research Laboratory. One by one a group of medical students and music graduate students entered a soundproof booth to listen to their favorite music over stereo headphones. Though their tastes ranged from Franz Liszt and Miles Davis to the raspy, whiskey-cured angst of Janis Joplin singing "Take Another Little Piece of My Heart," all of the students had something in common. When they heard their favorite musical passages they felt "thrills," or tingles, prickly feelings at the back of their necks or down their spines. By noting the hand signals the volunteers were asked to give every time they had this sensation, Stanford neuroscientist Avram Goldstein kept careful track of the frequency of the tingles.

Then he picked a few of the best "tinglers," gave them shots of either saline (a placebo) or a drug called *naloxone*, and repeated the experiment. This time the thrill was gone for the listeners who had been given naloxone—or at least, their tingles were fewer and less intense. Why? Naloxone blocked the action of endorphins, natural opiate-like substances in the brain. That suggested that sublime musical pleasure—something most of us would categorize as an aesthetic, even spiritual, joy—was a chemical experience. It depended on endorphins.

Experiments like this have taught us that everything from aesthetic thrills to existential despair is the product of minute chemical reactions in the brain. "The brain is just a little box with emotions packed into it," explains National Institutes of Mental Health (NIMH) pharmacologist Candace Pert, one of the pioneers of the pharmacologic revolution. "We're starting to understand that emotions have biochemical correlates. When human beings engage in different activities, neurojuices are released that are associated with pain or pleasure." About 50 different chemical messengers, or neurotransmitters, have been identified so far, and scientists estimate there are at least 200 in all.

In order to have an effect, a molecule of a neurotransmitter (or of a drug) must fit into a specially shaped receptor on the surface of a brain cell, rather as a key fits in a lock. In 1973 Pert, then an unknown 26-year-old graduate student at Johns Hopkins University, meticulously mixed radioactively labeled drugs into mashed mouse brain and discovered the opiate receptor. This was a customized "keyhole" in the brain cells for the opiate narcotics—morphine, heroin, and their relatives—and its discovery paved the way for the discovery, 2 years later, of the amazing endorphins. But the opiate receptor turned out to be just one of many specialized binding sites in the brain. Some two dozen have now been identified, including receptors for the popular antianxiety agent Valium (diazepam) and the street drug angel dust (phencyclidine, or PCP). Pain, hunger, moods, memories, and dreams are all the result of the intricate interaction of neurochemicals and receptors.

In the last 5 years brave new techniques for measuring brain receptors in test tubes have paved the way for "magic bullets," drugs that go directly to the intended receptors and bypass the others. Current drugs, such as barbiturates, do reach the proper targets, but on the way they set off dozens of inappropriate receptors, causing side effects. It's as if you sloshed a bucket of paint all over the floor to cover a 1-inch spot. "All our old drugs were discovered through one accident after another," explains pharmacologist Solomon Snyder of Johns Hopkins University. "And after we already had the drugs we went back and figured out how they worked. Now we have the molecular tools to design a whole new line of drugs."

With the discovery of the benzodiazepine (Valium) receptor in 1982, scientists began avidly to research the production of compounds that stick to only one subclass of the receptor, producing calm without fatigue. By tinkering with the six known subtypes of opiate receptors, they are designing new, nonaddictive super-painkillers. The receptors for adenosine, a sort of natural anticaffeine in the brain, have inspired the prototype of a drug with the wakeup power of a hundred cups of espresso but without the jitters.

Among the new "designer drugs" are experimental compounds that increase attention span, improve memory, sober you up the morning after, and quash the urge to gorge on potato chips. And in 1995, instead of worshipping at the feet of a Perfect Master, you may get 10 milligrams of transcendance in a pill. Research on two adenosine analogs, *EHNA* and *LPIA*, indicates that these compounds seem to put rats at the NIMH into a paradoxical state of "quiet wakefulness." "We may have hit on an altered state of animal consciousness," one of the researchers observed.

There are also hints of a suicide prevention pill. Recent experiments have shown that suicidal people have unusually low levels of a chemical messenger, serotonin. What's more, those who try to do away with themselves violently—using shotguns or leaps from tall buildings, say, rather than overdoses of sleeping pills—have the lowest serotonin levels. Very likely, then, the antidote to self-destruction will turn out to be a serotonin-boosting compound.

Brain Pills

Certain forms of violence have a peculiar chemical "fingerprint," as well. A few years ago scientists took blood samples from a group of mass murderers in a Swedish prison and found, to their astonishment, that all of them had low levels of a chemical called hydroxyindoleactic acid (5-HIAA), a metabolite, or breakdown product, of serotonin. Only one of the murderers had normal 5-HIAA levels, and he was a different sort of killer. A mild attendant in a nursing home, he had quietly performed mercy killings on some two dozen aged patients in his care. Low 5-HIAA appeared again among a group of murderers in Finland. They fell into two categories, psychopathic killers, who had murdered "totally out of the blue" for no discernible reason, and paranoid murderers, who had killed after long premeditation. Biochemical tests revealed that psychopaths had much lower levels of 5-HIAA than either paranoids or normals. The researchers concluded that low serotonin (once considered a mark of depression) is probably an index of general impulsivity that can lead to violence toward oneself or toward others.

What will happen when such blood tests enter the courtroom, bringing a new legal definition to the myriad faces of crime? What if the chemists design an "anticrime" pill capable of changing street gang leaders into wholesome, all American Rotarians? Who should be given such a drug and on whose authority? Who should decide what is antisocial behavior and what is not?

In 10 years such questions will not be hypothetical.

In another 10 years, too, a "Total Receptor Workup" will probably be more fundamental to psychiatry than free-association and dream analysis. With a PET scanner and some radioactively labeled compounds, a scientist will look into a patient's brain and see the problems in technicolor. Injecting the patient with a radioactive isotope to "light up" the receptors, the scientist will obtain a three-dimensional computerized map of the brain, in which the receptors are illumined like miniature galaxies. The computer will store the figures for each type of receptor on a separate floppy disk, and the patient will receive a printout of all the receptor densities. This isn't a pipe dream. Receptors were "photographed" inside a living human brain for the first time on May 25, 1983, when Dr. Henry N. Wagner, director of nuclear medicine at Johns Hopkins University, PET-scanned his own dopamine receptors. A year later the same Hopkins team PET-scanned human opiate receptors, and they are currently brewing a half dozen radioactive compounds to be used in visualizing other receptors.

When the results of the Receptor Workup are analyzed, the patient will get a prescription for four or five very specific compounds guaranteed to improve his or her inner life: a drug that dispels certain phobias, selectively erases traumatic memories, exorcises guilt, or curbs random aggression. There will be an antigrief pill, an antidote for lovesickness, a compound that controls the compulsion to shop, a capsule that helps you communicate openly with your spouse, a pill that makes familiar things (such as a mate of 20 years) seem novel.

"When we have a bacterial infection we go right in and treat it with a drug," observes David Nichols, a medicinal chemist at Purdue University in Indiana. "But psychiatry has this weightlifter's adage, 'No pain, no gain.' It's a very archaic attitude. Why shouldn't we develop chemotherapeutic agents that could quickly open up emotional problems and change them?"

The compounds Nichols tests happen to be *psychedelic* compounds. The word may conjure images of the Be-ins and freakouts of the 1960s, but Nichols is not alone among respectable, law abiding scientists in believing that refined descendants of LSD, mescaline, and the like could be tomorrow's psychiatric wonder drugs. Minor alterations in the mescaline molecule in the 1960s and 1970s, for instance, spawned a whole cafeteria of "neopsychedelic" analogs with very precise effects. While many of these drugs remained laboratory curiosities, one of them, MDMA—also known as Ecstasy, XTC, or Adam—leaked out to the street around 1984, gaining a wide circle of fans. A chemical blend of mescaline and amphetamine, Ecstasy has been touted as a "beginner's LSD" that "opens the heart." The prototype of the new "designer" psychedelic, it is said to produce a psychedelic high without the confusion and perceptual distortions of the classic psychedelics.

Nichols himself is brewing "second and third generation drugs" to treat minor psychiatric ills—phobias and the like. Following the law and testing his compounds on rat brains, not sophomores' psyches, he has just designed a promising new compound with "the same empathetic properties of MDMA but less of a high."

He hopes it will be more palatable to the establishment than MDMA/Ecstasy, which was recently banned by the Drug Enforcement Administration.

Perhaps, by using specific molecules to unlock specific compartments of the mind, twenty-first-century chemists will fulfill the ancient alchemical dream of turning base consciousness into gold. Psychiatric patients of the future will be taking Jungian drugs, empathy drugs, age regression drugs, telepathy capsules, Nirvana in a pill.

The Clocks within Us

For 10 years Gloria seesawed between midwinter gloom and summer elation. Between November and March every year she sank into some terrible Siberia of the soul. Exhausted and depressed, she slept 12 hours a night and was still tired. She gorged on sweets and starches, took more and more sick days from work, stopped seeing her friends, and derived pleasure from nothing. Then, miraculously, around late March or early April, she emerged from her doldrums. Her mood soared, she rejoined the human race, and her long dark night of the soul seemed a distant bad dream.

It was a weird form of depression, and it took Norman E. Rosenthal of the NIMH to diagnose it. He came across Gloria among a puzzling group of "atypical depressives" whose moods varied seasonally. These winter depressives, he noted, were distinct both from normal people (whose occasional January funks aren't incapacitating) and ordinary depressives and manic depressives. After giving the problem a name, seasonal affective disorder (SAD), Rosenthal proceeded to find a cure.

In the winter of 1981-82 he recruited a group of hard-core SAD patients, mostly women in their early to middle thirties who had suffered through 9 or 10 winters of discontent. Suspecting that their problems stemmed from an abnormal "light hunger," he tried prolonging their daylight artificially with bright, full-spectrum fluorescent lights, like the grow lights for plants. Every day, just before dawn and right after dusk, the winter depressives sat in front of a bank of lights that mimicked daylight. After 2 or 3 days their despair cleared up completely. Some discontinued the light therapy and plunged back into their winter funks, while those who kept up the regimen all winter long remained depression-free.

How did it work? The key appears to be an obscure hormone called melatonin, secreted by the pineal gland deep in the brain. Melatonin levels peak during the long nights of winter, while sunlight inhibits the chemical. In animals melatonin plays a role in coordinating internal biological rhythms to the external cycles of day and night. Hamsters injected with melatonin will go into hibernation even in the middle of summmer. "In most species," Rosenthal explains, "the seasonal rhythms governing such things as mating, food intake, hibernation, and migration are cued mainly by the light-dark cycle, which is largely invariant from year to year."

But humans, surrounded as we are by thermostats, air-conditioning, and one-stop shopping malls, don't hibernate, migrate, or build nests. Or do we? "I wish I were a bear," one of Rosenthal's winter depressives confided. "Bears are allowed to hibernate, but humans aren't." In fact, SAD may be something like a human version of hibernation. "Obviously, SAD patients don't actually hibernate, migrate, or go through the extreme temperature changes that many animals do," says Rosenthal. "But certain similarities are striking. They overeat, oversleep, change food preferences, and gain weight.

"Maybe SAD is an atavistic seasonal rhythm that might have been adaptive in some cultures. Or perhaps it is a pathology, a breakdown in the mechanisms that normally keep the internal environment constant despite changes on the outside."

In any case, the banks of super-bright artificial light (and *not* ordinary room light) had a "marked antidepressant effect" on the winter depressives, Rosenthal and his cohorts concluded. They believe light therapy works by altering the production of melatonin and serotonin, two brain chemicals known to be involved in regulating the body's internal "clocks."

This experiment and hundreds like it are revealing the importance of the biological timekeepers that rule our lives. Almost every system in the body—from the concentration of minerals, hormones, and infection-fighting cells in the blood to blood pressure and body temperature—oscillates over a period of hours, days, weeks, or months. By charting our internal rhythms, the fledgling science of chronobiology promises to revolutionize our lives in myriad ways. For instance, one new "rhythm" science, chronopharmacology, has shown that the effects of a medication vary with the time of day you take it, and that circadian (*from circa dies*, or "close to a day") rhythms influence both the effectiveness of and the amount of damage caused by anticancer drugs.

The closest thing to a "master clock" in the body is the *suprachiasmatic nucleus (SCN)*, a minute cluster of light-sensitive cells deep in the brain. The SCN appears to act as a sort of switchboard, cueing waking, sleeping, and activity patterns to external patterns such as the light/dark cycle. "Every neurotransmitter, every hormone, every tissue in your body has a rhythm," explains Joe E. Miller of the University of California at Riverside. "Usually the SCN coordinates all these rhythms." Our inner timekeepers, however, can be easily disrupted. Jet travel uncouples the internal rhythms from the rhythms of the external world, and manic depressives, as well as some people suffering depression, seem to have circadian clocks that run either too fast or too slow.

Recent experiments by Thomas A. Wehr and his colleagues at

the NIMH's sleep laboratory showed that depressives suffer from a sort of internal jet lag, their sleep/wake cycles out of phase with other circadian rhythms such as temperature. This gave Wehr the idea for a novel treatment for depression. Waiting until a patient was in the middle of a depression, Wehr shifted his sleep cycle by putting him to bed six hours earlier, at 5:00 p.m. instead of 11:00 p.m. After 2 days the patient's depression vanished completely. The reason, Wehr thought, was that the patient's sleep/wake cycle was jolted into phase with other body rhythms.

How nice if depression could be cured forever by simply moving someone's bedtime 6 hours ahead every night! Alas, after the third "phase advance," the patient remained depressed, probably because his temperature rhythm lagged behind the sleep/wake rhythm. But Wehr believes that a combination of shifts in sleep timing and drug therapy (antidepressants, for instance, alter circadian rhythms by acting on the master pacemaker of the SCN) will give us a long-lasting treatment for depression.

It's All in the Mind

A hay fever victim starts wheezing the moment he's shown a picture of ragweed. A hypnotized woman is told that the pencil in her hand is a lit cigarette, and within minutes her hand is covered in blisters. Entering a meditative state, a man with cancer of the colon visualizes his white blood cells as brave white knights, searching out and destroying every cancer cell in his body. His next checkup shows he's in remission.

We always knew intuitively that the mind could heal—or kill—the body, but in scientific circles the idea smacked of mumbo-jumbo, snake oil, and dubious south of the border cures. How, after all, does a belief translate into an ulcer? How can thoughts cure carcinoma? Well, a revolutionary new science called *psychoneuroimmunology*, or *PNI*, has the answer: The mind/brain and the immune system are wired together.

This is a radical departure from the standard doctrine of a totally independent immune system, and it all began with a group of mice at the University of Rochester in New York. In 1974 psychologist

Robert Ader put them through a standard behavioral conditioning experiment. Just as Pavlov conditioned his dogs to salivate at the sound of a bell, Ader trained his mice to be repulsed by the taste of water laced with saccharin. Every time they drank the sweetened water, he injected them with a drug, cyclophosphamide, that caused nausea. Before long the animals got sick whenever they tasted the sweet liquid, just as they were supposed to. Then something peculiar happened. Some of them started mysteriously dropping dead—just from drinking the saccharin-laced water. It turned out that the nauseating drug, cyclophosphamide, also suppressed the immune system. But the mice's mortality rate was proportional to the dose of *saccharin*, not the dose of cyclophosphamide.

"Because I didn't 'know' there was no connection between the brain and immune system, I was free to make up any story," Ader recalls. "I said it was possible that while I was conditioning the taste aversion I was also conditioning immunosuppression." Every time the conditioned mice drank saccharin, in other words, they *thought* they were drinking cyclophosphamide, and this belief was conveyed to their immune systems, with lethal results.

Needless to say, this was blasphemy. Most immunology textbooks *still* don't show any connection between the immune system and the nervous system, nor any way the mind could control immunity. But Ader followed up his accidental discovery with a meticulously controlled experiment that proved the mice had been killed by their "beliefs" and not by some mysterious toxin.

Since then, definite brain–immune system links have come to light. When brain chemicals are mixed with immune cells in laboratory dishes, they exert powerful effects on the white blood cells that make antibodies, for example. Receptors for many neurochemicals have turned up in different parts of the immune system. The mind does speak to the body, and at long last we're beginning to decipher the language.

"It's all one system!" says neuroscientist Candace Pert, who has recently teamed up with an immunologist to locate receptors for opiates and other "mood chemicals" on the surface of immune-system cells. "I can't relate to the mind/body dichotomy any longer. Is your consciousness in your head? No, it's in your whole body." Edwin Blalock, a microbiologist at the University of Texas Medical

Branch in Galveston, views the immune system as a kind of "sensory organ," sensing "those things that are not recognized by the central nervous system, those things you can't see, hear, touch, taste. . . ."

For years some forward-looking researchers have been charting connections between emotions and rheumatoid arthritis, breast cancer, and heart disease, and noting that people could literally die of grief. In 1964, author Norman Cousins claimed that positive emotions and "laughter therapy" cured him of a life-threatening disease. In Texas, cancer specialists Carl and Stephanie Simonton trained cancer patients to boost their immune response with mental imagery and meditation.

If the immune system is indeed an extension of the brain, then all medicine is psychosomatic medicine. Drugs that imitate brain chemicals will be used to bolster an immune system debilitated by grief or stress. A futuristic biofeedback apparatus linked to a blood analyzer could train patients to crank out more antibodies or mobilize their T-lymphocytes. Faith healing, the placebo effect, and laying on of hands will come out of the twilight zone.

As Candace Pert puts it, "I no longer believe in disease at all. Disease is a hundred percent mental. It's just your brain state being reflected in your body."

Pacemakers for Peace

In 1974 a 21-year old Louisiana librarian was shot in the head during a holdup, and a large portion of her frontal lobes had to be removed during surgery. After the operation she suffered frequent seizures, could barely talk, and had to be fed through a tube because she refused food. A year later she was in a continual frenzy, lashing out at anyone who approached her. Several times she attempted to stab her father. Complaining of constant, excruciating pain all over her body, she screamed in agony whenever she was touched. There seemed to be no hope for her until in November 1976, at Tulane University Medical School in New Orleans, she received a brain pacemaker.

Devised by the brilliant and controversial Dr. Robert Heath, the founding chairman of Tulane's department of psychiatry and neurology, the pacemaker is an array of 20 tiny battery powered electrodes that regulates the brain's electrical activity. It sits under the skull on the surface of the cerebellum, a large lobed structure at the very back of the brain, and its power source, a battery pack the size of a deck of playing cards, originally fit in the patient's pocket. Later it was miniaturized to the size of a matchbook; it is now implanted in the abdomen, and surgery is required for recharging it every 5 years.

The first recipient of a Heath pacemaker was "the most violent patient in the state," in Heath's words. The mildly retarded 19-year-old man had to be kept tied to his bed to prevent his savage outbursts. With a pacemaker installed in his brain, he stopped trying to slash himself and those around him and went home from the hospital. Everything was fine for a while, until he suddenly ran amok, he tried to murder his parents, severely wounded a neighbor, and narrowly escaped being gunned down by the sheriff in the process. When Heath x-rayed the man's brain, he quickly spotted the problem: The wires running from the pacemaker to the power source had broken. When the wires were reattached, the young man's rampages subsided, and he became pleasant and sociable. Today he is in vocational rehabilitation and doing well.

In the young librarian's brain an even more dramatic metamorphosis occurred. When the pacemaker was in place, her rage attacks waned. Her memory improved, she began eating again, and her doctors began to describe her personality as "pleasant" and "sparkling."

Brain pacemakers had been used to treat epilepsy, muscle coordination problems, and uncontrollable pain, but Dr. Heath was the first to apply them to behavioral problems. He claims the treatment works because the cerebellum is intimately connected with pleasure and pain centers deep inside the brain. Beginning in 1950 he implanted electrodes deep in the brains of some severely mentally ill people and recorded their brain waves as they talked, recalled the past, flew into rages, hallucinated, or had seizures. When his electrodes picked up abnormal electrical discharges in the limbic system (the emotional center) of these troubled brains, Heath began to suspect that mental illness sprang from a defective "pleasure system" and an overactive "aversive system." He found that by stimulating the pleasure circuits with electrodes, he could exorcise homicidal rages, depressions, suicide attempts, and delusions— sometimes for a long time. Eventually he determined that the same effect could be achieved with a pacemaker that delivers 3- to 6-volt pulses every 5 minutes to a precise half-inch of the cerebellum. Of the 40-odd recipients, about half have substantially improved, according to Heath—no mean feat, considering most had come from the ranks of the incurable. For some reason, the pacemaker has worked best with depressives, violent patients, and some epileptics, and least well with schizophrenics.

Heath, now retired, doesn't plan to oufit any more patients with cerebellar pacemakers. ("There are too many problems!") He proposes, however, that similar results could be achieved by stimulating the brain's pleasure center with an ultrasound device, which wouldn't require drilling holes through anyone's skull.

Electrotranquility

And there are other, less drastic forms of electrotranquility on the horizon. In the early 1980s, as part of a Soviet-American scientific exchange, Soviet scientists sent over something called a *Lida*, a crude machine made of vacuum tubes and other vintage parts. Scientists at Pettis Memorial Veterans Administration Hospital in Loma Linda, California, tested it by putting the Lida next to a nervous cat in a metal box. When the device began broadcasting radio waves in the frequency of deep-sleep brain waves, the cat slipped into a deep trance. "Instead of taking a Valium to relax yourself," concluded Pettis Memorial's Dr. W. Ross Adey, "it looks as if a similar result could be achieved with a radio field." The principle behind the Lida is a phenomenon called entrainment, meaning that a person's brain waves automatically fire in synchrony with the surrounding pulses. Soviet scientists claim they've used the Lida to treat insomnia, hypertension, anxiety, and neurotic disturbances, and there are rumors of a more-sophisticated version capable of controlling minds at a distance.

In this country, on the other hand, a wall of scientific skepticism will have to be overcome before Lida-like devices are sold at the corner drugstore. The traditional dogma is that low-intensity electromagnetic fields, unlike x-rays and other forms of ionizing radiation, have no biological effects. But Adey and his colleagues showed that very weak currents altered the way calcium ions bound to the cell membranes, setting off powerful chemical reactions within the cell. In experiments in Sweden, rabbits exposed to the electrical fields in railroad switching yards suffered stunted growth and grave neurological problems. Rats exposed in utero to the fields generated by video display terminals (VDTs) reportedly were born with birth defects, if they did not die first. Perhaps the Russians are right in taking these fields very seriously. Perhaps the electromagnetic waves flowing out of telephone lines, transmission towers, radar installations, and microwave appliances—as well as Lidas—can make us irritable, serene, alert, forgetful, anxious, or depressed.

Brain "Transplants"

> GOLDEN AGERS: Do you suffer from Parkinson's
> disease? Alzheimer's disease? Do you sometimes
> have trouble connecting your grandchildren's
> names with their faces? Would you like to
> throw away your walker and recover the
> physical agility of your twenties? If you
> answered "yes" to any of the above questions,
> you should seriously consider a BRAIN CELL
> TRANSPLANT. Call the FOUNTAIN OF YOUTH
> NEUROREGENERATIVE INSTITUTE for a FREE
> CONSULTATION today: 764-9986.

It may evoke images of Dr. Frankenstein, but in the year 2005 you could be reading such an ad, inviting you to replace your dead or diseased brain cells with fresh ones from a donor brain. Because the brain, like the eye, is an immunologically privileged organ, where the body's normally vigilant immunological defenders do not patrol against foreign invaders, tissue can be transplanted from one brain to another without the rejection problems that plague other organ transplants. In fact, this has already been done.

It began with rats. Using a toxin, scientists gave rats Parkinson's disease, a degenerative disease caused by the death of neurons that normally produce the chemical messenger dopamine, and marked by tremors, a masklike expression, and muscular rigidity to the point of paralysis. Then they took brain tissue from fetal rats and planted it in the brains of the rats with Parkinson's. Not only did the sick rats improve, but months later, when the scientists killed the animals and looked inside their brains, they saw the dopamine fibers, stained a fluorescent green, growing out from the graft and connecting to the target neurons in the host brain. "Somehow," one researcher remarked, "the nerves just know how to grow and they make the right connections."

In late 1985 the same feat was accomplished in the monkey brain, which in size and complexity approaches the human organ. Two separate research teams announced that they had induced Parkinsonian tremors and movement problems in a handful of adult monkeys and then reversed the symptoms with grafts of dopamine-rich cells from the brains of fetal monkeys. In the most dramatic case, a monkey lost its tremor and improved its movements a week after surgery and appeared altogether normal 2 weeks later. The implants reportedly survived in the host brain for at least 2 months.

Implants of specific clumps of brain have also made stumbling, elderly rats agile as youngsters; corrected various hormone deficiencies; cured a rat version of Alzheimer's disease; restored the memories of amnesiac, lobotomized rats; and reversed the "hypersexuality" of female rats with lesions of the hypothalamus, a part of the brain governing sexual appetite. Suppose you become senile around the year 2010. No problem. Surgeons will simply replace your dead "memory cells" (in an area of the brain called the hippocampus) with some good cells from a donor brain. If you're stricken with Parkinson's disease, Huntington's chorea ("Woody Guthrie disease"), or diabetes insipidus, or with blindess, deafness, or paralysis following a stroke, a brain graft will fix it. Maybe the right clump of neural tissue—a new set of frontal lobes, say—will even make you smarter or endow you with foresight.

In Sweden, four patients with severe Parkinson's disease have received brain grafts. The donors in this case were the patients' own adrenal glands, which happen to make the chemical dopamine. While the first two "transplants" were unsuccessful, two patients who had grafts in May 1985 reportedly improved temporarily, only to relapse 2 months later when the grafts presumably died.

Besides the technical difficulties posed by the sheer size and complexity of the human thought organ, the "brain transplant" is plagued by a number of ethical problems. The notion of harvesting fetal brains to repair aging ones stirs up such ethical heebiejeebies that this will probably never be done. Instead, donor brain tissue might come from baboons or chimpanzees (interspecies grafts have already worked between mice and rats).

The Biochip

While some scientists are working on brain grafts, a few Promethean souls are dreaming of a prosthesis for the entire apparatus of thought. Perhaps by the year 2086 your great-grandchildren, perusing the modern equivalent of matchbook covers or subway posters, will come upon the following advertisement:

Rather than acting like a computer, tomorrow's brain may actually be one, if biologist James V. McAlear has his way. McAlear, cofounder of EMV Associates, Inc., in Rockville, Maryland, is one of several forward looking scientists who are trying to make a "biochip," a computer chip made of organic molecules. Because it would be tiny and three-dimensional, a molecular computer chip could pack a million times the computing power of its solid-state equivalent. McAlear has already patented a technique for making a conductor out of a protein molecule—the first step, he says, in the creation of a VSD, or Very Small Device, capable of being implanted in a human brain.

What McAlear and colleague John Wehrung aspire to before the decade is out is artificial vision. A miniature television camera mounted on eyeglasses would serve as the "eyes," and the camera's signals would be converted to electrical pulses and sent to an array of miniature electrodes implanted in the brain. That part isn't so revolutionary, of course. What sets McAlear's device apart is that his electrodes would be coated with cultured embryonic nerve cells, which would actually hook up with the nerve cells of the visual cortex. And that's just step one of a truly audacious project.

The biocomputer of McAlear's dreams is a godlike instrument of thought that will wed the number-crunching power of electrons to the reasoning talents of neurons. It is an entire molecular computer that will set up residence in the human brain, sending out shoots of nerve fibers to grow into nerve cells. It will have a double helix so it can replicate itself. Biochip users will be able to store any sort of information on the biochip and use the neurons and thoughts to retrieve the entire Library of Congress. By mating nervous tissue to circuit switches 100 million times faster than synapses, the brain's "switches," the implant will evolve into "a superior, an omnipotent being," according to McAlear. What's more, he predicts that the being of the user will live on not in the central nervous system but in the biocomputer. In other words, when a person dies, the computer—storing memories and all knowledge—could be transplanted to a fresh host. "That pretty much fits the specifications for an immortal soul," notes McAlear.

Timeline

1987 • The brain's "natural Valium" is discovered, paving the way for a new line of no-side-effects tranquilizers.

1990 • A "perfect morphine," without the side effects of addiction, respiratory depression, and constipation, is developed, tailored to one subtype of the brain's many different varieties of opiate receptors.

1993 • In Stockholm, the first wholly successful "brain transplant" is performed on a 57-year-old woman with Parkinson's disease. Dopamine-producing cells from the woman's own body are implanted in her brain. Though totally mute, immobile, and bed-ridden for years, within a month of surgery the patient is taking walks, talking to friends on the telephone, and making plans to move into an apartment.

1994 • Hoffman-LaRoche markets a new drug, Pacifizine, as an "effective suicide prevention therapy."

1995 • Eli Lilly begins testing a drug that in 31 percent of normal subjects produces a "photographic memory" for ten days. The same compound reverses memory loss in demented patients.

1996 • The first ultrasound brain pacemaker transforms an uncontrollably violent paranoid schizophrenic into a "very pleasant, sociable guy."

1998 • Chronopsychiatrists at the University of Minnesota devise a "phototherapy and circadian alteration" program that is 98 percent successful in curing certain forms of depression.

1999 • A "Total Receptor Workup" is performed routinely on all new psychiatric patients. The test calculates the density and distribution of 47 different brain receptors and rates them against the age- and sex-matched norm.

2001 • Researchers discover the gene for depression. A simple genetic screen tells whether a person is a carrier of an affective illness (depression or manic-depressive disorder).

2002 • Agoraphobia, panic attacks, anxiety neurosis, and compulsions, are now totally curable by drugs.

2011 • In Rochester, New York, brain tissue from a fetal baboon is grafted into the brain of a 61-year-old man suffering from severe Alzheimer's disease. Although his memory improves temporarily, the graft is rejected after a month.

2012 • A second brain graft in an Alzheimer's patient, performed in Stockholm, is more successful. Two weeks after surgery, the patient recognizes his grandchildren for the first time in years.

2086 • The first Biochip, a supercomputer made of protein, is implanted into the brain of a 63-year-old Van Nuys, California, security guard.

Access Guide

New drug treatments for brain-related disorders such as Alzheimer's Disease and anorexia nervosa are experimental at present; however, research centers recruit volunteers with particular problems to take part in clinical trials of new drugs.

For more information contact one of the following institutions:

Eating Disorders

The Eating Disorders Research Unit
Dr. B. Timothy Walsh
New York State Psychiatric
 Institute
722 West 168th Street
New York, NY 10032
(212) 960-5751

Intramural Research Program
Dr. David Jimerson
National Institute of Mental
 Health (NIMH)
Building 10, Room 3S231
Bethesda, MD 20804
(301) 496-1945

Alzheimer's Disease

Dr. Dennis L. Murphy
NIMH
Building 10, Room 3D41
Bethesda, MD 20892

Phobias

Anxiety Disorders Clinic
Dr. Michael Liebowitz
New York State Psychiatric
 Institute
Columbia Presbyterian Medical
 Center
722 West 168th Street
New York, NY 10032
(212) 960-2367

Panic Disorder/Agoraphobia
Intramural Research Program
Dr. Tom Uhde
NIMH
Building 10, Room 3S239
Bethesda, MD 20205
(301) 496-6825

Obsessive-Compulsive Disorder

Intramural Research Program
Dr. Thomas Insel
NIMH
Building 10, Room 3D41
Bethesda, MD 20804
(301) 496-3421

(This clinical program is set up specifically for adults.)

Intramural Research Program
Dr. Judith Rapoport
NIMH
Building 10, Room 6N240
Bethesda, MD 20804
(301) 496-6081

(This program is set up specifically for children and adolescents.)

Depression

Depression Evaluation Service
Dr. Fredric Quitkin
New York State Psychiatric
    Institute
Columbia Presbyterian Medical
    Center
722 West 168th Street
New York, NY 10032
(212) 960-5734

Intramural Research Program
Dr. Robert Post
NIMH
Building 10, Room 3N212
Bethesda, MD 20804
(301) 496-4805

Schizophrenia

St. Elizabeth's Hospital
Dr. Richard Wyatt
2700 Martin Luther King, Jr.
    Avenue
WAW Building
Washington, DC 20032
(202) 373-7572

Intramural Research Program
Dr. David Pickard
NIMH
Building 10, Room 4N214
Bethesda, MD 20894
(301) 496-4303

Seasonal Affective Disorder (SAD)

Seasonal affective disorder is a recurrent winter depression interspersed with feelings of well being in spring and summer. For information on programs treating SAD with light therapy contact:

Seasonality Studies
Dr. Norman E. Rosenthal
Clinical Psychobiology Branch
NIMH
Building 10, Room 4S239
Bethesda, MD 20892
(301) 496-2141

Light Therapy Unit
Dr. Michael Terman
New York State Psychiatric
 Institute
722 West 168th Street
New York, NY 10032
(212) 960-5714

Light Ideas
Marc Zitelman
1037 Taft Street
Rockville, MD 20850
(301) 424-LITE

Zitelman supplies sun boxes and serves as an information network for any new light research.

Holistic Medicine

The role of the mind in healing is emphasized in Holistic medicine. Professional organizations of practitioners of alternative and nontraditional medicine include:

The American Holistic Medical
 Association
6932 Little River Turnpike
Annandale, VA 22003
(703) 642-5880

American Academy of Behavioral
 Medicine
12890 Hillcrest, Suite 200
Dallas, TX 75230
(214) 458-8333

International Academy of
 Biological Medicine
P.O. Box 31313
Phoenix, AZ 85046
(602) 992-0589

Society of Behavioral Medicine
P.O. Box 8530, University Station
Knoxville, TN 37996
(615) 974-5164

Academy of Psychosomatic Medicine
70 West Hubbard Street, Suite 202
Chicago, IL 60610
(312) 644-2623

Among institutions that teach techniques such as meditation, relaxation methods, and imaging are:

Interface
63 Chapel Street
Newton, MA 02158
(617) 924-1100

Association for the Development
  of Human Potential
P.O. Box 60
Porthill, ID 83853
(604) 227-9224

Esalen Institute
Big Sur, CA 93920
(408) 667-2335

East-West Center for Holistic
  Health
141 Fifth Avenue
New York, NY 10010
(212) 691-9107

Therapeutic Touch

In the Bible, it's called laying on of hands, and Western medicine has yet to come to terms with it. However, a hospital study in the early 1970s showed that patients given therapeutic touch by nurses had dramatic changes in their hemoglobin (the oxygen carrier in the blood) compared with routinely treated patients. For more information contact:

Dolores Kreiger
NYU Division of Nursing
429 Shimkin Hall
Washington Square
New York, NY 10003

Janet Quinn
College of Nursing
University of South Carolina
Columbia, SC 29208

Mind Over Matter Healing

At Yale University School of Medicine, surgeon Bernard Siegel heads an innovative cancer therapy program called Exceptional Cancer Patients (E-CAP). As an adjunct to surgery, radiation, chemotherapy, and other traditional cancer treatments, the program offers group therapy, guided imagery, meditation, lifestyle evaluation, and art therapy. For more information contact:

E-CAP
2 Church Street South
New Haven, CT 06519
(203) 865-8392

Biofeedback

By amplifying biological signs with a variety of machines, biofeedback trains you to become aware of and control autonomic nervous system processes. For information on clinics near you, contact:

Biofeedback Society of America
c/o Francine Butler, Ph.D
4301 Owens Street
Wheat Ridge, CO 80033
(303) 420-2889

Stress Management

Many companies have instituted stress management programs for their employees. The Department of Health Promotion at St. Louis University Medical Center has designed model stress programs, including such features as biofeedback training, nutrition management, physical fitness, executive renewal workshops, and stress assessment consultation. Companies or individuals interested in setting up such a program can contact:

Healthline Corporate Health Services
Ardith Grandbouche
1205 Carr Lane
St. Louis, MO 63104
(314) 577-8050

3

Super Tests: Diagnosis Enters the Space Age

The elderly New England homemaker could have used a consultation with Star Trek's Dr. McCoy. She was suffering from severe dizziness and nobody could figure out why. Dr. McCoy would have known. Whenever anyone was sick on the TV series he simply used his miraculous hand-held diagnostic device, the Feinberg, and got an instant readout of the patient's condition. But the woman from New England had gone in for an electroencephalogram, then a CAT scan, and nothing had shown up.

Finally she consulted a psychiatrist, who suggested she try something new—a technique know as brain electrical activity mapping, or *BEAM*. While she sat with electrodes fastened to her head, the BEAM scanner painlessly translated her brain's electrical signals into brilliantly colored patterns. The doctors read this topographical map—and concluded that there was something wrong with her neurological system.

The next step in the woman's diagnosis was a technique known as nuclear magnetic resonance testing (NMR). She was placed inside a large, cylindrical device that exposed her skull to a magnetic field and radio waves, causing her brain to send out signals that a computer translated into pictures. The NMR test revealed that the woman had multiple sclerosis. As a result of a confirmed diagnosis, she is now considering experimental treatment for the disease.

Today's testing techniques can't work miracles, and they aren't as magical as those used on the starship *Enterprise*. But they are, like that legendary craft, "boldly going where no man has gone before." Taking advantage of the latest developments in microelectronics, radiology, physics, and biochemistry, bioengineers are producing a new generation of diagnostic devices designed to provide detailed information on areas of the body that in the past were virtually inaccessible. Radio waves, radioactively tagged chemicals, precisely focused x-ray beams, and tiny silicon chips are slipping across boundaries even the surgeon's knife could not traverse. Computers are translating their journeys into color-coded maps and three-dimensional images that doctors can read with unprecedented ease and accuracy.

Laboratory testing devices are being scaled down so that physicians in remote locales can offer convenient, and in some cases life-saving, early diagnoses to their patients. A variety of home testing kits are also making this revolution in diagnostic services directly available to the public. Moreover, many of the new tests are far less intrusive than the painfully probing catheters, hazardous dyes, and exploratory surgery of the past, when often diagnosis was more dreaded than disease.

"There's been an explosion of technology," says Richard A. Robb, Ph.D, professor of biophysics and director of the research computer facility at the Mayo Clinic in Rochester, Minnesota. "It's a very exciting time to be in diagnostic medicine because we now have the capability to provide more definitive information about the patient than ever before. McCoy's little hand-held device is not so impossible to imagine now. That is the ultimate in diagnostic medicine. That is where we are going."

Nuclear Magnetic Resonance

Admittedly, some of today's super tests have to be scaled down quite a bit to fit in the hand. But that doesn't make them any less impressive. *Nuclear magnetic resonance testing (NMR)* is a good example.

The equipment involved in an NMR exam includes a 6-foot-long cylindrical tunnel, variously compared to a doughnut, a thermos bottle and the inside of a bongo drum. The tunnel contains a 7-to 8-ton magnet that can generate a field 30,000 to 50,000 times more powerful than the one on the surface of the earth.

"Nuclear magnetic resonance provides images of the human body as never seen before," says Manuel Viamonte Jr., M.D., professor of radiology at the University of Miami School of Medicine and chairman of the department of radiology at the Mt. Sinai Medical Center in Miami. "We see lesions that we don't see with other techniques." For instance, during a routine study of a hospital trustee, NMR detected a brain lesion. Recalls Dr. Viamonte, "He was asymptomatic. He said, I'd like to have a study. We found a lesion 1 centimeter in size. He went to surgery." A CAT scan of the same patient was negative. "We had a number of cases in which NMR has been a lot more informative than CAT scan," Viamonte adds.

The reason is that NMR sets up an ingenious form of communication with the body on an atomic level. NMR is based on the principle that when the nuclei of some atoms, particularly hydrogen, are exposed to certain conditions they give off radio waves. These signals are then read and interpreted.

To get the hydrogen atoms of the human body to send off this message requires several steps. First, the body is enveloped in a powerful magnetic field. To achieve this, the doctor slides the patient inside the tunnel on a special bed. In the presence of the electromagnetism, the nuclei of the hydrogen atoms align themselves with the axis of the field, like iron filings pulled into line by a toy magnet.

"That in itself does not generate a signal," explains Viamonte. To get the hydrogen atoms to "speak," a second magnetic field is introduced, perpendicular to the first. The hydrogen nuclei react by rearranging themselves along the axis of the new magnet. When the second magnetic field is removed, the nuclei flip back into alignment with the first magnetic field. "As the atom flips from the perpendicular position it will send out an echo, or radio frequency pulse," Viamonte says. A computer analyzes the message from the hydrogen nuclei and transforms it into an anatomical picture.

Hydrogen atoms send out various signals, depending on how densely they are concentrated and what type of chemical compound they belong to (water, fat, or amino acid, for instance). Viamonte compares their response to that of a sleepy army unit that is suddenly aroused. "You have a bunch of soldiers. You suddenly blow a horn," he says. "Not all of them will stand at the same time— some of the heavy ones will take longer."

NMR images show bone marrow and fat as light areas due to their high concentrations of hydrogen nuclei; tissues such as tendons and nerves, which have fewer of these nuclei, appear darker. Bones, very low in hydrogen, are invisible.

In addition to picturing concentrations of hydrogen, the NMR computer also analyzes the time it takes for the nuclear signal to fade away or "relax." This is a clue to local tissue conditions, including their temperature and viscosity. It can also signal malignancy. In cancerous tissue, for instance, relaxation tends to take longer.

Because the NMR scanner is sensitive to hydrogen-containing tissues, it can penetrate areas of the body difficult for other scanning devices to reach. NMR is not blocked by bones and thus is an excellent device for examining the brain and nervous system. Some experts believe NMR will be able to detect the earliest signs of brain cancer. One of the first signs of malignancy in the brain is the water (edema) that collects around the site of a tumor, even before the lesion is visible. Hydrogen-sensitive NMR will be able to locate the edema and diagnose brain carcinoma early; it may also prove useful in early diagnosis of hydrocephalus (accumulation of cerebrospinal fluid around the brain.) Researchers further expect it to be helpful in diagnosing diseases of the fatty myelin sheath covering the nerves, including multiple sclerosis and perhaps some forms of dementia. Doctors hope NMR will be useful in exploring physiological causes of psychiatric disorders.

NMR applications aren't limited to the nervous system. For instance, it can detect concentrations of fat on the walls of the arteries, signaling possible atherosclerosis. It can also pinpoint disc disease: A normal disc will give off a high signal, a dehydrated disc an attenuated signal. Experts in sports medicine hope that NMR's soft tissue sensitivity will make it a valuable tool in treating athletes' injuries and studying the effects of physical activity on the musculoskeletal system.

Despite its current expense, NMR is clearly a promising diagnostic tool for the future, and its capabilities are expanding. Experts are working on developing scanners that will measure reactions of other atoms besides hydrogen, such as phosphorus and sodium. Phosphorus distribution is key in diagnosing myocardial infarction, while tracking of sodium concentration casts light on the activity of cancer cells.

Positron Emission Tomography

While nuclear magnetic resonance sets up a form of communication with the cells of the body, *positron emission tomography* (*PET*) actually penetrates them. In a PET scan, radioactive molecules are dispatched to enter the bloodstream, participate in the body's processes, and report back to the diagnosing physician.

"The technique gives you detailed physiologic and metabolic information you can't obtain with any other technology," Viamonte says. In PET, natural substances integral to body function, such as sugar, oxygen, amino acids, and fats, are mixed with radioactive isotopes (radioactive forms of carbon, oxygen, and nitrogen). The combination is then injected into the patient or inhaled.

Disguised as natural substances, the radioactive isotopes ride into the body like spies slipping across a border. Soon they begin signaling their whereabouts and reporting on body conditions. They do this by emitting positrons which collide with electrons and produce photons. The photons are picked up by the PET scanner.

PET goes beyond the observation (however detailed) of CAT scans and x rays and the communicative capabilities of NMR. Instead, PET actually participates in the body's metabolic processes providing a insider's look at what is going on. "The ordinary x ray shows us structure," observes Thomas Chase, M.D., chief of experimental therapeutics at the Neurology Institute of the National Institutes of Health in Bethesda, Maryland. "PET allows us to look not only at structure but also function."

In a typical PET exam, a patient lies on a padded steel tray with his or her head (or other body part being observed) encircled by the doughnut-shaped scanner. After the injection or inhalation of the radioactive chemical, the scanner starts to pick up the photon signals. The tiny bursts of light strike detector crystals inside the doughnut. Then devices called photomultiplier tubes amplify and convert the signals to electrical impulses. The computer translates these impulses into maps of brain activity (or the activity of another body part being observed) by reconstructing the location of the isotopes and their reactions with the tissues.

Areas of the brain that are taking up a lot of glucose and hence emitting a lot of photons, for example, are probably more active than areas not using as much sugar. A weak photon signal indicates diminished activity.

The maps are color-coded to indicate areas of greater and lesser concentration of the isotope, which signals greater or lesser activity. Areas of heightened activity are bright whites, reds, or oranges. Diminished activity comes across as a darker color, perhaps a deep russet.

Although a PET scan can be used on many areas of the body, it is particularly useful for looking at the brain. Because the brain depends on glucose for fuel (it gets 80 percent of its energy from it), glucose concentrations are key in revealing how well various brain areas function. Injecting subjects with radioactive glucose, PET researchers have been able to study and diagnose a number of brain disorders.

It is now believed, for instance, that schizophrenia can be identifed with the scanner. Patients with the disorder show a lack of glucose in the frontal cortex, an area experts believe plays a role in emotions. When the National Institutes of Health compared a group of schizophrenics to a group of nonschizophrenics, they found that a normal subjects scan showed bursts of orange in the frontal lobe, while their schizophrenic's frontal cortex was dimmer. With their eyes closed, the controls had no coloration in the vision centers of their brains. The schizophrenics showed brilliant colors in their vision centers even with eyes shut, because they were hallucinating.

PET is also proving useful in helping epileptic patients. A seizure shows up as an explosion of color in a PET scan as glucose rushes to the area of heightened activity. At the University of California at Los Angeles, doctors use PET to determine which areas of the brain produce epileptic seizures and to pinpoint those areas for surgical removal.

Other brain disorders being studied with PET are Huntington's Chorea, amyotrophic lateral sclerosis (Lou Gehrig's Disease), and Parkinson's Disease. Doctors also take PET scans of stroke patients in order to observe the brain's use of oxygen. These patients are asked to inhale radioactive oxygen so their brains can be scanned by PET for damage. (The affected areas don't take up oxygen, so the radioactive signal from these parts is negligible.)

PET can also be helpful in studying the circulatory system. For instance, by having the patient inhale a minute amount of carbon monoxide labeled with radioactive carbon 11, doctors can measure certain circulatory problems. Carbon 11 attaches to blood platelets, and as it rides with them through the bloodstream, it can track problems such as blood vessels blocked by atherosclerosis. PET helps measure blood flow to specific parts of the body and determines how well tissues use it. Doctors at UCLA have placed the PET device over patients' hearts to monitor blood flow, a vast improvement over painful and risky cardiac catheterization. And PET can show the scope of damage wrought by a heart attack.

PET may prove a boon to cancer patients. It can show how much oxygen a tumor is using, and studies have indicated that tumors absorbing more oxygen are more vulnerable to radiation treatment. Furthermore, it can identify various types of tumors by determining what types of amino acids they ingest. Finally, it can even reveal which tumors are growing most rapidly, because fast-growing lesions use more glucose.

Researchers are still trying to figure out what all the signals PET produces mean. Sometimes the photons detected by PET are exact clues to where the glucose is at any given moment because they are emitted at the moment and place of positron emission. At other times, however, the positron travels a short distance before colliding with an electron and creating a photon, thus skewing the picture slightly.

Another question plaguing PET's proponents is which radioisotopes produce the best image. Sugar works slowly, giving a slow-exposure picture of brain chemistry over a half-hour period. Experts are trying to find a way to produce snapshots of the brain showing moment-to-moment thought processes—"real time" images. Despite those lingering questions, PET remains a very promising technology. "With PET we're able to map out the brain the way Columbus mapped out the New World," Dr. Chase says. "I see PET evolving quickly. This type of technology allows us to go the next step." One day, he conjectures, PET will help scientists "understand the cause of alcoholism, the cause of depression, things today that plague us. The imagination and the technology are there."

Evoked Potentials

The middle-aged man from Massachusetts was having trouble walking and his doctor wanted to figure out why. Finally the man went in for a highly sensitive nervous system test known as an *evoked potentials* test. This revealed a problem with his spine, cervical spondylosis, in which an overgrowth of bone presses on the spinal cord. He was treated for this disease and eventually was able to walk again.

Evoked potentials tests were discovered in Britain by Dr. Richard Katon in 1877. The first testing equipment was pioneered in the 1950s and was used routinely by the 1970s in London at the National Hospital. Evoked potentials tests measure the electrical signals (also known as waves or potentials) the brain gives off in response to external stimuli. The timing and configuration of the waves may indicate normal or abnormal body conditions. "These tests provide us a very reliable objective look at functional anatomy," explains Keith Chiappa, M.D., assistant professor in the department of neurology at Harvard Medical School. "They tell us if a sensory tract is functioning or not, and whether the anatomy of that tract is intact."

During an evoked potentials test, specific channels of the nervous system are stimulated to see how effectively they respond. For instance, to test the part of the nervous system that processes visual stimuli, the patient is shown light patterns—shifting checkerboards or flashes. "It doesn't sound like much of a stimulus but it produces a nice response," Dr. Chiappa observes. Electrodes attached to the head pick up the brain wave response. If the nervous system pathways are healthy or unobstructed, the signals will be normal. Certain abnormalities—such as growths or diseases of the nervous system—cause disruptions in the signal. Doctors look for a variation in the amount of time it takes signals originating in one part of the body to reach the brain. Another clue to body conditions is the specific form of the wave.

In addition to visual stimuli, doctors expose patients to clicks (to test hearing channels) and administer shocks to various nerves to test motor function. "People get anxious when they hear we're going to shock them," Dr. Chiappa says, "but it's not painful. Often people doze off."

Dr. Chiappa emphasizes that EP exams are most helpful when used in conjunction with other diagnostic procedures. Although EP tests can reveal "roadblocks" in the nervous system pathways, they cannot identify a specific disease. "These tests are best thought of as very sensitive, objective extensions of the neurological examination," he says. Even so, evoked potentials have many uses. Because they can test eye and ear disorders without relying on a patient's testimony they can be indispensable aids in diagnosing nonverbal patients, including very young children and infants. Evoked potentials testing can also help determine if a complaint is all in the patient's mind or is genuine.

At the University of Missouri, Columbia, visual evoked potentials are used to diagnose intracranial pressure caused by head injuries or hydrocephalus (water on the brain). Abnormal visual EPs can also be a clue to optic neuritis, ambylopia, glaucoma, tumors obstructing visual pathways, and other nervous system disorders, including Friedrich's ataxia, pernicious anemia, and Parkinson's disease. Visual EP tests are important in following the development of children's visual systems and determining the effectiveness of treatment for children's eye disorders.

Brain stem auditory EPs, which test hearing channels, are the most sensitive way to detect tumors of the ear. "The earlier you find the tumor, the more chance you have of saving hearing," says Dr. Chiappa, recalling the example of a young female patient whose hearing was preserved as a result of early detection. Brain stem auditory EPs can also reveal multiple-sclerosis-related lesions that don't show up in other tests, as well as tumors of the brain stem. And EP testing can help to detect autism in children and determine which infants are at risk for sudden infant death syndrome.

People plagued with back pain are also benefitting from EP testing. At the Loyola University Medical Center in Maywood, Illinios, Dr. Timothy B. Scarff has develped an evoked potentials test for slipped discs. First the doctor applies an electrical stimulus to the skin on the patient's leg. The physician then measures how long it takes for the signal generated by the stimulus to travel via the spinal cord to the brain. In the event of a slipped disc, the length of the EP signal is somehow altered and this shows up in the EP test.

Other hospitals use evoked potentials tests to monitor the brain and spinal cord during operations such as those to correct scoliosis or remove spinal cord tumors. By frequently administering EP tests during surgery (which can be done without bringing the patient out of anesthesia) doctors can spot nervous system problems and correct them as they come up. The wave of the future, Dr. Chiappa says, will include magneto evoked potentials, which will measure the magnetic fields of the brain in response to a stimulus and add a wealth of new information on brain function.

Mapping the Brain

Imagine a weather map of the mind, a color chart that, with the help of an EEG, displays an array of emotions from depression to elation, and physical abnormalities from epilepsy to brain tumors. Called *brain electrical activity mapping (BEAM)*, this technology was developed by electrical engineer David Culver and Dr. Frank Duffy, a physician with Children's Hospital in Boston.

What brain mapping does is enhance EEG testing with the aid of a computer. In fact, the raw material for the map is gathered through an EEG, by placing 20 electrodes on the scalp to record the waves generated by brain cells. The BEAM computer complements this information by converting it into a topographical map of brain activity. With BEAM, the physician sees brain waves represented as waves of color—and color-coding helps the doctor pinpoint problem areas. (Before BEAM, physicians had to read between squiggly lines on the pages of EEG printouts.) Among other things, BEAM was instrumental in the charting of those brain waves associated with dyslexia: "It can indicate the neurophysiological underpinnings of dyslexia before it shows up when a child starts to read," says Dr. Duffy.

Scientists are also looking into the usefulness of BEAM in exploring possible physiological causes of mental illness, senility, and criminality. Researchers at New York's Upstate Medical Center are interested in using BEAM to search for evidence of organic brain impairment in criminals. Dr. Duffy explains that EP testing helps define brain abnormalities noninvasively in mental illness. "We use it daily to search for evidence of organic impairment in patients who are emotionally disturbed," he says. EP tests also demonstrate the chemical changes of Alzheimer's disease. Sometimes the symptoms of depression and dementia are similar, but the BEAM test can distinguish between them and help detect early signs of dementia.

Office Testing

While lofty projects involving such space-age technology as BEAM, PET, and NMR are being pursued at the nation's top medical institutions, there is also a diagnostic revolution occurring at the grassroots level. Physician office testing is bringing laboratory technology to remote areas and speeding up diagnosis for anxious patients.

Recent technological advances have produced scaled down and simplified diagnostic devices doctors can use right in their offices. Consequently, thousands of physicians are becoming part-time lab technicians. Using desktop analyzers, disposable dipsticks, and other convenient devices, physicians can now perform their own serum chemistry, urinalysis, hematology and microbiology tests. They can test for strep throat, meningitis, colon cancer, and venereal disease, among other ailments, and in some cases give results in minutes. They can monitor for toxic effects of medications used to treat patients with heart problems, lung disease, and epilepsy.

"Patients love it," says William Beshlian, M.D., attending physician at St. Joseph's Hospital and Medical Center in Patterson, New Jersey. Not only are they spared unnecessary prescriptions and multiple office visits, but patients can also have their tests performed in a familiar setting. "They don't have to go to a strange place or a large institution," he says.

For patients, this can mean faster test results, fewer office visits and less anxiety. "The main thing for the patient is convenience and savings," says Dr. Beshlian. "In one visit the exam and the diagnostic test are done. The patient can get an answer and get therapy."

For doctors, office testing can mean increased income. Recent regulations have severely restricted Government reimbursement to physicians for tests done at outside laboratories. But office testing is reimbursed at a better rate: 60 percent of the prevailing charge.

The possibility of profit, considerations of convenience to the patient, and new technology have conspired to radically alter the diagnostic process. A survey of the members of the American Society of Internal Medicine (ASIM) showed that 70 percent of them do in-office lab testing. Doctors now spend $300 million a year for equipment and supplies for in-office testing.

Office testing can also help improve medical care in remote areas far from laboratories and large hospitals. "If you're in the middle of an Indian reservation, you may want to do certain things you wouldn't do in an urban setting," points out Dr. James D. Barger, senior pathologist at Humana-Sunrise Hospital in Las Vegas.

Dr. Barger and other pathologists, however, are worried that physicians are not qualified to perform all the tests now available to them. Studies have shown that in some cases physician testing is less reliable than independent laboratory testing. "My concern is a question of expertise," Barger says.

Many pathologists feel that it is all right for physicians to perform basic blood and urine tests and simple bacteriology procedures, such as the test for strep throat. They are more cautious, however, about complicated biochemical tests, such as those for acquired immune deficiency syndrome (AIDS), particularly because there is very little in the way of uniform quality control of physicians' labs.

As of this writing, the majority of states are not regulating office labs. But efforts are underway to introduce more control over physician office testing. Dr. Barger heads an office lab assessment committee established jointly by ASIM, AAFP, and the College of

American Pathologists, which is talking about establishing some type of certification for physician office labs. In the meantime, pathologists in many states are playing a consulting role to help physicians improve the quality of their office lab testing. And experts believe that recent advances in office lab technology are making it easier for physicians to do a good job.

For his part, St. Joseph's Dr. Beshlian says he expects regulation—and will welcome it. "I think in the future office testing is going to be targeted for regulation," he says. "Proficiency is going to be required. Pathologists are correct. This is the way that you're going to eliminate poor testing. We will be happy to have it."

Field Effect Transistors

Researchers in the U.S., Great Britain, and Japan are developing tiny electronic diagnostic tools that doctors can use to instantly analyze a patient's blood chemistry. Known as Field Effect Transistors (FETs), these minute transistor chips are injected into the body, just as a serum would be. But their purpose is quite different from a drug's: These powerful signal amplifiers are specially coated with materials that seek out certain substances, such as calcium and potassium. The FETs attach themselves to their targets, and this union produces electrical signals that are picked up by the transistor, processed by the chip and sent to the doctor's monitoring equipment. FETs can measure the levels of glucose, hydrogen, sodium, and other substances in the blood.

Scientists have yet to determine the perfect substance to coat the FET chips with—currently, they are experimenting with silicon, polyurethane, and cellulose. And, to date, the accuracy of these tiny reporters is not what it should be. Changes in body temperature can alter their messages. Doctors are also concerned about the risk of infection and blood clotting.

Despite these drawbacks, more-sophisticated FETs are in the offing. Researchers envision implantable chips that will transmit radio signals to remote receivers: An ulcer patient resting at home would swallow an FET that would broadcast the patient's stomach pH to an instrument on a physician's desk. Within the next several years, FETs could be performing such feats as monitoring antigens and antibodies in a patient's blood to see if the immune system is fighting an infection. These transistors may even be useful in cancer treatment, reporting on the effectiveness of radiation or chemotherapy.

Home Testing

While physicians are working on speeding up office diagnostic procedures, patients are also taking matters into their own hands with home tests.

The dramatic news of President Reagan's colon cancer focused attention on the booming new market in home health tests. Among the many devices now available for home use is a fecal occult blood test, an important first step in diagnosing colon cancer.

Other devices that have come on the market in recent years is a test for pregnancy, menopause, gonorrhea, diabetes, and urinary tract infections. Someday, people may even purchase kits that detect genital herpes, strep throat, kidney disease, asthma, hepatitis, and glaucoma.

"Home testing is going full blast," observes Diana Woods, director of the division of consumer affairs at the Food and Drug Administration's (FDA's) Center for Devices and Radiological Health, which regulates home test kits and approves them for marketing. "It is probably the fastest-growing health market out there." Sales of home tests topped $80 million in 1984, up from $60 million in 1983, and industry experts expect a 30 percent growth rate annually for the near future.

Introduced in the late 1970s, pregnancy tests now account for the biggest share of home test sales. Among the newest tests are a device that tells a woman when she is ovulating and a test that indicates whether or not patients with high blood pressure are sticking to their low-sodium diets.

Experts attribute the growth in test kit sales to the interest in home health care. One advantage to the home testing devices is that they may save some money by ruling out certain conditions. They may also bring some people into the health care system who otherwise might not have gone for treatment.

But experts are concerned about the shelf life of devices as well as the adequacy of instructions and labeling. They also worry that patients may misinterpret test results. Experts stress, for instance, that the hidden blood test is an important step in detecting colon cancer but does not in itself constitute a diagnosis of malignancy. A positive pregnancy test should be confirmed by a physician's pelvic exam and cannot distinguish ectopic pregnancy, a serious condition that requires immediate medical attention.

The V.D. home test kits raise other issues. Health professionals are concerned that a person using a V.D. test may ignore a positive result or not tell his sexual partners about it. Or he may have a false negative and continue to spread the disease.

There is also the possibility of quackery. "We hope our review process is keeping products off the market that have potential for misuse," says Dr. Jerome Donlon, a director in the division of device evaluation at the FDA's Center for Devices and Radiological Health. In a few instances, however, the FDA has taken products off the market.

"We took action against a device called a urinometer a few years ago," Dr. Woods says. "It was a diagnostic device to test urine sugar for diabetics—an oversized eyedropper with plastic dropper. How many balls floated or sank determined how much sugar was in the urine. It didn't work and it was obviously dangerous so it was taken off the market."

The FDA also intercepted a urine test designed to detect the gender of a pregnant woman's baby. It was known as "the gender reacting agent," Woods says. "You were supposed to take urine and put it in the vial with the reacting agent. Then you were to compare the color to a color spectrum chart. If it was blue or brown it indicated you were carrying a boy. Shades of green denoted a girl. The manufacturers claimed 99 percent accuracy." However, she adds, "There is no scientific basis for anything in the urine that would tell you whether you're carrying a boy or a girl. We took it off the market."

With the home test business growing, Woods fears an increasing number of abuses. "With more and more home use devices there will be more opportunities for these things to happen," she says. "We're concerned about people selling kits to detect or even cure AIDS."

The FDA is working on special guidelines for regulating home diagnostic kits. Yet with all the concerns, doctors and scientists seem to have a positive feeling about the do it yourself diagnostic tools especially if they are used in conjunction with a doctor's care. "Home testing may encourage people to have an interest in their health and reinforce their need to get medical attention," Dr. Donlon says. "Positive results give them the added incentive they need to check things out."

Will the day come when most tests will be done by the consumer in the comfort of his or her own home? It's not likely, but the selection of home tests on drugstore shelves will continue to grow. As Woods points out, "Any test that's done in a lab is likely to be considered for the open market."

3-D Vision

Imagine being able to perform exploratory surgery without laying a hand on a patient and you've understood the beauty of the *Dynamic Spatial Reconstructor* (*DSR*), an experimental device recently developed at the Mayo Clinic in Rochester, Minnesota, by Richard A. Robb, Ph.D., and his associates.

"The DSR is a three-dimensional imaging machine," Robb explains. "Using DSR, we are able to view organs inside the body while they are moving."

DSR is based on the same principles as the CAT scanner. A kind of glorified x-ray machine, it takes multiple pictures of the body from many angles and sorts them out with the help of a computer. But DSR snaps even more pictures than CAT, so many, in fact, that it can create three-dimensional images. Instead of the CAT's single x-ray tube that rotates around the body, DSR has 14 tubes, each firing 60 times a second. "It collects information 500 times faster than the CAT scanner," Robb says. "The entire heart can be imaged 60 times per second."

The 14 x-ray tubes also mean that rather than imaging a single two-dimensional slice of the body (which the CAT scan does) the DSR can image volumes of the body. "We can image any 24 centimeter by 24 centimeter by 24 centimeter cube of the body dynamically, Robb says. "You get 240 cross sections, like a stack of pancakes."

Like other imaging devices, the DSR is ring-shaped and is mounted on one end of a long cylinder. During the exam, the patient, lying on a bed, slides into the cylinder, with the ring surrounding the part of the body the doctor wants to investigate. The 14 tubes are turned on and begin their firing as the circle rotates. The tubes are mounted on one half of the ring, while the cameras are mounted on the other half. As the x-ray beams pass through the body, the cameras record their journey. The DSR generally uses less radiation than other clinically accepted diagnostic procedures, says Dr. Robb. For instance, in a CAT scan the typical dosage is 10 to 20 rads. The most a patient receives in DSR is 10 to 15 rads.

"The camera picks up the differential absorption pattern of the x ray," says Robb, "and converts it into an electrical signal. This then goes into a computer which converts it to numbers which represent the brightness at each location on the image. The computer then reconstructs from these projections. It asks itself: 'What must the body have looked like to form these projections? What must have been in the way to create this pattern?' The result is a series of cross sections of the body."

The next step is to take these images and "display them, analyze them, make measurements," Robb explains. He compares looking at the DSR video display screen to "looking into a box. You don't see a cross section It's a three-dimensional image."

Using an electronic pointer, the doctor can move the image around in order to view all sides of it, erase a part of it, cut into it, take it apart and put it back together. "We perform mathematical surgery, if you will, or numerical biopsy. We have the capability to noninvasively study the body like a surgeon or pathologist would. Not only can we take the body image apart and look, but we can cut it open and focus in on the region of interest and peel away parts of it."

Still in the research stage, the DSR has been used mainly in heart studies. "We're studying the normal physiology and patho-physiology of the heart," Robb says. "We're looking at coronary artery disease and measuring how severe it is so physicians can decide on surgery. The greatest thing it's been used for clinically is heart disease."

But Rob envisions that the number of applications for the DSR will grow as its use becomes more widespread. DSR has proven to be invaluable in improving the state of the art in clinical diagnosis. "You don't need to go back very far in history to get a perspective on what's happening today in diagnostic medicine," Robb continues. "The x ray was discovered in 1895. For 85 years the technique remained basically the same until the 1970s when the CAT came out. All of a sudden the computer gave us this new dimension—a reconstruction from projections. This led to an explosion in new medical technology in diagnostic medicine. It's going to be fun to be around in the year 2000 because I think there are going to be instruments used that we haven't even thought about yet."

Robb views the DSR and other super tests as only the forebears of future generations of even more advanced diagnostic devices. The revolution spawned by the marriage of medical testing and computer technology will work even greater miracles in years to come. On the horizon, Robb envisions an imager that determines the chemical properties of all the tissues in the body. The machine would be able to tell not just where a tumor was, but exactly what the chemicals were in that region of tissue.

"We will be able to do the things we now do in autopsy and surgery with a noninvasive imaging device," he says. With contin-ued computer advances as well as the growing possibility of min-iaturization, doctors may well hold diagnostic instruments like the Feinberg in their hands.

"There's no reason to believe that that's not possible." Robb adds. "We're going to have fantastic new tools. We will evolve from year to year with improved instrumentation. It's a continuum."

Timeline

1988 • Sales of home tests reach $250 million.
• Worldwide market for NMR testing reaches $750 million.

1990 • Motor-evoked potentials tests widespread.
• DSR-like machinery installed in major medical institutions around the world.
• Doctors spending $600 million annually on office testing, double what they spent in 1985.
• Three to four times more office testing than in 1985; 400,000 physicians doing 2.7 billion tests on outpatients annually.
• Most EEG labs using BEAM or BEAM-like devices to augment their testing.

1995 • In-home diagnostics market tops $1 billion.
• Magneto-evoked potentials testing in use.

2000 • All diagnostics except for those requiring very sophisticated equipment available in physicians' offices.
• Chemical imagers in use.

2100 • Miniaturized diagnostic instruments similar to the Feinberg in use.

Access Guide

Nuclear Magnetic Resonance

A typical NMR exam ranges in cost from $500 to $1,000, depending on the type of equipment used and how extensive the exam is. It is covered by Medicare and an increasing number of private insurance carriers. Some 200 U.S. hospitals now have NMR equipment. NMR exams are also offered at 160–170 other locations around the country, including clinics, imaging, centers and the offices of radiologists.

Among the medical institutions offering NMR: The Cleveland Clinic, Cleveland, Ohio; The Mayo Clinic, Rochester, Minnesota; The Medical College of Wisconsin, Milwaukee, Wisconsin; Mount Sinai Medical Center, Miami Beach, Florida; New York Hospital-Cornell Medical Center, New York, New York; Scottsdale Memorial Hsopital, Scottsdale, Arizona; Temple University Medical School, Philadelphia, Pennsylvania; The University of Alabama, Birmingham, Alabama; The University of California at San Francisco. For more information write to:

Otha Linton
The American College of Radiology
1891 Preston White Drive
Reston, VA 22091
(703) 648-8900

Positron Emission Tomography

Since PET is still classified as an experimental procedure, it is generally cost-free. To date, less than a dozen institutions nationwide have fully equipped PET centers. Since the device is still experimental, patients are limited and carefully screened. Among the medical institutions equipped with PET are: The UCLA School of Medicine, Los Angeles, California; The National Institutes of Health, Bethesda, Maryland; The Brookhaven National Laboratory, Upton, New York. For more information write to:

The National Institute of Neurological and Communicative Disorders
    and Stroke
National Institutes of Health
9000 Rockville Pike
Bethesda, MD 20205
(301) 496-4000

Evoked Potentials

Cost of testing ranges from $100 to $250 per exam and is usually covered by insurance. Evoked potentials tests are given at most large medical centers around the country as well as some smaller county hospitals. For more information, read *Evoked Potentials in Clinical Medicine*, Keith Chiappa, M.D., Raven Press, New York, 1982

Brain Mapping .

Testing ranges in cost from $150 to $700, depending upon the type of exam involved, and is covered by insurance. BEAM is offered at 12 institutions around the country including: University of Utah Medical Center, Salt Lake City, Utah; Children's Hospital, Boston, Massachusetts; Encino Neurological Medical Group, Encino, California; Dallas Neurosciences, Dallas, Texas. For more information write to:

BEAM Laboratory
Childrens Hospital
300 Longwood Avenue
Boston, MA 02115
(617) 735-6000

Office Testing

Ranges in price from around $5 for a single test to measure blood sugar to around $20 for drug therapeutic monitoring, although costs vary around the country. Covered by insurance. Availability is widespread especially in remote areas. For more information write to:

College of American Pathologists
5202 Old Orchard Road
Skokie, IL 60077
(312) 966-5700

Field Effect Transistors

FETS are not available yet to doctors, but when they are it is estimated that a typical scan will cost the patient $200 to $300. Currently in the research and development stage. Integrated Ionics Incorporated of Dayton,

New Jersey, expects to be marketing a device similar to the FET by the late 1980s. For more information write to:

John Patterson
Vice President, Commercial Development
Integrated Ionics Incorporated
2235 State Route 130
Dayton, NJ 08810
(201) 329-9555

Home Tests

Ranges from around $3 for a home test for urinary tract infection to around $275 for an electronic home blood glucose meter. Most simple tests cost between $3 and $10. For more information write:

Division of Consumer Affairs
Center for Devices and Radiological Health
FDA
Rockville, MD 20857
(301) 279-7511

Dynamic Spatial Reconstructor

There are presently no charges for DSR studies since the DSR is still regarded as an experimental device. When doctors start charging for testing with DSR-like devices, anticipated in a couple of years, the cost will probably be around $500 per exam. The DSR is currently only available at the Mayo Clinic, where an average of four to five scans a week are performed. Patients are screened by a review board and by and large are those with cardiovascular problems. For more information write to:

Richard A. Robb, Ph.D
Biodynamics Research Unit
Department of Physiology and Biophysics
Mayo Foundation
Rochester, MN 55905
(507) 284-2511

4

The Real Bionic Man

"Don't quit." These two words, mouthed by the first artificial heart recipient, Barney Clark, to Dr. Robert Jarvik on December 20, 1982, articulated completely the critical role of artificial organs.

Not that doctors and researchers need encouragement to continue their work. Artificial organ development—or bionics—continues at a feverish pace. The mechanical heart is only the beginning: Already, artificial ears bring the sounds of the world to the deaf; manmade skin, applied over massive burn wounds, helps regenerate real skin and nerves; and a unique genus of coral replaces some of the body's most delicate bones. Children once crippled by kidney disease play and go to school with an artificial kidney in their pocket. Bionic developments over the last few years have made what was yesterday's science fiction today's medical reality.

By the middle of the next decade many of the organs in our body will have an artificial counterpart. Fashioned from Teflon, carbon, graphite, titanium, aluminum, silicone rubber, dacron and nylon, microchips, biochips, and minute computers, these manufactured parts may help extend our lives.

"The use of artificial body parts has a very long and accepted history," Dr. Warren Reich of Georgetown University has said. "The wooden leg is a marvelous prototype. It is an artificially constructed part from a pretechnological era. It shows that we quite eagerly accept artificial parts that support our life and bodily functions." Transplantation is also a well-accepted procedure used to replace diseased or damaged body parts.

Not all organs can be transplanted, however. Those that can—heart and kidneys, for example—may be rejected by the recipient's body. In some cases the human body adapts better to artificial organs. Researchers have developed a synthetic material, made chiefly of teflon and graphite, called Proplast, that coats the artificial organ. The body's healing tissues actually grow into and around the Proplast, which is strong, flexible, and highly porous. The tissues then protect the artificial materials from rejection. Used mostly in artificial joints now, Proplast looks very promising for all facets of bionics.

Not only medical doctors but bioengineers, mechanical engineers, chemists, and physicists are involved in bionics. Breakthroughs in medicine have never before encompassed so many disciplines. The dozens of changes occurring daily in the field indicate that we are getting closer and closer to assembling a "bionic man"—one with tiny electrodes in the brain to give sight, a titanium heart driven by implanted motors, plastic arms and hands operated by mere thought, hollow fiber chambers that act as a pancreas.

Skin

Margaret Dawson, a 52-year-old Massachusetts homemaker, was cleaning her kitchen floor with a petroleum based solvent when some of the solvent splashed on the stove's pilot light. A devastating explosion and fire erupted. Dawson's body became a human torch: more than 85 percent of her body surface was burned. But rather than administering conventional treatment, doctors covered nearly half of her body's surface with an artificial skin product. Without it, she would have suffered, at minimum, severe and permanent disfigurement—if she had survived.

At present, artificial skin is used only on an experimental basis. As MIT physical chemist Ionnis V. Yannas, one of the skin's developers, says, "In *performance* artificial skin has totally replaced conventional autografting techniques. In *practice*, no." But full FDA approval is expected by 1987, and Yannas predicts that artificial skin will completely replace autografting as the remedy for burns.

The skin is the body's largest organ, weighing up to 50 pounds on the average sized adult. It is also the body's principal defense against bacteria. The top layer of skin, the epidermis, can regenerate, as it does for instance, after a sunburn. The second layer, the dermis, houses the sweat glands, the lower portions of hair follicles, and nerve endings. Once the dermis is destroyed, it never regenerates; the site simply scars.

The standard procedure has always been to cover the burn wounds with skin taken from pigs or human cadavers. To prevent rejection of this foreign tissue, doctors administer drugs that suppress the immune system; this further weakens the patient's ability to fight other infections.

Following this treatment, autografting is done. This involves taking small pieces of the patient's own skin and grafting them onto burn sites. Autografting prevents infection and fluid loss as well as skin contraction and scarring. A very painful procedure, it must be repeated many times.

In 1979 Drs. Yannas and John F. Burke, a surgeon affiliated with Harvard University began treating patients with their artificial skin. The results were so promising that the FDA has allowed more than 60 patients to be treated since then.

The artificial skin, only a few thousandths of an inch thick, is made of silicone plastic and a combination of collagen (a natural polymer found in animal and human tissue) and another natural polymer, called chrondroitin 6-sulfate. Burke and Yannas have been using collagen derived from cowhide and chrondroitin from shark cartilage, which have proved to be a perfect match for human skin. After a special mixing, heating, and cooling process that takes about 4 days in the MIT lab, several 6- by 10-inch sheets of artificial skin are produced. The skin looks and feels real, down to the pores.

When the man-made skin is affixed to burns, a new dermal layer begins to grow almost immediately, a physiological phenomenon once thought impossible. Sweat glands and hair don't grow back but that doesn't seem to cause any major problems for the patient, Yannas says. What does grow back with the dermal layer, though, is nerves. Not only does "our product cause regeneration of the dermis, but it has the ability to regenerate two organs, nerves and skin," Yannas adds.

Because the product regenerates two wholly different tissues, it may be capable of regenerating other organs as well. "We can only leave it to the speculators to decide which ones," Yannas says. "We

will use the principle of inducing a wound to give you back what
was there before the wound."

Bones

To remake portions of the human skeletal structure, researchers
are going back to our most rudimentary, atavistic ancestors—the
creatures of the sea. A particular genus of coral from the warm
South Seas is modeled to replace bones in humans.

Dr. Kenneth E. Salyer, a reconstructive surgeon at the Texas
Cranial Facial Center in Dallas, has been one of the first surgeons
to work with the coral product, called *Interpore*. To rebuild bone,
especially delicate facial and cranial bone, he says, "We use the
catacomb structure of coral. We take this same structure and put
it into the patient."

The standard procedure for replacing certain facial and cranial
bones is to borrow pieces of the hip, elbow, and ribs. Unfortunately,
not much bone tissue can be spared. Silicone bones can also serve
as replacements, but they are seldom used since they are frequently
rejected by the body.

Procuring—and preparing—the coral for use is no small task.
The coral is harvested in large quantities and then cut and sliced.
Next, it undergoes a hydrothermal process, a standard chemical
procedure in which, in this case, the coral is transformed into calcium triphosphate, a principal material of bone.

The surgeon can then carve pieces of the coral for tailor-made
fits. Once the coral is implanted, its pores act as a natural bed for
real bone tissue. Real cartilage and bone tissue actually grow into
the pores. And because the coral biodegrades, in time a real bone
will grow in place of the coral. To date, doctors have used Interpore
for spinal fusions and for reconstructing jaw bones and other parts
of the skull and face. Sayler contends that Interpore will be a common replacement by 1987.

Early in 1985 Salyer rebuilt Cindy Fleming's entire left cheek
using coral. An automobile accident had obliterated the lower left
side of her face. Her appearance today is normal, and beneath her

skin there is now real bone. In another operation, Salyer was able to reconstruct the face of a toddler born without some of his facial bone. "We can cut the bones of the face now and move facial parts around like pieces of a puzzle," Salyer says.

A system called Computer Aided Design–Computer Aided Manufacturing (CAD-CAM) allows for the very accurate fashioning of the coral needed for these procedures. The computer system takes a two-dimensional CAT scan and makes it into a three-dimensional image. The system can "massage the data" so that a surgeon can custom build the bone replacements.

The doctor feeds digital data into the computer and draws the replacement part on the computer screen. The computer produces a tape that is fed into a milling machine, which produces a mold. Using this as the model, the surgeon sculpts a new bone, one as unique as the patient's original bone.

Despite its versatility, the coral won't replace all artificial bone substitute materials because it cannot be used in areas where bones must support the body's weight. The artificial hip, for example, will continue to be made of plastic and teflon.

Blood Brother

By 1990 countless stroke, heart attack, and trauma victims will have coursing through their vascular systems a combination of whole blood and a synthetic blood substitute. Duplication of all of the functions and components of whole blood in an artificial substance is still doubtful. But researchers are developing two major products that perform one of blood's chief functions—transporting oxygen.

Robert Geyer of the Harvard School of Public Health noted in the mid 1960s that fluorocarbons, derivatives of petroleum and other inert organic chemicals, had an inordinate capacity for absorbing and carrying oxygen. Together with Drs. Leland Clark of the University of Cincinnati and Henry Sloviter of the University of Pennsylvania, Geyer developed the formula for *Fluosol-DA 20%*, a *perfluorochemical (PFC)*. The milky white substance, with roughly the same viscosity as whole blood, can carry large amounts of oxygen to cells and body tissues. Because Fluosol molecules are one-seventieth the size of red blood cells, the fluid can "slip around" blood clots. The molecules can also slide by the more massive red blood cells that might otherwise block the flow of oxygen to the heart, brain, or other vital organs. Fluosol typically would comprise about one-third of a patient's blood volume.

Though Fluosol lacks many of real blood's critical components —clotting factors, platelets, immunoglobulins, antibodies, and hormones—its potential uses are widespread. For the 533,000 Jehovah's Witnesses in the U.S., a religious group that refuses any blood transfusions, Fluosol is very promising. One of the first people treated with Fluosol in the U.S. was an Akron, Ohio, man struck by a car in March 1982. A Jehovah's Witness, the man refused to have any life-saving blood transfusions. Over a 3-week period he received 16 pints of Fluosol. His body was able to regenerate enough new red blood cells to keep him alive.

For victims of heart attack and stroke—conditions in which tissues are starved for oxygen—Fluosol can also be lifesaving. Dr. Kenneth Waxman, a surgeon at the University of California at Irvine Medical College, has been conducting clinical trials with Fluosol and other PFCs. "We can infuse PFC directly into coronary arteries to try to limit the size of the heart attack," he has said. The same could be done for stroke victims.

PFCs are also attracted to tumor sites, thus helping doctors locate deeply embedded tumors. And because massive doses of oxygen seem to break apart tumors, theoretically, PFCs could be aimed right at a tumor, and destroy it. Because it bears a concentrated amount of oxygen, the PFC Fluosol can also quickly detoxify the blood of a carbon monoxide poisoning victim. Also, there is no risk of contracting hepatitis or AIDS from Fluosol.

Unlike whole blood, which has a shelf life of 3 weeks (24 hours unrefrigerated), Fluosol can be stored for 2 years (in refrigeration), and one substance can be used for all blood types.

In Japan, more than 1 in a 1,000 people suffering from ailments ranging from carbon monoxide poisoning to major burns have been successfully treated with Fluosol to date. But the FDA is more cautious. The fluid has undergone many tests in the U.S., most notably those carried out on four patients by Dr. Karl Swann at

Massachusetts General Hospital in 1983. He and other American investigators found that PFCs change white blood cell counts and cause decreases in blood pressure, allergic reactions, and lung complications. Dr. Waxman admits that "it's not clear how big the risks are. But in exactly the right circumstance, PFCs may save a life." Dr. Sloviter is currently developing a new Fluosol solution that carries even more oxygen than the original. Clinical trials of his product will begin around 1988.

In Chicago, a race is on between the Rush-Presbyterian-St. Luke's Medical Center and the Michael Reese Hospital to develop *artificial hemoglobin solutions*. Dr. Ljubomir Djordejevich, one of the original developers at Rush, takes hemoglobin from outdated supplies of blood. He mixes the hemoglobin with lecithin and cholesterol to form a fatty membrane that encapsulates tiny droplets of hemoglobin, so-called liposomes. The liposomes transport oxygen just as red blood cells do but have a shelf life of 6 months and are 50 times smaller than red blood cells, and can get around virtually any blockage. Also, the lab-produced cell walls are stronger than real ones and can better withstand the pressure exerted by blood pumps during open-heart surgery.

Meanwhile, at Michael Reese, developers are working on a hemoglobin-based blood substitute that has no cell walls. Hemoglobin is mixed with a polymer that loosens the fluid's bind on oxygen, so that it is released evenly and quickly in the body.

Before human trials can begin, the prohibitively expensive filtration process required to sterilize hemoglobin must be modified so that it is less expensive. Hopefully by 1992 researchers will have found an answer.

Blood Vessels

Artificial blood vessels with diameters as tiny as paper clip wire have begun to replace the body's miles of arteries and veins. After close to two decades of lab research, Dr. Donald J. Lyman of the University of Utah has created plastic vessels that behave like their natural cousins, dilating and contracting in response to changing blood flow.

The human body has three types of vessels that transport blood: the arteries, veins, and capillaries. Arteries carry the blood away from the heart through a series of smaller conduits, including the capillaries. Oxygen, food, and wastes pass from the blood and body cells through the semipermeable capillary walls. And after the capillaries absorb oxygen, the blood, now rich in carbon dioxide, flows into the veins. It's the veins that carry the blood back to the heart and lungs, through a number of increasingly larger vessels.

An estimated 300,000 Americans could benefit from Dr. Lyman's artificial blood vessels, including those in need of coronary bypass surgery. He is currently conducting experiments to see if his vessels can be made to substitute for the common bile duct, ureter, and bladder. Meanwhile, Dr. Malcolm Herring, a vascular surgeon at the Indiana University School of Medicine, has tried seeding artificial blood vessels with living cells. Seeding the artificial tubes with cells produces a smooth, natural surface that is accepted by the body and resists clotting.

"What we'd like to do in the future is to create even smaller artery grafts," Herring says. The tiny grafts he envisions could be useful in brain operations.

Ear

On November 29, 1984, the FDA approved Dr. William House's cochlear implant, making it the first bioelectronic device to replace a human sense. It is estimated that some 200,000 of the nearly 2 million deaf and hard of hearing people in the U.S. could benefit from the remarkable gadget. "It has been very rare that we have had any patients in whom we could not produce some sensation of sound. Certainly not more than 3 percent," says Karen Berliner, director of hearing service research at the House Institute.

For some patients, like 22-year-old Kristen Cloud, the cochlear implant has done much more than that; it has transformed their lives. Kristen Cloud began regular visits to the House Institute when she was 6, already suffering from severe hearing impairment. By the time she had reached high school, her world was truly silent. At that point, Dr. House's implant required bulky, unsightly glasses, a headband, and coiling wires. But within a few years the implant had been dramatically refined and miniaturized and Kristen agreed to try it. Her life was saved recently, when having stepped into a busy street, she heard the siren of an approaching ambulance.

In normal ears, sound waves enter the ear canal and strike the eardrum. Vibrations ripple along the three tiny fragile bones of the middle ear to the cochlea, a snail-shaped organ also known as the inner ear. Hair cells within the cochlea convert the sound waves to electrical impulses that flow to the brain's auditory nerve. When these hair cells are destroyed or impaired, that link with the brain is cut. The cochlear implant can duplicate the electrical signals the auditory nerve registers as sound. (A standard hearing aid simply transmits a highly amplified sound.)

A tiny microphone worn on eyeglasses or in the patient's clothing picks up sound and converts it to electrical impulses. These are transmitted to a signal processor (about the size of a small transistor radio) that can be tucked in a pocket or clipped to a belt. The signals then travel along a slim wire to a coin-sized transmitter tucked behind the ear. By means of magnetic induction, the signal is sent through the skin to an implanted internal receiver. Finally, the impulses or signals travel by wire to the inner ear, where the auditory nerve fibers are stimulated. The brain registers sound.

For House's patients the device means being able to hear spoken words, to distinguish music from conversation, sirens from doorbells, telephones from horns. Many of the patients describe hearing sounds like those that come from a mistuned radio—static-filled, tinny, metallic. In conjunction with lip reading, the patient is able to participate in and follow conversation much more easily. Kristen Cloud admits that "I am getting more out of my implant than I ever expected."

So far about 450 adults and more than 190 children have been fitted with the implant. The youngest recipient is 28 months old. In children younger than this the degree of deafness cannot be accurately determined. "What makes our device so appealing?" Berliner asks. "It's the simplest one of all and the only one for children." The 3M House Design implant (named for the company that manufactures it), works best in those patients who become deaf later in life than for the congenitally deaf.

Another promising device, and one which used a multielectrode system as opposed to House's single one, is *Ineraid*, developed at the University of Utah in cooperation with Symbion, Inc. (the same firm that has licensed the Jarvik-7 artificial heart). Its developers foresee FDA approval shortly.

Dr. Donald K. Eddington, director of the Cochlear Implant Research Laboratory says that about 35 patients have been fitted with Ineraid. They can identify random two-syllable words without any lip reading 70 to 80 percent of the time.

This multichannel system has six electrodes implanted along the cochlea. The difference between single and multielectrode implants is in the kind of signal processing used and the particular sound that reaches the cochlea. The debate continues as to whether single or multielectrode implants are the most effective and safest for the patient.

Over the next few years, several other firms will be manufacturing cochlear implants, each claiming to be better than the other. Their common goal at this point, though, is to produce a totally implantable device that will make speech completely recognizable without lip reading.

Eye

The ultimate triumph of bioengineers may be the bringing of light into a world of darkness. Tests have now been done on an artificial eye, or what the leading researcher in the field, Dr. William Dobelle, calls electronic vision.

Dr. Dobelle, who heads the Institute for Artificial Organs on Long Island began his astonishing research in the late 1960s while at the University of Utah. He teamed up subsequently with Dr. John Girvin at the University of Western Ontario, and together they have performed several human trials of their artificial vision system. Their first experiment took place in the early 1970s with Craig, a 33-year-old man who was blinded in a freak hunting accident.

In an unprecedented operation surgeons removed a 2-by 3-inch piece of bone from the back of Craig's skull, exposing his visual cortex. There they implanted a thin, 1-square-inch sheet of Teflon with a grid of 64 platinum electrodes. A bundle of wires connected the electrodes to a computer, which in turn hooked up to a TV camera. The visual image recorded by the camera was then translated by a computer into electrical impulses, which were sent to the visual cortex.

With each minute electrical impulse or shock, Craig saw a "distant star," a white point of light known as a phosphene. The computer created a phosphene pattern of Braille characters right "in the mind's eye." Craig was able to distinguish a vertical line from a horizontal one. Dobelle wrote simple Braille sentences like "He had a cat and ball," which Craig could "read" five times faster than the standard tactile Braille alphabet. Craig said the pattern of lights looked like the scoreboard pictures we see at a sports stadium.

In 1982, the same surgical procedure was performed on Doug, who had lost his sight in 1966 after stepping on a land mine in Vietnam. He was also able to see the scoreboard-like lights.

Dobelle and Girvin realize that 64 electrodes are simply too few to create a real semblance of vision. The next step is to use a Teflon sheet containing a minimum of 256 electrodes. Given enough electrodes and the ability to brighten and mute an individual phosphene, a blind person might be able to see an image similar to the cartoons produced on a sports scoreboard.

In conjunction with the 256-electrode implant, Dobelle and Girvin envision a fingernail-sized camera that would be implanted in an artificial eye. A microcomputer small enough to rest on eyeglasses would then be able to stimulate certain electrodes to produce particular and recognizable images of phosphenes. Before the turn of the century this goal may be realized.

James McAlear, who heads Gentronix Laboratories in Rockville, Maryland, believes that making electrodes from fiber optics instead of metal is the key to an artificial eye. This new technology which involves bonding protein onto biocompatible polymer surfaces, is called molecular electronics. It could mean a sizeable increase in the number of effective electrodes able to be implanted in the brain. McAlear sees the technology as the answer to 20/20 by the year 2020.

Heart

In many ways, the notion of a bionic person didn't really seem plausible until December 2, 1982, when Barney Clark received the Jarvik-7 heart. The replacement of a human heart by metal, dacron, and plastic was one of the most amazing developments in medical history. As of this writing, artificial hearts have been placed in the chests of 16 persons since 1969. Some of these were temporary replacements, until a suitable human heart could be found. In others, the hearts were meant to be permanent. The best known artificial heart, the Jarvik-7, kept recipients Murray Haydon and William Schroeder alive for more than 1 year. The Penn State Heart, developed by Dr. William S. Pierce, has only been used as a stopgap measure.

Bian Que was a Chinese doctor who reputably performed two human heart transplants in 500 B.C. If that is true, then it took over two millennia for us to hear about heart transplants again. In the mid 1960s heart transplants became a history-making medical accomplishment. Today they are relatively common, and scores of people lead normal lives with transplanted hearts.

In the U.S. alone, 600,000 people die of heart attacks each year, two-thirds of them before even reaching the hospital. The National Heart, Lung, and Blood Institute estimates that up to 35,000 people would be candidates for an artificial heart. And bioengineers predict that by 1991, a wholly self-contained artificial heart will be available.

Structurally, the heart is among the body's simplest organs and the easiest to copy. Its purpose is to pump blood through the body—10 liters, pulsating at 80 beats per minute, 115,000 times per day, 42 million times per year. The right side of the heart has the easier job of pumping blood from the veins into the lungs where it picks up oxygen. The function of the left side is more complicated, because it must pump the oxygen-rich blood through the arteries to the rest of the body. The left side is the one that most frequently fails.

The Jarvik-7 is made largely of polyurethane, titanium, and dacron. (A smaller version is called the Jarvik-70; in December 1985, it was implanted in the first female artificial heart recipient.) It has two chambers rather than four as in a real heart, and dacron cuffs attach the artificial heart to major blood vessels. The left and right polyurethane ventricles are inserted into the cuffs. The power for the heart comes from an external air-driven system to which the patient is tethered. Once the machine is turned on, a steady 60 beats per minute results.

There have been major problems with the Jarvik-7. Blood clots have formed on the titanium valves. The body regards the inert surfaces as foreign invaders and platelets accumulate on them. The opening through which the tubes leave the patient's chest to connect to the external driver is a chronic area for bacterial infection. Four of the first six recipients suffered strokes, and being tethered to a machine caused them to become depressed. Fortunately, the 323-pound system has been reduced to a briefcase-sized portable 11-pound unit.

As Jarvik has said, the next step for the artificial heart is that "it must be forgettable." In other words, it must be both self-contained and self-sufficient. Dr. Donald Olsen, director of the Utah Artificial Heart Research Lab, implanted a totally self-contained heart, the UTAH 100, in a calf at the end of 1985.

To make the UTAH 100 self-contained, though, Olsen is seeking to implant between the ventricles a brushless dc motor with a hydraulic pump. Olsen has eliminated valves and the diaphragm, which have been the two main areas of failure so far. The diaphragms in an artificial heart must fold and unfold a total of 80 million times per year, and no material can withstand such stress over several years. The UTAH 100 that Olsen implanted in the calf has a small blood pump that runs in one direction. It has a fixed speed, pumps all the hydraulic fluid out that it receives, and has no valves or flexing membranes.

The Cleveland Clinic was the first institution to found an artificial organs department, and the department's director, Dr. Yukihiko Nosé, plans on implanting the world's first self-contained heart in humans in 1991. "At this stage of development, any permanent artificial heart would leave the patient with tubes sticking out of his chest connecting him to an external power source the size of a suitcase. We do not believe this is humane. The patient must have a totally implantable artifical heart so that he can live the same as you or I," Dr. Nosé explains.

Several versions of Nosé's self-contained heart have been implanted in calves. Just as it would be in humans, an internal battery pack is implanted along the ribcage. A wearable external belt-pack battery provides current that simply passes beneath the skin and recharges the pack, which drives the heart's motor. Patients would wear the battery pack for most of the day. The battery belt could be removed for short periods, but the power stored in the internal battery would last only 40 minutes. That is enough time to "take a shower or have sex," Nose says, but by 1990 he plans to have a thermal pump that will last 8 hours before needing to be recharged.

Lung

In 1947, Drs. Willem J. Kolff and Donald B. Effler developed the first, and only, crude artificial lung. To mimic the real function of lungs, a membrane and pump acted to introduce oxygen into the blood and draw carbon dioxide from it. It was designed to assist during open-heart surgery when a patient's heart and lungs are incapacitated. Ultimately, the artificial lung was not useful. The "membrane oxygenator" design, however, did pave the way for similar open-heart assist devices used today.

Since then, little work has been done toward development of an artificial lung, which many researchers consider to be a remote possibility. But Dr. Pierre Galletti has designed a device that consists of a coiled bundle of microporous tubes with a common inlet and outlet through which blood circulates. In the early 1980s, he implanted the device in sheep, where it functioned well for several hours at a time. He implanted it in the thorax between the pulmonary artery and vein. Blood flows through the tubes, absorbing oxygen and releasing carbon dioxide.

"My objective is not to see how well it [the lung] works, but if it works," Galletti says. He will continue to refine the device so that it will function longer in sheep. If his tests prove successful, human trials could begin in the early 1990s.

Kidney

Artificial kidneys are among the oldest of all artificial organs, and a constant refining of the original design has meant dramatic improvements. A new technique called *continuous ambulatory peritoneal dialysis* (*CAPD*) requires no bulky machines, and allows patients to treat themselves.

The kidneys are astonishingly efficient organs; indeed, most people need to have only 10 percent of their kidney tissue in healthy condition to stay alive. The 4-inch-long kidneys, which lie on either side of the lower spine, act as the body's filtering system, disposing of metabolic wastes, salt, and excess water as urine. They also adjust the body's fluid volume, blood composition, and blood pressure.

Acute kidney failure is largely a reversible condition. Patients are hooked to conventional dialysis machines that enable damaged kidneys to regenerate and heal. Chronic kidney disease, however, is incurable. More than 15 million Americans suffer from kidney and urinary tract diseases. An estimated 78,000 die each year and more than 70,000 depend on an artificial kidney to stay alive.

Basically, there are two kinds of artificial kidney systems: *hemodialysis* and *peritoneal dialysis*. Hemodialysis, the first practical system for taking over the kidney's function, was developed in Holland during World War II by Dr. Willem J. Kolff, now the director of the Utah Institute for Biomedical Engineering. Greatly refined in the 1960s, the system requires that the patient be hooked up via catheters to a dialysis unit the size of a washing machine. Blood flows from an artery in the arm into the machine, where on one side there is a semipermeable membrane, and on the other, a cleansing fluid. The blood's wastes, salt, and water pass through the membrane into the fluid. Healthy blood components, such as cells and proteins, cannot cross the membrane. The cleansed blood returns to the body through a vein in the arm. Patients must undergo the expensive treatments three to four times per week, for 4 to 6 hours each time.

The *Wearable Artificial Kidney* (*WAK*) was developed at the University of Utah in 1976. "One of the great things about WAK is that it changes the psychological effects of the illness," says Barry Hanover, one of the original developers. WAK is a portable, miniaturized hemodialysis unit that requires no plumbing or electrical outlet. It weighs only 8 pounds, and is worn in front of the body with belts. Unlike conventional 120-quart hemodialysis units, the WAK system uses 20 quarts of fluid.

The Wonderland Travel Program has taken advantage of this portability by sponsoring exotic trips for kidney disease patients. The company has dialyzed more than 300 patients "in every kind of location, on everything from river banks, tropical isles, to desert tents, and remote mountain cabins," says John Warner, the director of the program.

Peritoneal Dialysis (PD) is the newer artificial kidney system, introduced in the mid 1970s. This system uses the patient's abdominal cavity (peritoneum) and the blood vessels that line it. The lining acts as the membrane, and the washing fluid is pumped in and out of the abdomen by a machine. Wastes pass through the stomach lining into the solution that fills the cavity.

Continuous Ambulatory Peritoneal Dialysis (CAPD) is an extension of this technology. CAPD completely frees patients from a machine. A patient has a catheter surgically implanted into the peritoneal cavity. A plastic bag containing about 2 liters of dialyzing solution is hooked to the catheter. When the patient raises the bag of solution to shoulder level, gravity pulls the solution into the abdominal cavity. The empty container is simply rolled up and placed under the clothing. The patient goes about his or her daily activities while toxic wastes and excess water pass through the abdomen's network of tiny blood vessels and into the solution.

The exchange process is completed every 4 to 8 hours. The patient unrolls the plastic container and holds it below the abdomen, allowing the toxin-bearing solution to drain out. The bag is discarded and a new infusion process is begun.

Dr. Richard Fine, a pediatric nephrologist at UCLA, has adapted CAPD for children. Since 1980, when he received FDA approval, he has had more than 100 children fitted with the artificial kidney device. One of the severe side effects of kidney disease in children is stunted growth, but early use of CAPD prevents this. Also, dietary restrictions are less severe with CAPD than with standard hemodialysis.

CAPD requires great care and meticulousness on the patient's part. Peritonitis (inflammation of the peritoneum), can be fatal. Edward Andrulee of the Baxter Travenol Laboratories, which pioneered PD in the 1970s, sees "a lot of new advances in CAPD in the next few years. Researchers are currently looking for ways to simplify the treatment and to reduce all risks of infection."

Pancreas

Two different routes are being pursued in the quest for an artificial pancreas. *Implantable infusion pumps*, which take over the insulin-producing function of the pancreas, are used widely today, and their success grows yearly. The second method for reproducing the function of the pancreas involves a microencapsulation of insulin-producing cells.

The pancreas' major role is to produce insulin. Digestive juices flow from the pancreas into the first part of the small intestine, the duodenum. These juices contain enzymes and salts that break down and digest proteins, starches, sugars, and fats. The islets of Langerhans are special clusters of cells in the pancreas that secrete insulin into the bloodstream. Without insulin, body cells can't absorb and use glucose from the blood. Glucose fuels cells, and when there is too little insulin, diabetes results.

Glucose is either instantly used by the body or stored for future use. In diabetics, the glucose is not used properly in the body and many diabetics require daily injections of insulin to keep their glucose metabolism functioning. Long-term complications of the disease can include blindness, ketoacidosis (diabetic comas), kidney disease, and circulatory problems.

In 1970, Dr. Henry Buchwald, professor of biomedical engineering at the University of Minnesota, and a team of doctors and engineers designed a titanium and silicone implantable insulin pump. What followed was a greatly refined series of pumps. The several types of pumps, now scaled to the size of a deck of playing cards, all use a simple vapor pressure system. They are implanted either in the abdominal or chest wall. The hollow titanium metal canister is refilled with insulin percutaneously (through the skin) every 7 to 10 days. A mechanical flow pump and an electronically controlled programmable pump deliver steady dosages of insulin into the bloodstream.

One of Buchwald's most dramatic case histories involves five women in their twenties with diabetes so severe that insulin injections were totally useless. They suffered from DRIASM—diabetes with resistance to insulin administered subcutaneously or intramuscularly,—and "had life-threatening episodes virtually every day," Buchwald says. Between 1983 and 1984, Buchwald implanted pumps in the women. Within 4 to 6 months of her operation, each woman's diabetic comas were reduced 90 percent. The nightmare of intravenous catheters and frequent confinement to the hospital had ended.

Buchwald projects that within the next decade the majority of insulin-dependent (Type I) diabetics will be treated with an insulin pump containing a built-in glucose sensor. Instead of delivering a constant stream of insulin, the pump will sense the body's insulin needs and deliver appropriate amounts. The needs of Type II patients (those who secrete some insulin) are met by the pumps that exist now.

Already, Dr. Robert Fischell of the Johns Hopkins University has invented a pump with a built-in alarm system that looks for flaws and tickles the patient if something goes wrong. His pump, called the *Programmable Implantable Medication System* (*PIMS*), can be read by telephone, and the drug dosage can even be reprogrammed over the phone. Using radiotelemetry, the doctor will be able to instruct the 3½-inch-diameter pump to deliver specific doses of insulin. Dr. Fischell expects to receive FDA approval imminently.

Another—still experimental—method for coping with a nonfunctional pancreas or poorly functioning pancreas involves wrapping pancreatic islet cells in a semipermeable plastic. This allows body fluids to flow in and insulin to flow out. When these "capsules are injected into the stomach, the cells act almost like free islets," says Dr. Anthony Sun of the University of Toronto Medical School. The capsules tend to remain in the stomach cavity, releasing insulin into the bloodstream. Because the system has worked for up to 9 months in rats, researchers have begun experiments on dogs.

Dr. Pierre Galletti and Dr. William Chick of the University of Massachusetts are working on similiar systems. They are experimenting with seeding pancreatic islet cells into hollow fiber chambers implanted in the abdomen. Blood circulates through the network of chambers—artificial capillaries, in a sense—and picks up released insulin. As with the cells encapsulated in plastic, the hollow fiber system prevents immune rejection of the foreign cells—a buffer exists between implanted tissue and the patient's own antibodies. The Chick-Galletti system has functioned well in dogs, and tests will begin in larger animals in 1986.

Liver

The most promising artificial liver devices have been those that combine synthetic parts with living cells—that is, they have been what have come to be known in medicine as bioartificial organs.

The liver is the body's largest internal organ and among its most complex. Basically, the liver is the body's refinery. All of the blood that leaves the stomach and intestines passes through the liver before being distributed elsewhere. Among a myriad of functions, the organ converts food into vital chemicals, processes drugs, detoxifies and excretes poisonous substances, and regulates hormones. Even more remarkable, though, is the liver's unparalleled ability to regenerate much of its own tissue should it be damaged or diseased.

Unlike the heart or ear, for example, organs whose form and action are based more on structure than on biochemistry, the liver's principal functions are accomplished at the cellular level. In a sense, each liver cell is a microcosm of the entire organ; each cell is its own factory. That characteristic, along with the liver's great regenerative powers, has caused researchers to concentrate on developing external support systems that take over, temporarily, some of the functions of the liver until it can repair itself.

Paul Malchesky, a chemical engineer at the Cleveland Clinic, has developed a device called a hepatic assist that filters out toxins that cause painful symptoms. Activated charcoal naturally attracts toxic substances to its surface. Malchesky's device treats the blood plasma "just as you would treat water in your own home—with softeners, resins, or maybe even a charcoal filter right on the water line." The patient's blood is drawn into a system similar in size, function, and design to a kidney hemodialysis unit. The plasma is separated from other blood elements in a process called *membrane plasmapheresis*. Thin plastic tubes with microscopic pores act as filters. The plasma then passes through compartments where resins and activated charcoal process out toxins. The cleansed plasma reunites with blood cells and other components and is returned to the body.

Plasmapheresis' principal use has been to treat chronic itching (which characterizes a certain kind of liver disease). While this system cannot reverse organ damage, it continues to be helpful in determining many causes of liver disease.

Drs. Pierre Galletti and Hugo Jauregui are using a hollow fiber system like the one Galletti is working on to replace pancreatic function, to create an "artificial liver." The liver will be used in clinical situations for a comparatively short period while the patient is in the hospital. Liver cells will be attached to fibers (the fibers are made of a material similar to acrylic) in an implanted hollow chamber. Blood will circulate through the semipermeable fiber where the liver cells will remove toxins. Because the cells are receiving constant nourishment, they will grow; in a sense, a new liver mass will begin to form in the fibers. Galletti and Jauregui are currently working to replace single fibers with a matrix. This will result in a three -dimensional liver culture, which would perform a greater variety of liver functions.

Fallopian Tubes

For many of the women suffering from infertility, artificial fallopian tubes hold out great hope. A first-year medical student at the University of Utah, Steven Hunter, has been working on the development of artificial tubes since 1984, and successful animal tests point to their use in women in less than 10 years.

The fallopian tubes are the pair of narrow ducts in the abdominal cavity through which an egg passes on its journey from the ovary to the uterus. Fertilization takes place in the tubes, which are only 10 to 13 centimeters long and 0.5 to 1.2 centimeters in diameter. Elaborate muscular contractions along the walls, in conjunction with mucous membrane secretions, help move the egg or sperm along.

Hunter explains that "to mimic all of the functions of fallopian tubes would be impossible." Instead, his goals are to "provide an environment where fertilization can take place, a means to keep the egg and sperm viable, and a means to transport the embryo to the uterus at a time when implantation into the uterine wall is possible. Our animal tests indicate that we can probably achieve all three goals." Hunter is also designing a *programmable micropump*, similar to those used for insulin delivery. This will provide the eggs captured from the ovaries with essential nutrients and transport them to the uterus.

Hunter's work is, as far as he knows, the only research of its kind. He points out, though, that if in vitro fertilization techniques improve significantly, they may eliminate the need for artificial fallopian tubes. But he adds that an artificial fallopian tube capable of providing a suitable environment for fertilization "will eliminate the moral and legal problems" associated with test tube babies. "We will have devised a sort of in vivo, in vitro fertilization," he adds.

Hunter's tests have progressed from implants in rabbits to implants in sheep, but no real attempts have been made yet to get any of the animals pregnant using an artificial tube. Ongoing testing in sheep will help determine the ideal design for humans as well as which type of plastic will be most compatible with human body tissue.

Arm

Developments in artificial limb technology have been as encouraging and speedy as any in medicine. Indeed, courses in orthotics and prosthetics were not even offered in medical school until the mid-sixties. But by 1981 the medieval system of hooks, pulleys, and rubber bands that served as artificial arm replacements was thrown away for good. Dr. Stephen Jacobsen's *Utah Arm* or "thinking arm", gave patients the ability to move the prosthesis toward or away from the body, and to perform four other movements. When an amputee thinks of a movement, an electrical signal travels along nerve pathways. Electrodes implanted in the artificial arm detect the impulses and, via wires and tiny motors, move the limb. In the near future the artificial arm will be able to perform more of the human arm's 27 movements.

In 1983 two new developments gave the amputee a totally electric elbow and hand. The *Otto Bock Hand*, originally developed in West Germany and adapted to the graphite-and-fiber-reinforced plastic Utah Arm, now means that "we're essentially controlling two degrees of freedom, motion in the elbow and grasping of the hand, with the same control sites," Dr. Jacobsen says. The hand weighs only 1 pound. Implanted within it are the electric motors and reduction systems that control the speed with which the patient moves the fingers and the amount of grip force exerted. The hand has a maximum grip force of 22 pounds, slightly more than that of a real hand, but the artificial hand can easily hold a styrofoam cup without crushing it, open jars, even be used to apply makeup. The metallic fingers are given a lifelike appearance with a cosmetic glove.

The first person fitted with the full arm, elbow, and hand system was Alice Olson, who lost her own arm in an industrial accident. The design of the Utah Arm is ultimately so simple that when there is a mechanical problem, "generally, I can handle any problem over the phone, or the manufacturer will send me a part through the mail and I replace it myself," Olson says. A screwdriver and pair of pliers are often the most elaborate tools needed to make repairs.

Jacobsen is currently working to improve the touch sensors, which allow amputees to "sense" how tightly they are clutching something. Multiple electrode sites will be implanted, enabling simultaneous movements to occur, such as elbow and humeral rotation, wrist and hand, hand and elbow. All Utah Arms are tailored to the individual amputee's needs; specific rotations, movements, speeds, grasp forces are geared to the individual's work and play needs.

Neurophysiologist Dr. Richard Stein of the University of Alberta, in conjunction with electronics technologist Dean Charles, wants to go beyond the myoelectric arm. The two researchers recognize that many amputees are left with little or no remaining muscle; for them the myoelectric arm is largely useless. So Stein and Charles have invented a system called *biotelemetry*.

A radio transmitter reprocesses a nerve's electrical signal into a radio wave, and back to an electrical signal which drives small motors implanted in the arm. The transmitter's power is provided by a second transmitter in the prosthesis. It is hoped that this system will give amputees an even greater range of movement capabilities than they will have with artificial limbs that use only muscle signals. Stein has tested the system in a cat over a period of 1 year and hopes by late 1986 to try it on humans.

Foot

The so-called *Seattle Foot* is as beautifully sculpted as any by Michelangelo, and so it's not surprising that it was one of the the 12 winners of the first Presidential Awards for Design Excellence in 1985. But form does indeed follow function, and its applications for amputees are as equally impressive as its looks. Paddy Rossbach, a member of the Achilles Track Team, ran the 1985 New York City Marathon with a Seattle Foot.

Dr. Ernest M. Burgess, director of Seattle's Prosthetics Research Foundation, and Don Poggi, a Boeing engineer, have designed a foot flexible and springy enough to absorb gravitational energy. A cantilevered plastic spring keel manages to store energy and release it in such a way that there is a lift and thrust forward. The feet on old wooden legs and even contemporary polyurethane ones are crudely fashioned to vaguely resemble real feet, or else are shaped like a shoe. The wearer has to use remnant upper leg muscles to move the foot along, ploddingly. With the Seattle Foot, the wearer can walk at a near normal pace, even jog.

Dr. Burgess was inspired to create a usable, lifelike foot when he saw many of the amputee veterans coming home from Vietnam. They "tended to be very young, and some of them were having a very bad time. We wanted to improve their recreational activities," he has said. The ordinary wooden foot "was not filling the bill. The [veterans] could walk and climb stairs, but not much else. They couldn't run, fish or play golf. It was pretty discouraging," Burgess has commented. Jim Mayer, who lost both legs in Vietnam in 1969, has said that with the Seattle Foot "I can feel the earth move. It's an incredible asset. That dead effect is gone." Nebraska Governor Bob Kerrey is another of those veterans who has been fitted with the Seattle Foot. Ted Kennedy, Jr., the senator's son who lost a leg to cancer when he was a young boy, wears it, as does former Senator Warren Magnuson.

For many of the some 600,000 leg amputees in the U.S., the Seattle Foot will mean changes in their lives. Professor Jim Clark at the University of Washington received the artificial foot in 1985, and "the first jump I made with it was like a dream," he says. "Instead of the floor beating me to a pulp, I felt as though I was springing on a diving board. That night, I went dancing."

Tendons

A three-person team at the University of Medicine and Dentistry of New Jersey has found a material that encourages torn ligaments and tendons to regrow. Like coral that biodegrades, allowing for real bone to grow back, carbon tendons and ligaments soon yield to new real ones. Scores of people have had limbs saved as a result of this discovery. The technology has been used also to rebuild ligaments in heels, hips, shoulders, elbows, knees, and hands.

Ligaments connect bone to bone, while tendons connect muscle to bone. Both are tough, fibrous tissues that can be easily torn in falls or sports or simply by stepping wrongly. In the majority of cases, a surgeon can sew back together the torn ends of a ligament or tendon. If the rupture is especially severe, though, the surgical procedure will not work, and the limb can then become useless. For patients with this type of rupture, of whom there are an estimated 100,000 annually in the U.S., artificial ligaments and tendons are working wonders.

Only a couple of years ago surgeons had few choices. The body frequently rejects ligament and tendon grafts from cadavers. Taking grafts from elsewhere in the patient's body means transferring the problem. The few synthetic replacements that have been tried have not been biocompatible and often cause abnormal growth in surrounding tissue.

The New Jersey team's tendons consist of a three-foot carbon rope, one-eighth of an inch thick, and composed of 10,000 filaments of pure carbon. This cable is sewn in and around the ripped tissue. A biodegradable, nontoxic acid coats the carbon rope to make it pliable.

The developers, materials engineer John Parson, mechanical engineer Harold Alexander, and orthopedic surgeon Andrew Weiss, have topped the body's own healing process. Because carbon is among the most biocompatible of materials, the fibers attract fibroblasts, cells that produce collagen. As the carbon and polyactic acid are biodegrading, collagen is forming in and among the implant fibers. Often within 9 months connective tissue has completely filled in the rupture in the ligament or tendon. The carbon fibers act as a sort of scaffold for the regrowing tissue.

Already 1,500 people in the U.S. have been implanted with the artificial tendons and ligaments. The success rate has been very high. As Dr. Weiss has said, "Many patients were unable to walk. Now they are jogging again."

That we will achieve immortality through artificial hearts, carbon tendons, camera-and-computer eyesight, and coral bones is doubtful. This does not, however, diminish their import. These tributes to human ingenuity promise the millions who will receive them the greatest gift we know of: a longer, healthier, more productive life. The development of artificial skin will spare the thousands who suffer severe burns each year untold agony and disfiguration. Carved coral "bone" will permit surgeons to sculpt new visages for victims of auto accidents, for children born without jawbones. No fewer than 35,000 Americans would benefit from the unalterable beat of a mechanical heart. Already, more than 70,000 people depend on an artificial kidney to keep them alive. The hundreds of thousands who have been made whole again through the efforts of technology and medicine repeat Barney Clark's simple message: "Don't quit."

Timeline

1986 to 1990
- Artificial skin approved by FDA as standard procedure for burn treatment.
- Interpore (coral) in wide use as bone replacement material.
- Synthetic blood substitutes (PFCs) used in transfusions, open heart surgery, for stroke victims.
- Multichannel artificial ear in use.
- UTAH 100 replaces Jarvik-7 as artificial heart.
- Computerized programmable insulin pump changes lives of many diabetics.
- Tendons and ligaments made of carbon approved by FDA.

1991 to 1995
- Biotelemetry used to power artificial limbs.
- Total artificial ear implant enables deaf to understand speech without any lip reading.
- Self-contained artificial heart implanted.
- Human trials with artificial lung begin.
- Hemoglobin solutions substituted for blood.

1996 to 2000
- Infertile women implanted with artificial fallopian tubes.
- Hollow fiber liver and pancreas become common in humans.
- Pancreas islet cells injected in human gut cure diabetes.
- PFCs obliterate tumors.

2001 to 2020
- Artificial eyes run by biochips see the world.
- Total movement gained in artificial arms and legs.

2100
- Every organ and tissue able to be replaced—the Bionic man?

Access Guide

Skin

The Massachusetts General Hospital
Fruit Street
Boston, MA 02114
(617) 726-2000
(Also for blood, blood vessels)

Bones

The Texas Cranial Facial Center
3600 Gaston Avenue
Dallas, TX 75235
(214) 826-1000

CAD-CAM
Phoenix Data Systems
80 Wolf Road
Albany, NY
(518) 459-6202

CAD-CAM
Contour Medical Systems, Inc.
1931A Old Middlefield Way
Mountain View, CA 94043
(415) 969-2983

Blood

The University of California at
    Irvine Medical Center
101 The City Drive
Orange, CA 92668
(714) 634-6011

The Michael Reese Hospital
Lake Shore Drive and 31st Street
Chicago, IL 60616
(312) 791-2000

Rush-Presbyterian St. Luke's
    Medical Center
1753 West Congress Parkway
Chicago, Il 60612
(312) 942-5000

Blood Vessels

Vascular International, Inc.
4750 Wiley Post Way
Salt Lake City, UT 84116
(801) 537-7137

The St. Vincent Hospital and
   Health Care Center
The Indiana University School of
   Medicine
Indianapolis, Indiana 46202
(317) 871-2345

Ear

The House Ear Institute
256 South Lake Street
Los Angeles, CA 90057
(213) 483-4431

The 3M Company
Public Relations Department
P.O. Box 33600
St. Paul, MN 55133
(612) 736-0876

Symbion, Inc.
825 North 300 West
Salt Lake City, UT 84103
(801) 531-7022
(Also for heart)

The University of California at San
   Francisco
Public Information
532 Parnassus Avenue
San Francisco, CA 94143
(415) 666-2557

Eye

The Institute for Artificial Organs,
   Inc.
145 Rome Street
Farmington, NY 11735
(516) 293-3630

The University of Western Ontario
   Hospital
P.O. Box 5339
Terminal A
London, Ontario, Canada N6A
   5A5
(519) 663-3000

Heart

The Cleveland Clinic
9500 Euclid Avenue
Cleveland, OH 44106
(216) 444-2549
(Also for pancreas, kidney, and
   liver)

The American Heart Association
205 East 42nd Street
New York, NY 10017
(212) 661-5335

The University of Utah Medical
　Center
50 North Medical Drive
Salt Lake City, UT 84132
(801) 581-2121

The Humana Hospital Audubon
1 Audubon Plaza Drive
Louisville, KY 40217
(502) 636-7111

The University of Utah
Department of Public Relations
308 Park Building
Salt Lake City, UT 84112
(801) 581-7931

Kidney

The National Kidney Foundation
2 Park Avenue
New York, NY 10016
(212) 889-2210

The Baxter Travenol Laboratories
1425 Lake Cook Road
Deerfield, IL 60015
(312) 948-2000

The University of California at Los
　Angeles Medical Center
10833 Leconte Avenue
Los Angeles, CA 90024
(213) 825-9111

Pancreas

The American Diabetes
　Association
2 Park Avenue
New York, NY 10016
(800) 223-0179

The University of Minnesota
　Medical School
420 Delaware Street, Southeast
Minneapolis, MN 55455
(612) 373-2851

The Johns Hopkins University
　Hospital
600 North Wolfe Street
Baltimore, MD 21205
(301) 955-5000

Liver

The American Liver Foundation
998 Pompton Avenue
Cedar Grove, NJ 07009
(800) 223-0179

Lung

The American Lung Association
1740 Broadway
New York, NY 10019
(212) 315-8700

Foot

Model and Instrument Works
1103 Ranier Avenue South
Seattle, WA 98114
(206) 325-0715

Arms

Motion Control, Inc.
1005 South 300 West
Salt Lake City, UT 84101
(801) 364-1958

Tendons and Ligaments

The University of Medicine and Dentistry of New Jersey
The New Jersey Medical School Hospital
100 Bergen Street
Newark, NJ 07103
(201) 456-4300

5

Childbirth 2000

On July 25, 1978, Louise Brown—the first "test tube baby"—was ushered into the world in an otherwise unremarkable delivery in England. Serving as midwives were two British doctors, Patrick Steptoe and Robert Edwards, who have developed a process in which a female egg is mated with a sperm in a petrie dish, a technique known as *in vitro fertilization.*

Millions of couples with incurable infertility problems now have their first real shot at becoming biological parents, and since Brown's arrival an estimated 800 to 1,000 children worldwide have been conceived in a lab dish. At the same time, scientists have been pushing forward the frontiers of reproductive technology so rapidly that couples now may choose from many childbearing alternatives that were unimaginable just a decade ago.

If the husband is infertile, the wife's eggs can be fertilized with sperm donated from another male using artificial insemination or in vitro techniques. If the wife can't ovulate, her husband's sperm can be united with an egg donated by another woman. The embryo is then transplanted into the wife's womb—a still experimental technique known as embryo transfer. Or the husband could artificially inseminate another woman, who could carry the baby to term or have the embryo removed and transplanted to the wife's womb. If both partners are infertile, donated sperm and eggs can be mated in the lab, and the resulting embryos can be placed in the womb of the wife or surrogate. In the future, men might be able to have embryos transplanted into their abdominal cavity, making male pregnancy possible.

These breakthroughs have come none too soon. The record number of abortions has led to a precipitous drop in the number of newborns available for adoption. Also, the incidence of infertility has more than doubled in the past two decades; it now afflicts close to 10 million Americans.

The good news is that significant advances in the diagnosis and treatment of infertility with drugs and microsurgery mean that "roughly 75 to 85 percent of infertile couples can have a baby with appropriate treatment," says Dr. Edward E. Wallach, professor and director of the department of gynecology and obstetrics at Johns Hopkins Hospital. "For the remainder, in vitro fertilization and other approaches may be hopeful last resorts."

It's also possible to successfully select the gender of an unborn child almost 80 percent of the time. And thanks to a process called *cryopreservation*, semen and embryos can now be frozen indefinitely and thawed out when a couple is ready to have children—even when the parents are 40 or 50 years old.

Ironically, this reproductive revolution has spawned a back to basics movement in childbirth. More and more women are choosing alternative methods of having their babies—midwives, birthing centers, and at-home births. New technologies allow the vast majority of premature babies—many of whom had they been born 20 years ago would have died or have been severely handicapped—to not only survive but lead normal lives. Startling breakthroughs in fetal surgery, in which delicate operations are performed to correct defects on the fetus while still in the womb, are paving the way towards drastically reducing the number of babies born with fatal or severely debilitating maladies.

These advances have stirred up a hornet's nest of disturbing legal and ethical dilemmas. What happens to those unused embryos that are kept frozen in storage? Should they be destroyed, used for research, or implanted in a surrogate? Who is financially responsible if a surrogate mother gives birth to a child with serious defects? When embryo transfer becomes widespread, will the "rent-a-womb" business skyrocket? Will a class of women breeders emerge who are hired by the wealthy to carry their offspring?

Some states have proposed legislation to regulate our growing reproductive powers, but as it stands, our legal system has no guidelines to clarify these controversies. "These developments are pushing us to ask some of the most difficult and profound questions about life that we've ever considered," said Clifford Grobstein, professor of biological science and public policy at the University of California at San Diego. "We are poised at a major watershed of human development. At this point there are no answers, just countless questions."

Despite these questions scientific progress will dramatically transform childbirth in the 21st century. Prospective parents will exercise unheard of control over the circumstances in which they conceive and bear their offspring. "In the Bible, Sarah had her baby when she was 90," noted Dr. Landrum Shettles, a pioneer in the field of infertility. "The day when such a miracle actually comes to pass, when a modern day Sarah—retired on her social security pension—has a child, may be very near."

Combatting Infertility

Infertility is medically defined as the inability of a couple to conceive after a year of unprotected intercourse, or to carry pregnancies to a live birth. Ironically, the trend toward postponing parenthood among career-minded couples has doubled the incidence of infertility over the past twenty years. Close to 20 percent of married couples in the United States—totaling more than 10 million people—cannot conceive children.

"We know that as time goes on couples expose themselves to more potential causes of infertility," explains Dr. Wayne H. Decker, executive director of the Fertility Research Foundation in New York. Difficulty in ovulating increases with age, and the chances of miscarriage, which is triggered at least 60 percent of the time by chromosomal defects in the fetus, increase dramatically after age 35.

What was once a rare problem in a society that began parenting in its twenties, has become a highly charged ordeal for the growing number of couples who have deferred childbearing until their thirties or forties, only to discover that something has gone awry in their reproductive systems. And contrary to the popular myth that infertility is *always* the woman's problem, infertility afflicts both sexes equally.

"Infertility rips at the core of a couple's relationship," says Betty Orlandino, who counsels infertile couples in Oak Park, Illinois. "It affects sexuality, self-image, and self-esteem. It stalls careers, devastates savings, and damages associations with friends and family."

But the nightmarish trauma of infertility may soon end, thanks to new diagnoses and treatments. Four out of five infertile couples can have a baby with the aid of fertility drugs, artificial insemination, intricate microsurgeries to repair damaged reproductive organs, or hormonal regimens to prevent miscarriages. The remaining 15 percent of couples also have a good chance of becoming parents as a result of breakthroughs in reproductive science, including in vitro fertilization, embryo transfers, and surrogate gestation.

What's fueled these advances? In the past decade researchers have identified many of the factors that produce infertility—the first step toward discovering treatment or methods of prevention. The most common causes of infertility among men are physiological. For instance, varicocele, which is a varicose vein within the scrotum and is responsible for nearly 40 percent of all cases of male infertility. Other abnormalities, such as injuries or infections in the male organs, as well as exposure to toxic chemicals, poor health, stress, or drug abuse, can drastically diminish the numbers of normally shaped, fast-moving sperm available to fertilize eggs.

Physicians have made strides devising remedies that can be as simple as timing intercourse with ovulation cycles or making minor lifestyle changes, such as limiting the consumption of alcohol, drugs, and tobacco, or not wearing tight-fitting jeans or underwear, which can inhibit the production of healthy sperm. A therapeutic regimen of various types of drugs, such as hormones to stimulate sperm production, antibiotics to control prostate infections, and steroids to decrese antibodies that hamper sperm motility, can also boost fertility.

Probably the most significant breakthrough has been the development of microsurgical techniques. For example, varicocele, a condition that causes low sperm count, can be corrected with minor surgery that boasts more than a 50 percent success rate. Similarly, more than half the men who undergo a "reverse vasectomy"—a procedure in which the scar tissue is removed from the ends of the tied-off duct which is then repaired—can father children. (The prospects of restoring fertility more than 10 years after a vasectomy is not good, however.) Both procedures can be done in a doctor's office and require only a local anesthetic.

Another recent advance by an Australian research team headed by Dr. Alan Trounson, the IVF pioneer, holds out hope even for men with irreversible vasectomies or significant damage to the vas deferens (the tube that transports the sperm to the penis). In preliminary experiments using microsurgical techniques, researchers were able to recover sperm directly from the epididymis, the ductal system that drains the testes.

In the future, surgery may not even be necessary to correct varicocele. Last year, a new device, the *Repro-Med THD*, which lowers testicular temperature (heat reduces sperm production), received FDA approval and is available from physicians or by prescription. In clinical tests on groups of men who were diagnosed as "hardcore" infertility cases, the production of healthy semen improved 73 percent, even when surgery had failed.

New artificial insemination techniques can also increase the chances for infertile men to become fathers. By using a "split ejaculate" procedure, doctors can isolate the semen with the highest sperm count, which is then used to inseminate the wife. When all else fails, wives can be artificially inseminated with either fresh or frozen sperm from a donor. There isn't any reliable data on how many children are born each year by artificial insemination, but estimates range anywhere from 10,000–100,000 births in the United States annually.

Startling progress has also been made in the treatment of female infertility. The most common causes of infertility in women are blocked fallopian tubes; endometriosis, which is the presence of extra tissue that lines the uterus and interferes with conception; excess cervical mucous, which acts as a barrier against sperm; irregular ovulation; hormonal imbalances and deficiencies, which can trigger miscarriages; and tubal ligations, a form of voluntary sterilization in which the tubes are tied.

Advances in microsurgical procedures to repair or untie fallopian tubes, correct damaged reproductive organs, and remove endometrial adhesions have doubled the birth rate in those who've had these operations. But the biggest news has been the development of several drugs, such as *Clomid*, *Serophene*, *Profasi*, and *Pergonal*, that induce ovulation. In fact, at least 80 percent of women who ovulate sporadically or not at all could become pregnant if they used fertility drugs. Out of the more than 40,000 women who've taken Pergonal since 1980, more than 20,000 have given birth. Fertility drugs also increase the risk of multiple births, but better understanding of the delicately balanced hormonal process that leads to conception has enabled physicians to reduce the likelihood of woman's conceiving more than one child. Pergonal stimulates the development of an egg in the ovary, but Profasi, which is another hormone, must be taken so that the ovum is released from the ovary. By constantly monitoring estrogen levels, and examining the pelvis and cervix, doctors can detect the possibility of multiple conception and not administer Profasi. The result: "Fewer than 2 percent of all women who received Pergonal last year delivered three or more children," says Dr. Gary D. Hodgen, a professor in the department of obstetrics and gynecology at the Eastern Virginia Medical School in Norfolk.

On other fronts, medical researchers have made excellent progress in preventing miscarriages. Thanks to the recent development of a very sensitive hormone test, doctors now can accurately detect pregnancy within a week of ovulation. They speculate that many women who are considered infertile may be conceiving but spontaneously aborting embryos at such an early stage that the women never suspected they were pregnant.

Dr. Alan Beer, a professor of obstetrics at the University of Michigan, believes these spontaneous abortions could be the result of a quirky biochemical reaction. The mother's immune system rejects what it perceives as a foreign invader—the fetus. After their immune systems had been desensitized with injections of their husbands' cells, close to half of Dr. Beer's patients, all of whom had had at least four miscarriages, were able to finally deliver healthy babies.

Less than a generation ago, infertility was often dismissed as a psychological problem. Today, we know this isn't so, thanks to the development of diagnostic tools that show 90 percent of infertility cases have a physical cause. Physicians are confident that reproductive research will conquer infertility and end the frustration and anguish of infertile couples.

In Vitro Fertilization

When Jennifer Blair was born, her arrival represented more than the typical blessed event. Her mother had undergone a tubal ligation that couldn't be reversed after she changed her mind about having children. But that didn't stop the Blairs.

The latest addition to their family is just one of approximately 200 babies across the country that have been conceived via in vitro fertilization since the first American IVF baby, Elizabeth Carr, arrived in 1981. This technology offers the first real hope of becoming parents to an estimated 1 million Americans with fertility problems that can't be cured by conventional treatment.

It's not surprising that 121 medical centers specializing in IVF have sprung up across the country, and that these centers now number more than 200 worldwide. An IVF baby is born almost daily. By the end of this decade, predicts Clifford Stratton, director of the IVF Laboratory in Reno, Nevada, "there will be a successful IVF clinic in every U.S. city."

Essentially, IVF involves retrieving an egg from the woman's body, uniting the egg and the sperm outside of the womb, then inserting the fertilized egg into the uterus. Besides bypassing the damaged tubes or lumps of endometrial tissue that impede the normal reproductive process, the IVF technique uses the most active sperm, which can compensate for low sperm counts.

The actual process is costly ($5,000 per attempt with couples averaging three attempts), time-consuming, emotionally and physically draining, and often disappointing. IVF only has an overall 30 percent success rate, although America's premier IVF center, the Jones Institute for Reproductive Medicine in Norfolk, Virginia, reports a 45 percent pregnancy rate when two mature eggs can be transferred.

Prospective mothers are evaluated and tested to find those who are so damaged that there is no hope. If accepted into the program, patients are given hormone injections twice a day for a week to stimulate the production of several mature eggs. The women are monitored with blood tests, ultrasound, and pelvic exams, so doctors can pinpoint the precise moment when ovulation occurs and remove the eggs (using a technique known as laparoscopy) at the best time for conception. The eggs are placed in a petrie dish, fertilized with sperm, allowed to mature for about 48 hours, then put into the uterus, where, if everything goes perfectly, the embryo will attach itself to the uterine wall.

IVF is still far from an exact science, but techniques have come a long way since Louise Brown, the first test tube baby, was born in 1978. Drs. Patrick Steptoe and Robert Edwards, who developed the IVF procedure, operated under the mistaken notion that the sperm and the egg must be joined within minutes. "Now it is customary to wait 5 or 6 hours before insemination," says Dr. Howard Jones, founder of Norfolk's IVF clinic. He adds that the two IVF pioneers made so many incorrect assumptions that "the birth of Louise Brown now seems like a fortunate coincidence."

Improvement in IVF pregnancy rates at first proceeded at a snail's pace due to one of nature's inflexible rules: Only one egg is released during a woman's menstrual cycle. This meant that there was only one embryo per cycle, hence only one chance per month to achieve pregnancy. In 1980, a research team headed by Dr. Alan Trounson of the Monash University in Melbourne, Australia, hit upon a solution that ultimately transformed IVF. By using fertility drugs during menstruation, they induced ovaries to release several eggs, a feat that vastly upped the odds for achieving a pregnancy. "Suddenly, we had eight pregnancies that went to birth," said Dr. Trounson. "So other researchers switched to superovulation instead of using the women's natural cycle."

This advance generated problems, however. Implanting more than one embryo in the uterus greatly increases the possibility of multiple births, which is not only dangerous to the mother's health, but can drain the parents' financial and emotional resources. Equally important: What to do with the extra embryos? Indeed, the first problem has yet to be satisfactorily solved. But Trounson and his colleagues developed a process, known as cryopreservation, for freezing unused embryos, which can be kept indefinitely or later thawed out. To date, three in vitro babies have come from frozen embryos.

The rapid pace of these scientific advances has outstripped the legal system's ability to regulate them. The depth of this confusion was brought into focus when Mario and Elsa Rios were killed in a plane crash in 1983. The American couple left behind an estate valued at over $1 million, one grown son, and two embryos that were in cold storage in an Australian IVF clinic.

Did these embryos have rights under the law? Should they be destroyed or given to their "half-brother"? Were they entitled to a share of their parents' estate? Australian officials eventually decided the embryos should be implanted in surrogates and then surrendered for adoption, but many IVF clinics now require parents to choose what should be done with any unused embryos.

Here in the United States, experiments that could provide significant insights into which embryos are more viable, or identify effective methods of reducing the risks of multiple births, have been plagued by a 1975 federal ban on funding for research on human embryos. The moratorium has stalemated and stigmatized experimentation, forcing American investigators to rely heavily on the findings of British and Australian scientists.

"Society has always been leery of innovation and change, particularly at the scientific level," notes Dr. Howard Jones. "Before research can go forward in a meaningful way, society must reach, if not a consensus, at least a majority view about these issues. Scientific endeavor does not flourish without popular support." Nor does the anguish of infertile couples disappear simply because the moral and legal dilemmas haven't been ironed out. Witness the *16-year* waiting list for entry into the Norfolk program.

Perhaps even by the year 2000, Dr. Alan Trounson predicts, "people will have a much freer choice about the type of reproductive options that will suit them." Today, sex is no longer necessary for conception. Within the next 30 to 40 years, it's quite likely that the only role men and women may play in the reproductive process is to furnish the sperm and the eggs—the rest may be done in the laboratory.

Embryo Transfer

In January of 1984, history was made at a hospital in southern California: The first child produced by embryo transfer was born.

A woman who donated her ovum was artificially inseminated with the sperm from the husband of an infertile woman whose fallopian tubes were blocked. Five days after conception, the embryo was flushed from the donor's uterus, and implanted into the infertile woman, who became the mother of a healthy boy 9 months later.

This feat was repeated less than a month later when the second child, a girl, delivered by an infertile woman was born. "This second birth is significant because it established the viability of this procedure," says Dr. John Buster, head of the embryo transfer research team at Harbor-UCLA Medical Center in Torrance, California, that developed this technique.

This nonsurgical procedure, which can be performed in a doctor's office, requires no anesthesia. Likely candidates for embryo transfer are couples who've failed with IVF or artificial insemination, carriers of genetic defects, and women who've experienced premature menopause or have blocked fallopian tubes. This procedure may soon be more popular than in vitro fertilization. "It's simple and may have a higher success rate—perhaps 50 percent," predicts Dr. Duster, who anticipates performing 4,000 to 5,000 embryo transfers by the end of this decade. Plans are in full swing to franchise 20 to 30 embryo transfer clinics across the country under the auspices of Fertility & Genetics Research Inc., Chicago. More than 2,000 couples are on the waiting list.

The key stumbling block in launching a nationwide embryo transfer program is developing a pool of donor women "who can be genetically matched with recipients," says Dr. Roger K. Freeman, medical director of Women's Hospital at Memorial Medical Center of Long Beach, which is the scheduled site of the first commercial embryo transfer center. One way FGR officials plan to attack this problem is by setting up a computerized list of donors across the country.

By the end of this decade, the refinement of techniques should make this experimental procedure a common medical practice. What's perhaps more significant is that embryo transfer could free women from the tyranny of the biological clock. It won't be long before corporate fast trackers simply stow several embryos in the deep freeze during their fertile twenties and thaw them out when they're ready to have children—even if they're past menopause.

Scores of scientists are searching for ways of successfully freezing unfertilized eggs. For years, frozen sperm and embryos have been routinely stored, but researchers have been unable to discover why the same process destroys eggs. Once this problem has been solved, a woman will no longer be forced to select the father of her child in her twenties.

"In the far future, it may be possible to cut out a wedge of the ovary with hundreds of eggs in it," says Lucinda Veeck, a researcher at the Jones Institute for Reproductive Medicine in Norfolk, Virginia. "By maturing the immature eggs one would recover from such a wedge, and then by freezing them, the woman could become pregnant whenever she chose, simply by transferring a fertilized, mature egg into her uterus."

As we move into the twenty-first century, embryo transfers may liberate women from the chore of carrying babies. John Money, professor of medical psychology and pediatrics at Johns Hopkins medical school, speculates that *men* might carry children. There's already considerable scientific evidence that suggests male pregnancy is possible. How? There have been 24 documented cases worldwide in which women become pregnant *after* having hysterectomies. The most notable case was that of a New Zealand woman who had an embryo migrate from her abdominal cavity and attach itself to her small intestine. Nine months later, she delivered a healthy 5-pound girl by caesarean section.

If a woman without a uterus can bear a child, it's certainly feasible that embryos could be transplanted into the abdominal cavity of a man, theorized Money. The man would be primed with hormones so that his body could nurture the fetus.

In fact a male baboon was made pregnant in this fashion in a controversial experiment conducted in the mid-1960s. The baboon carried the fetus well past four months (the normal gestation period for a baboon is seven months); similar experiments have been conducted with mice and other animals. Scientists tend to agree that the best site in a male for attaching an embryo is the omentum, a fatty tissue loaded with blood vessels that hangs down in front of the intestines like a protective apron. Whether a human male can be made pregnant using this technique remains to be seen, and as of this date, no live births have ever resulted from male pregnancy, even in animal studies. On the other hand, test-tube babies were also considered to be in the realm of science fiction only a decade ago. Can the possibility of pregnant males be dismissed out of hand?

Surrogate Mothers

When Sherry King gave birth to a healthy girl, there was nothing unusual about the delivery—except that the child was Sherry's niece, not her daughter. This confusing case represents the latest wrinkle in the birthing revolution—Sherry King was a surrogate mother.

King had been impregnated by artificial insemination with her brother-in-law's sperm and, in her view, was simply providing a womb for her sister, who had had a hysterectomy when she was 21 years old. "We want infertile couples to realize that this is a real and inexpensive option for them *if* they have a loving friend or relative willing to be a surrogate mother," says King. "What was unthinkable yesterday is acceptable today."

With long waiting lists at American adoption agencies and the expense and hassle of foreign adoptions, more and more of the estimated 3 million infertile married women in the United States are now considering surrogate mothers as a not so awful last resort. Since the late 1970s, an estimated 100 to 150 babies have been borne by surrogate mothers.

Unlike King's, the vast majority of these births have been arranged through the 20 or so agencies across the country that match infertile couples with women who are willing to be surrogates—at an average cost of $22,000–$25,000, which includes a $10,000 fee for the surrogate. Agencies screen potential surrogates, who sign a contract pledging to surrender the child and to have their health habits—no smoking, drinking or taking nonprescription drugs—monitored during pregnancy.

But women's groups fear that as this practice becomes more widespread it will spawn an underclass of women who serve as breeders for the wealthy. No regulations are on the books to protect couples, surrogates, or their babies from exploitation. Nor is the law clear as to whether surrogates' fees are an illegal form of buying a child. "How can you be sure the surrogate won't take drugs or liquor during the pregnancy? What if she reneges and wants to keep the child? What if a retarded child is born?" asks Doris Jonas Freed, a New York lawyer and former chairperson of the American Bar Association's Custody Committee.

The upshot is that if something goes wrong, couples can find themselves entangled in a legal quagmire that will take years to get out of. Perhaps the final word on surrogate parenting comes from Albert Gore, Jr., who heads a House science subcommittee that has been attempting to clarify these issues. "There is something unnatural, even violent, about a procedure that takes a newborn from its mother's arms and gives it to another by virtue of a contract," says Gore. "But the touching search for children may justify a great many things that make others of us who are more fortunate uncomfortable."

Sex Selection

Sean Greig was the answer to his parents' prayers. John and Maureen Greig, who already had two daughters, decided to use a new technique of sperm selection that boosts the normal 50-50 chance of having a boy to almost 80 percent. "Some people say, 'How unnatural and bizarre,' " said Maureen. "But I wanted to do every thing humanly possible to have a boy."

This innovative method of "male order" sex selection was invented by Dr. Ronald Ericsson, a research biologist and founder of the Montana-based Gametrics Limited, which oversees the application of his technique at 46 licensed clinics worldwide. Since 1981, 79 percent of couples who've paid $250–$300 fees to conceive a boy have succeeded. Gametrics' track record for girls is about the same, and Ericsson predicts that in 20 years the method will be 90 percent successful.

Ericsson's procedure for male sex selection is based on the fact that Y-bearing (male-producing) sperm swim faster than X-bearing sperm. His technique involves filtering of sperm through layers of human serum albumin in a glass column. Approximately 80 percent of the sperm at the bottom of the column are the speedier, male-producing Y sperm, which are then used to artificially inseminate the would be mothers.

To select a girl is a little more complex. A similar process sifts out the X chromosomes, but perspective mothers must also take clomid, a fertility drug that stimulates ovulation and tilts the odds in favor of conceiving a female.

On the immediate horizon, fertility researchers are working on over-the-counter sex selection kits that could be used by couples in the privacy of their bedrooms. The scientific community, however, has been reluctant to sanction sex selection. The potential consequences of this procedure have ignited a storm of controversy. Once this practice is widespread, "you have to be concerned about the future of all women," says Roberta Steinbacher, a psychologist at Cleveland State University. "There's no question that there exists a universal preference for sons," she adds, particularly in Third World countries where infanticide of female babies is common.

Many fear sex selection would cement the second-class status of women. Others think a shortage of marriageable females would result, which could increase prostitution and homosexuality. Some maintain that picking the sex of offspring reduces children to little more than commodities. And a few worry that after a few generations, this technique could significantly alter—and possibly harm—the genetic pool.

Advocates point out that sex selection could be a potent weapon in the war against the more than 200 sex-linked genetic disorders that severely debilitate or kill thousands of infants annually. Parents with a family history of such male diseases as hemophilia or Duchenne's muscular dystrophy could opt to have only female children.

One of Ericsson's dreams is to separate sperm that may carry abnormalities—Down's syndrome, multiple sclerosis, Tay-Sachs disease, or other genetic problems. "Instead of using the whole damn shootin' match, let's figure out a method to take only the sperm we want," says Ericsson. "The rest we're going to pour down the sink. I don't think the egg ought to have to accept every blind date, should she?"

Cloning

In the film *Starman*, the alien hero, who hails from a civilization that is 100,000 years more advanced than Earth's, transforms himself into a clone of a man by using a strand of the man's hair. Clearly, the technology necessary to accomplish such a feat is perhaps hundreds of generations away, but scientists have taken the first steps toward cloning humans.

Of course, the idea of cloning humans conjures up chilling visions of mad scientists churning out armies of little Hitlers, but ever since the 1978 publication of *In His Image: The Cloning of a Man*, by David Rorvik, the possibility of human cloning has become the subject of intense scientific debate, even though the controversial book eventually turned out to be a hoax.

"There is nothing to suggest any particular difficulty about accomplishing this [cloning] in mammals or man," says Joshua Lederberg, a Nobel-Prize-winning geneticist, "though it will rightly be admired as a technical tour de force when it is first accomplished."

The first successful cloning of a mammal, in this case a mouse, was done in 1981 by Drs. Karl Illmensee, of the University of Geneva, Switzerland, and Peter Hoppe, of the Jackson Laboratory in Bar Harbor, Maine. They used a variant of a technique, known as nuclear transplantation, which has been used for years to clone frogs, toads, fruit flies, and salamanders.

During this procedure the nucleus from a cell of a mice embryo is removed and transferred to another embryo whose nucleus was also removed. The altered embryo is implanted in the womb of a surrogate, who gives birth to several genetically identical mice. There has been some scientific dispute as to whether these offspring were actually clones, and both Illmensee and Hoppe readily concede that it will be many years before this method can produce a human clone.

But it is "twinning," which is another type of cloning, that could prove to be a useful medical tool. The process that spawns identical twins, a process in which a human embryo divides in half in the uterus, is an example of a very rudimentary form of twinning. It has long been used in animal husbandry, where the embryos of prized cattle or racehorses are split and transplanted into surrogates.

Although debates over cloning rage, human embryos may someday be routinely altered in the womb, as Aldous Huxley envisioned in *Brave New World*. The extra embryo could be frozen and thawed out later to breed genetically matched organs and tissues. This technique could end the problem of organ rejection and save countless lives.

Neonatology

Roni Handler went into labor with her first child 3 months before she was due. She gave birth to a boy, but his next 12 weeks of life were punctuated by several crises.

Clinging to life in an intensive care nursery at Children's Hospital National Medical Center in Washington, D.C., the infant suffered from many of the complications that afflict the 300,000 babies born prematurely in the United States each year: hyaline membrane disease, in which clogged lung passages deprived the baby of oxygen; severe intestinal problems; and lowered breathing and heart rates.

Handler's son survived thanks to a new subspecialty of pediatrics that deals with the critical first 28 days of life: neonatology. The medical progress in this field, which has been largely responsible for the 37 percent decline in U.S. infant mortality rate since 1970, has made it possible for the vast majority of premature infants who couldn't have survived a decade ago to now lead relatively normal lives.

Until the late 1960s, little progress has been made in keeping such babies alive. Their lungs—the last organ to develop in the womb—couldn't function and they died. The development of a ventilating machine that would keep a tiny newborn's lungs inflated led to a dramatic drop in the number of infants who died from respiratory distress syndrome.

More recently, researchers have zeroed in on the underlying cause of this syndrome. Studies on infants who died from respiratory failure revealed that the infants lacked surfactant, a substance that lubricates the lung's air sacs so they can expand and contract easily. Scientists are developing a synthetic surfactant.

For even smaller "preemies," the development of a procedure called *extracorporeal membrane oxygenation* (*ECMO*), which uses special machines to support hearts and lungs, has more than tripled the survival rates for tiny newborns who couldn't use conventional respirators. As these devices are refined, physicians speculate that they will save more preemies as young as 16 weeks old.

Research teams are making excellent progress in treatments for brain hemmorhages, which can be lethal and are the prime cause of mental retardation and cerebral palsy. Moreover, the FDA recently approved the use of *Indocin I.V.*, a drug that effectively controls ductus arteriosus, a circulatory condition that afflicts more than 17,000 infants annually and can cause heart failure.

Probably the biggest advance in neonatology has been the development of the nation's 600 intensive care nurseries with state of the art equipment that is designed to simulate the critical functions of the womb. There, fragile infants are connected to probes and tubes, and surrounded by monitors that flash heartbeats and vital signs around the clock.

These impressive advances have not come without hidden costs. Half of the babies born weighing less than 1,000 grams born in the U.S. now survive. But each year at least 3,000 of these babies are sentenced to a life with severe handicaps: mental retardation, epilepsy, cerebral palsy, and blindness. This figure has more than doubled in the past 20 years, and another 4,000 babies suffer from moderate impairments. Understandably, many parents are less than ecstatic about the prospect of their child's illness, its cost, and damage done to marriage and family life. Perhaps the thorniest question of all concerns abortion. Some hospitals are saving preemies in one wing while aborting fetuses that are only a few weeks younger in another. As Supreme Court Justice Sandra Day O'Connor recently noted, our abortion laws are on "a collison course" with the steady march of technology.

Fetal Surgery

When Ali Thomson was a 7-month-old fetus, a catheter was inserted into her chest by a team of specialists at St. Luke's Regional Medical Center in Boise, Idaho. The doctors drained a cyst that had developed on the fetus. The day after Ali's birth by caesarean section, the cyst was removed, and 11 days later, the healthy infant was discharged from the hospital.

Fetal—or in utero—surgery remains mostly experimental, but it offers the first real hope for the more than 30,000 infants that are born each year with serious defects. Research is proceeding at an explosive pace thanks to sophisticated *ultrasound* techniques that can be used in a doctor's office. (The ultrasound device bounces high-frequency sound waves off the fetus, and the returning waves provide a detailed picture of the inside of the womb. It's now possible with ultrasound to detect a whole array of ailments and defects in utero.

Armed with this knowledge, physicians have been laying groundwork towards transforming highly risky fetal surgical procedures into common medical practices. These include inserting a catheter into the bladder of a fetus to drain a urine buildup that endangered the lungs and kidney; inserting a shunt to drain the skull of a fetus with hydrocephalus (the buildup of fluid in the brain, which can cause severe brain damage and mental retardation); and partially removing a 5-month-old fetus from the womb to correct a kidney defect.

"I became interested in this field because it got to be too frustrating dealing with newborns with devastating birth defects," says Dr. Michael Harrison, a member of the University of California at San Francisco research team that performed the first successful surgery on a fetus outside the womb, "defects that you knew could be prevented if you could operate on the fetus."

Several recent experiments on lab animals have helped surgeons expand the repertoire of procedures for human fetal surgery. Surgery was performed on a rat fetus to correct malformations in the brain and spinal cord. Working with rhesus monkey fetuses suffering from limb malformations, surgeons discovered that a limb could be removed as late as the beginning of the second trimester, and often a normal limb would develop in its place.

Medical researchers are also close to overcoming the major hurdles to removal of fetuses from the womb for operations. Surgical procedures could damage the fetus and trigger a spontaneous abortion, but new drugs that halt premature labor have been found. What's more, scientists have discovered in experiments with animals that when the fetus is asleep, it is unharmed by surgery.

Physicians are confident that congenital heart defects, neural tube defects, and numerous neurological disorders could be corrected in utero. By the end of this century, machines may routinely scan embryos for possible genetic or physiological defects. It may be possible, even within the first 6 weeks of life, to remove the embryo, repair it, and then return it to the womb for a normal gestation.

Alternative Birthing Techniques

When Jane Textor arrived at her sister's home to watch her give birth, she had no idea the event would change her life. "It was a beautiful, energizing experience," Jane recalled. "I decided right then that I wanted to have a home birth." Indeed, Jane's two children were born at home in what she euphorically characterized as celebrations.

Unhappy with the strict rules and impersonal atmosphere of the traditional hospital maternity wards, an increasing number of expectant mothers are choosing home births, along with a whole array of other alternative birthing methods. They range from midwives, and natural birthing centers, to the use of birthing chairs or even delivering infants while immersed in water.

This movement is fueled by a growing desire among prospective parents to find a more personal way to give birth, and to share that experience in an intimate setting with family members. Also, alternative birthing is less costly. For example, fees for midwife-assisted births range from $500 to $1000, including lab tests, follow-up visits, and hospital or clinic costs. In contrast, physicians charge $1000 to $2000 for their services alone.

Many suspect that medical intervention—IVs, forceps, internal fetal monitors, caesarean sections—can be dangerous and unnecessary. "Many procedures that doctors use are merely time savers, such as speeding up labors chemically and performing caesareans," says Dr. Don Creeyy, clinical assistant professor of obstetrics and gynecology at Stanford University School of Medicine.

Ironically, until the 1940s giving birth at home was the norm, but today almost 97 percent of children are delivered in hospitals. Why? Physicians believed that the more sterile, controlled conditions in a hospital would reduce the number of deaths among newborns and mothers. There's no question that mortality rates have declined, but there's some debate as to whether this is directly attributable to hospital births.

There are, of course, certain high risk groups who aren't good candidates for home births, such as women under 16 or over 40 years old, those who are having their first baby, or women in poor health. But the available data indicates the vast majority of women can give birth safely at home.

A 1980 North Carolina survey found that over a 3-year period the neonatal mortality rate of planned home deliveries was 4 per 1,000 with a midwife present versus 12 per 1,000 in hospitals. But home birth advocates most frequently cite statistics from the Netherlands, which has the highest percentage of home births of any industrialized country. About 1,000 trained obstetric specialists, or midwives, perform most deliveries. In 1982, the Netherlands had the seventh lowest infant mortality rates of all countries measured, while the U.S. placed a distant seventeenth.

Despite these impressive statistics, the American medical fraternity has consistently discouraged home births and midwifery. Laws governing the practice of midwifery are vague in some states, virtually nonexistent in others, while a few states have taken steps to ban the practice. What's not in dispute, however, is that this age-old profession is in the midst of a renaissance.

There are now almost 2,400 certified nurse midwives (CNMs) in this country. CNMs who undergo extensive training in nursing and obstetrics, and handle about 1 percent of all births in the United States. There are also at least 4,000 of the more controversial "lay" midwives, unlicensed practitioners who get their education on the job. The tremendous demand for midwives has been spurred by their reputation for competent, personal, and compassionate care.

"Relinquishing the responsibility for your birth to a doctor is a cultural thing in this country," explained Genna Withrow, a Gainesville, Florida, midwife who's helped bring over 300 children into the world. "But with a midwife, you can be certain that there will be very little interference, such as the routine rupture of membranes, to complicate the birth process, and that the ultimate control and responsibility will belong where they should—with the parents."

There is another place for parents who are reluctant to have their child delivered at home in the event of complications, yet are uncomfortable in the rigid confines of a hospital: the alternative birthing center. Since 1975, when the first birthing center opened its doors in New York City, these centers have become quite popular, and there are now more than 115 of them nationwide.

Some centers use birthing chairs, which permit mothers to sit in an upright position, and improve the efficiency and comfort of the mother during labor. Another method these centers may use is underwater birthing. The baby is delivered in a tub filled with water heated to 101 degrees Fahrenheit to simulate the womb; this method, which advocates say, spares the child the trauma of a conventional birth.

In the future, changing attitudes should quell the debate about alternative birthing. "It is not the place of birth but the management of birth that makes the difference," says Tonya Brooks, founder of the Association for Childbirth at Home International (ACHI). "I believe our society is on the verge of a big decision, and we can go either way: Toward greater intervening technology, where a good outcome simply means an alive baby and mother, or a combination of the best of technology with the traditional values of human caring and concern."

Hundreds of dedicated scientists around the globe continue to study the intricate mechanisms that govern human reproduction with the aim of helping millions of infertile couples. Other researchers are racing to devise more effective, safer, and reliable methods of correcting birth defects in the womb. Researchers are confident that infertility will be conquered, ending the heartbreak of couples who want to have children, and that scores of genetic disorders will be eradicated as new techniques are perfected.

Startling advances in reproductive technology have already transformed our traditional notions of birth and parenthood, and this trend should accelerate as we move into the twenty-first century.

New technology will liberate women from the confines of their biological deadlines, freeing them from making choices between family and career. Postponing childbearing to their forties and even fifties will become commonplace. As more women pursue careers, they will share parenting responsibilities with men more often. This, coupled with the growing popularity of alternative methods of birthing and refinements of techniques that could make male pregnancy possible, means that men will become much more intimately involved with childbearing.

In the distant future, sex may only be for pleasure, not procreation. Prospective parents would simply drop their eggs and semen off at reproductive centers, list any preferences for gender, personality traits, or physical attributes, and pick up a healthy baby 9 months later. Embryos will be incubated in carefully monitored artificial wombs, where developing fetuses will be routinely scanned for any impairments, which, of course, are corrected immediately. And infertility, genetic defects, and unwanted children will be relegated to the dustbin of history.

Timeline

1987 to 1990
- In vitro fertilization and embryo transfer clinics open in every major city.
- Congress lifts ban on human embryo research.
- Technique developed to freeze eggs.
- Scientists can identify less viable embryos.

1991 to 2000
- 55-year-old woman gives birth to her biological child from an embryo frozen for 12 years.
- Egg banks open across the country.
- FDA approves over-the-counter sex selection kits.
- Sperm successfully injected directly into eggs, making in vitro fertilization virtually 100 percent reliable.
- Fifty percent of all U.S. births now assisted by nurse-midwives.

2001 to 2010
- Full-service reproductive centers open across the country.
- First male pregnancy.
- FDA approves over-the-counter device that induces daily ovulation.
- First successful surgery to correct a genetic defect in the womb.
- Women routinely undergo ovarian sections to store hundreds of eggs.

2011 to 2030
- Government approves limited human cloning research.
- Artificial womb developed.
- First child to be conceived and gestated outside of the human body is born.
- Birth defects conquered.
- Transplant organs no longer needed from donors—clone breeding farms now provide genetically matched organs.

Access Guide

Infertility

The American Fertility Society
2131 Magnolia Avenue, Suite 201
Birmingham, AL 35256
(205) 251-9764

Founded in 1944, the Society currently has 9,500 members, who are medical professionals in the field of obstetrics and gynecology. Resource lists are maintained to help direct the patient to the most appropriate source of help, which includes referrals to members in various parts of the world as well as alternative programs to aid in conception.

RESOLVE, Inc.
P.O. Box 474
Belmont, MA 02178
(617) 484-2424

Founded in 1973, this national nonprofit agency serves as a counselling, referral, and support system for infertile couples and offers education and assistance to associated professionals. RESOLVE has chapters in over 40 cities around the country; the chapters sponsor support groups and educational programs.

In Vitro Fertilization

The following is a list of the major centers around the country which are actively engaged in in vitro fertilization. However, costs and success rates vary greatly. Contact the American Fertility Society to find out your local clinic's record and it they meet standards set by the Society.

University of Alabama-
  Birmingham Medical Center
Laboratory for IVF-ET
547 Old Hillman Buiding,
  University Station
Birmingham, AL 35294
(205) 934-5631

Arizona Center for Fertility Studies
IVF-ET Program
4614 East Shea Boulevard D-260
Phoenix, AZ 85028
(602) 996-7896

Alta Bates Hospital
IVF Program
3001 Colby Street
Berkeley, CA 94705
(415) 540-1416

Central California IVF Program
Fresno Community Hospital
P.O. Box 1232
Fresno, CA 93715
(209) 439-1914

University of California at Los
  Angeles School of Medicine
Department of Ob/Gyn: IVF
  Program
Los Angeles, CA 90024
(213) 825-7755

University of Southern California
  School of Medicine
IVF-Embryo Replacement Program
Hospital of the Good Samaritan
637 South Lucas Avenue
Los Angeles, CA 90017
(213) 226-3421

University of California at San
  Francisco
IVF Program
Department of Ob/Gyn and
  Reproductive Sciences
Room M 1480
San Francisco, CA 94143
(415) 666-1824

University of Colorado Health
  Sciences Center
IVF Program
4200 East 9th Avenue, Box B198
Denver, CO 80262
(303) 394-8365

Mount Sinai Hospital
Department of Ob/Gyn
Division of Reproductive
  Endocrinology and Infertility
675 Hartford Avenue
Hartford, CT 06112
(203) 242-6201

Yale University Medical School
Department of Ob/Gyn: IVF
  Program
333 Cedar Street
New Haven, CT 06510
(203) 785-4019

Geroge Washington University
  Medical Center
Department of Ob/Gyn: IVF
  Program
901 23rd Street Northwest
Washington, D.C. 20037
(202) 676-4614

Memorial Medical Center of
  Jacksonville
IVF Program
3343 University Boulevard South
Jacksonville, FL 32216
(904) 391-1149

University of Miami
Department of Ob/Gyn: D-5
P.O. Box 016960
Miami, FL 33101
(305) 547-5818

Atlanta Center for Fertility and
  Endocrinology
Northside Hospital
5675 Peachtree-Dunwoody Road
  Northeast
Atlanta, GA 30342
(404) 256-8000

Medical College at Georgia
Humana Hospital-IVF Section
Augusta, GA 30912

Pacific In Vitro Fertilization
Institute
Kapiolani Women's and Children's
Hospital
1319 Punahou Street Suite 1040
Honolulu, HI 96826
(808) 945-2226

Michael Reese-University of
Chicago
IVR-ET Program
31st Street at Lake Shore Drive
Chicago, IL 60616
(312) 791-4000

Mount Sinai Hospital Medical
Center
Department of Ob/Gyn: IVF
Program
California Avenue at 15th Street
Chicago, IL 60608
(312) 650-6727

Rush Medical College
IVF Program
600 South Paulina Street
Chicago, IL 60616
(312) 942-6609

Indiana University Medical Center
Department of Ob/Gyn:
Reproductive Endocrinology
926 West Michigan Street, N 262
Indianapolis, IN 46223
(317) 264-4057

Kansas University Gynecological
and Obstetrical Foundation
University of Kansas
College of Health Sciences
39th and Rainbow Boulevard
Kansas City, KS 66103
(913) 588-6246

Norton Hospital
IVF Program
601 South Floyd Street, Room 304
Louisville, KY 40202
(502) 562-8154

Tulane Fertility Program
IVF Program
1415 Tulane Avenue
New Orleans, LA 70112
(504) 588-2341

Baltimore IVF Program
2435 W. Belvedere Avenue, No. 41
Baltimore, MD 21215
(301) 542-5115

Greater Baltimore Medical Center
IVF Program
6701 North Charles Street
Baltimore, MD 21204
(301) 828-2484

The Johns Hopkins Hospital
IVF Program
600 North Wolfe Street
Baltimore, MD 21205
(301) 955-8759

Brigham and Women's Hospital
IVF Program
75 Francis Street
Boston, MA 02115
(617) 732-4239

In Vitro Fertilization Center of
Boston
Boston University Medical Center
75 East Newton Street
Boston, MA 02115
(617) 247-5928

Blodgett Memorial Medical Center
IVF Program
1900 Wealthy Street Southwest
Suite 330
Grand Rapids, MI 49506
(616) 774-0700

Hutzel Hospital
Wayne State University
IVF Program
4707 St. Antoine
Detroit, MI 48201
(313) 494-7547

William Beaumont Hospital
IVF Program
3601 West 13 Mile Road
Royal Oak, MI 48072
(313) 288-2380

University of Minnesota VIP
  Program
Department of Ob/Gyn
Mayo Memorial Building, Box 395
420 Delaware Street Southeast
Minneapolis, MN 55455
(612) 373-8852

Mayo Clinic
Department of Reproductive
  Endocrinology and Infertility
200 First Street Southwest
Rochester, MN 55905
(507) 284-3188

University of Mississippi Medical
  Center
IVF Program
Department of Ob/Gyn
Jackson, MS 39216
(601) 987-4662

Missouri Baptist Hospital
IVF Program Room 301
3015 North Ballas Road
St. Louis, MO 63131
(314) 432-1212

UMD: Rutgers Medical School
Department of Ob/Gyn: IVF
  Program
Academic Health Science Center,
  CN19
New Brunswick, NJ 08903
(201) 937-7635

Childrens Hospital of Buffalo
IVF-ET Program
140 Hodge Avenue
Buffalo, NY 14222
(716) 878-7232

Cornell University Medical College
IVF Program
515 East 71st Street 2nd Floor
New York, NY 10021
(212) 472-4693

Mount Sinai Medical Center
IVF Program
One Gustave Levy Place
Annenberg 20-60
New York, NY 10029
(212) 650-5927

North Shore University Hospital
IVF Program
300 Community Drive
Manhasset, NY 11030
(516) 562-4470

Columbia-Presbyterian Medical
  Center
IVF-ET Program
622 West 168th Street
New York, NY 10032
(212) 694-8013

Norrh Carolina Memorial Hospital
IVF Program
Chapel Hill, NC 27514
(919) 966-5438

Duke University Medical Center
Dept. of Ob/Gyn: IVF Program
Durham, NC 27710
(919) 684-5327

Akron City Hospital
IVF-ET Program
525 East Market Street
Akron, OH 44309
(216) 375-3585

Jewish Hospital of Cincinnati
IVF Program
3120 Burnet Avenue Suite 204
Cincinnati, OH 45229
(513) 221-3062

University of Cincinnati Medical
   Center
IVF Program
Department of Ob/Gyn
231 Bethesda Avenue
Cincinnati, OH 45267
(513) 872-6368

Cleveland Clinic Foundation
IVF Program
2105 Adelbert Road
Cleveland, OH 44106
(216) 844-1514

Miami Valley Hospital
IVF Program
1 Wyoming Street
Dayton, OH 45409
(513) 223-6192

Hillcrest Infertility Center
1145 South Utica No. 1209
Tulsa, OK 74104
(918) 584-2870

Albert Einstein Medical Center
Department of Ob/Gyn
York and Tabor Roads
Philadelphia, PA 19141
(215) 456-7990

Hospital of the University of
   Pennsylvania
Department of Ob/Gyn: IVF
   Program
3400 Spruce Street Suite 106
Philadelphia, PA 19104
(215) 662-2981

The Pennsylvania Hospital
IVF-ET Program
Eighth and Spruce Streets
Philadelphia, PA 19107
(215) 829-5095

Magee-Women's Hospital
IVF Program
Forbes Avenue and Halket Street
Pittsburgh, PA 15213
(412) 647-4000

Medical University of South
   Carolina
IVF Program
171 Ashley Avenue
Charleston, SC 29425
(803) 792-2861

Vanderbilt University
IVF Program
D3200 Medical Center North
Nashville, TN 37232
(615) 322-6576

St. David's Community Hospital
IVF-ET Program
P.O. Box 4039
919 East 32nd Street
Austin, TX 78765
(512) 397-4107

The University of Texas/
   Southwestern Medical School
IVF Program
5323 Harry Hines Boulevard
Dallas, TX 75230
(214) 688-2784

University of Texas Medical
   Branch
IVF Prgram
Galveston, TX 77550
(409) 761-3985

Baylor College of Medicine
IVF Program
1 Baylor Plaza
Houston, TX 77030
(713) 797-0322

Texas Woman's Hospital
IVF Program
7600 Fannin
Houston, TX 77054
(713) 795-7257

Genetics and IVF Institute
Fairfax Hospital
3020 Javier Road
Fairfax, VA 22031
(703) 658-7355

Eastern Virginia Medical School
Jones Institute for Reproductive
  Medicine
825 Fairfas Avenue 6th Floor
Hoffheimer Hall
Norfolk, VA 23507
(804) 446-8935

University of Washington
Department of Ob/Gyn: IVF
  Program
RH-20
Seattle, WA 98195
(206) 543-8483

University of Wisconsin Clinics
IVF Program
600 Highland Avenue H4/630
  CSC
Madison, WI 53792
(608) 263-1217

Waukesha Memorial Hospital
IVF Program
725 American Avenue
Waukesha, WI 53186
(414) 544-2722

Sex Selection

There are close to 40 licensed Gametrics Limited clinics in the United States. Contact either one of the following for the name of the center in your area.

Gametrics Limited
Colony (Wyoming) Route
Alzada, MT 59311
(307) 878 4484

Gametrics Limited
324 South Third Street
Las Vegas, NV 89101
(702) 384-1049

Alternative Birthing Methods

American College of Nurse-Midwives
1522 K Street Northwest, Suite 1120
Washington, D.C. 20005
(202) 347-5445

Founded in 1955, with 2,000 members who have completed a program of study and clinical experience in recognized midwifery schools. Publishes a membership directory and registry of services and practices.

Association for Childbirth at Home, International
P.O. Box 39498
Los Angeles CA 90039
(213) 667-0839

Founded in 1972 with 10,000 members currently nationwide, this organization offers a variety of educational seminars, as well as resource and referral services.

Center for Humane Options in Childbirth Experience (CHOICE)
2862 Johnstown Road
Columbus, OH 43219
(614) 476-1474

Founded in 1977 with 1,200 members currently nationwide. Services include medical referrals, childbirth education classes, and supplementary prenatal care.

Childbirth Education Foundation (CEF)
P.O. Box 37
Apalachin, NY 13732
(607) 625-4133

Founded in 1972, with 5,200 members nationwide. Promotes home births, birthing centers, certified nurse-midwife pregnancy management and delivery. Provides referrals, educational material, and statistical information to childbirth educators and childcare organizations.

The Cybele Society
414 Peyton Building
Spokane, WA 99201
(509) 838-2332

Founded in 1988, this organization acts as a national clearinghouse for information on family-centered maternity care.

International Association of Parents and Professionals for Safe
  Alternatives in Childbirth (IAPSAC)
P.O. Box 428
Marble Hill, MO 63764
(324) 238-2010

This organization promotes education concerning the principles of natural childbirth; acts as a forum to facilitate communication and cooperation among parents, medical professionals, and childbirth educators; and assists in the establishment of maternity and childbearing centers.

National Association of Childbearing Centers (NACC)
Route 1 Box 1
Perkiomenville, PA 18074

Founded in 1883, this organization acts as a national information service on freestanding birth centers for state health departments, insurance companies, physicians, certified nurse-midwives, and families.

Embryo Transfer

Fertility and Genetics Research, Inc. (FGR)
135 South LaSalle, Suite 616
Chicago, IL 60603
(312) 236-5492

Plans are underway to franchise embryo transfer centers across the country. Contact FGR for the names of clinics in your area.

6

The Biochemistry of Desire

Today we have a social climate in which we can indulge almost any and all of our sexual fantasies—if we are willing and able. Yet in one of history's typically ironic turns, more than 10 million men suffer from chronic impotency (cannot sustain an erection adequate for intercourse), and much of the nation is plagued with yet another malady, one which *Time* magazine ranks as the chief sexual problem of our time: lack of desire. In this chapter, we'll address both of those concerns: desire and performance.

What happens biochemically when one person becomes attracted to another? It may all begin with sex scents called pheromones that initiate attraction, even across a crowded room. Then a series of neurochemical reactions occurs within the body. Messengers of desire race along neural pathways—sometimes at a speed of nearly 100 feet per second—to a tiny part of the brain called the hypothalamus. The hypothalamus collects these messages and, provided the thinking part of the brain gives the okay, orchestrates the release of sex hormones from the pituitary and sex glands. Positive sex signals then move back down the neural pathways from the brain, prompting excitement in the sex organs.

For centuries human beings have searched for the ultimate aphrodisiac to artificially induce sexual desire. Not content with the divine ability to have sex wherever and whenever we pleased—all other mammals must await the fleeting female estrus periods to mate—humans have concocted innumerable faunal and floral "love potions" to increase their sexual appetites. From rhinoceros horn, bees' wings, camel's hump fat, and reindeer genitals to ginseng root, sarsaparilla, and pego palo leaves, we haven't missed a trick. Many would-be Casanovas have even claimed that chocolate has aphrodisiac powers, and in fact the eighteenth century superlover himself craved hot cocoa.

But some psychiatrists maintain that these substances, as well as most street drugs—including marijuana, cocaine, and LSD—engender responses too subjective and inconstant for them to be considered true aphrodisiacs.

Perhaps the most heralded of all aphrodisiacs is Spanish fly. Rubbed on the genitals, it causes rapid erection, lubrication, and orgasm. But this dried green beetle is not an aphrodisiac, but an irritant of the mucous membrane of the urethra that prompts a painful and unnatural reaction. In 1984, a scientific panel of the FDA dismissed Spanish fly and a host of other folk remedies including those listed above as giving "no evidence of aphrodisiac action." The panel warned manufacturers against the use of hormones, such as testosterone, in oral drugs, claiming such hormones are not safe for use except under the supervision of a physician. ("Androgen" and "estrogen" are generic terms for male and female sex hormones respectively. Testosterone is an androgen, while progesterone and estradiol are estrogens.)

Injections of sex hormones for inhibited sexual desire are still experimental. It is clear that androgens are necessary for normal sexual desire in both males and females, and for ejaculation. But, initial studies have shown that increasing the level of these hormones in the body has no behavioral effect. Also injections of androgens only last a short period of time. As reported on ABC's 20-20, a shot of testosterone will elicit an immediate sexual response, but the effects will last only two or three hours. And a patient can receive only 10 shots per month.

There *is* help at hand for those who find their sexual appetites waning. A large corps of determined neurologists, research psychiatrists, physiologists, sexologists, pharmacologists, and urologists are working on new ways to treat low sexual desire. Pretty soon, we may be able to set our own "sexostat." Researchers are also taking a closer look at impotence and its causes and cures.

African Aphrodisiac

African tribes have been using it for centuries to reduce high fever. But the drug *yohimbine* might be just the medicine to cause sexual fervor. Originally extracted from the sap of the tropical tree *Coryanthe yohimbe*, the drug is now available by prescription. In a 2-year study funded by the National Institutes of Health, physiologists at Stanford University Medical School found that sexually active male rats injected with yohimbine mounted females up to 45 times in 15 minutes—almost twice as often as they normally would. Half of the impotent and virgin rats injected with the drug copulated. Although the female rats were given sex hormones to make them more receptive to the males, researchers have yet to quantify female reactions to yohimbine. The reason yohimbine—known on the street as "yo-yo"—works is still a mystery. But scientists believe the drug stimulates the flow of norepinephrine, a natural chemical in the brain that may control sex drive. Will yohimbine produce sex-crazed humans? Willing volunteers are now being tested, but "please, please, please make it clear that we don't need any more volunteers for this study," says Dr. Julian Davidson, professor of physiology at Stanford. "We have more than we can handle right now."

Stud Drug

The remedy for feeling undersexed may be yet another drug, one called *naltrexone*. Naltrexone is an oral version of naloxone, a drug used to curb heroin addiction. In a series of experiments conducted by David Margules of Temple University in Philadelphia, rats injected with naloxone, like those treated with yohimbine, copulated continually. Apparently naloxone blocks the actions of opioid peptides, natural hormones that latch onto receptor molecules in the sperm duct and halt ejaculation.

A recent study of the effects of naloxone on female orgasm showed that while the drug increased sexual pleasure dramatically for some women, it diminished it for others. Conducted at the South African Brain Research Institute by Drs. Mark Gillman and Frederick Lichtigfeld, the study revealed (as have many other studies) that female sexuality seems to be far more complicated than male sexuality.

Four women ranging in age from 22 to 39 were given small doses (2 milligrams or less) of either naloxone or water just prior to orgasm. The women weren't told which of the two liquids they were receiving. One subject reported that the orgasms achieved after doses of naloxone were "the best she could remember." In two subjects, high doses (as much as 4 milligrams) inhibited sexual desire, while low doses (as little as 0.4 milligrams) enhanced it. The fourth subject's desire was inhibited regardless of the dosage. None felt any change with doses of water.

Why naloxone excites some women and not others is not known. But women shouldn't lose hope: In another study, Gillman and Lichtigfeld found that nitrous oxide, commonly known as "laughing gas," heightened sexual desire in all seven of the women tested. The researchers believe that nitrous oxide may trigger the release of the body's natural opiates.

Sexy Hormones

Hormonal effects in women sometimes may be unpredictable, but hormones certainly do affect female sexual function. In general, female hormones—with the exception of progesterone—increase sexual desire.

It's a bit surprising, however, that androgens, the male hormones produced in varying amounts by women's ovaries and adrenal glands, appear to make women randy. Researchers at the University of Pennsylvania and the Marriage Council of Philadelphia discovered that women with high androgen levels make love more often and enjoy it more. Dr. Harold Persky and his associates at Penn analyzed blood samples from 11 young married women and 19 postmenopausal women. The younger women made love more often and enjoyed more overall gratification than the postmenopausal women, probably because testosterone production in the ovaries slows down after menopause, says Persky.

Will women with waning sexual desire feel desire reawaken with regular doses of androgens? "That's the big question," Persky says. "How hormones influence sexuality remains one of the gray areas of science." But studies now in progress may soon provide an answer.

Ultimate Aphrodisiac?

Our own bodies may contain the ultimate aphrodisiac. It is a chemical released by the hypothalamus called luteinizing hormone-releasing hormone, (LHRH). LHRH stimulates the release of a particular sex hormone from the pituitary glands of both men and women; but it may do more than that. In rats, LHRH seems to function as a sex stimulant even when the rodents' sex glands have been removed.

Dr. Robert Moss, a professor of physiology and neurology at the University of Texas Health Science Center in Dallas, injected rats missing their ovaries and pituitary glands with ten-billionths of a gram of LHRH and a touch of estrogen as primer. The rats engaged in sexual activity for up to 8 hours.

In animals, LHRH seems to be responsible for activating the brain during ovulation, so that mating will occur. In humans, LHRH affects the brain at all times, irrespective of ovulation.

Why the difference? The work of anthropologist Helen Fisher, formerly associate researcher with the American Museum of Natural History, may provide a clue. According to Fisher, in our transformation from four-legged creatures to two-legged creatures, the female's birth canal shrank considerably. As a result, smaller and weaker babies were born. To keep such weaklings (and themselves) alive, women needed help. So females began to lure men into domesticity with frequent offers of sex.

To do this, Moss contends, women developed brains directly affected by LHRH (and possibly other hormones), so that they would not have to wait for the brief estrus period to mate. Hence, evolution did away with the estrus cycle in humans so that, unlike all other mammals, we can have sex whenever and wherever we please. (Well, almost.) Direct hormonal stimulation of the brain is also the reason why women with their ovaries removed will still feel as sexy as those with their sex glands intact, says Moss.

Will shots of LHRH affect humans as dramatically as they do the rats? Moss administered LHRH to 50 men with psychological (as opposed to physical) impotence. About 60 percent found some improvement in sexual function, though the intensity and duration of effect varied dramatically.

More studies are in order, but an LHRH pill could be in stores by the end of the decade.

Neurosexuality

Other chemical messengers, or neurotransmitters, not directly involved with hormone release, may play a large role in regulating sexual desire. Two of these, *dopamine* and *serotonin*, are gaining a lot of attention.

Dopamine, a neurotransmitter necessary for psychomotor activities, falls to pathologically low levels in victims of Parkinson's disease. When elderly patients with the disease were treated with the drug *L-dopa*, a chemical forerunner of dopamine, they began to make bold sexual advances towards their nurse. After further tests, doctors found that the drug heightened sexual desire in about half the men and one in five of the women.

Dopamine affects men and women differently, according to neuropsychologist James Prescott of the Institute of Humanistic Science in West Bethesda, Maryland. Men depend more on dopamine because sex for them is a reflex, a psychomotor activity. When dopamine levels drop in Parkinson's disease, sex is curtailed in men, but not in women. Researchers believe that sexual activity in women is directed through different neural pathways. Another neurotransmitter, serotonin, seems to inhibit sexual desire. Rats treated with *(PCPA) parachlorophenylalanine*, a serotonin reducer, showed a dramatic increase in sexual activity. PCPA seems to have some unpleasant side effects on humans—including vertigo, headaches, and mental dullness—but researchers are in the process of developing other serotonin reducers.

Neuroscientists and pharmacologists are working together to produce safe and inexpensive drugs to regulate the actions of these and other neurotransmitters.

Aroma Arousal

Pheromones, odiferous substances long known to be sex attractants in insects and lower mammals, may draw humans together. The scent chemical androstenone, which is more prevalent in men than in women, is reputed to attract women. A synthetic form of this, called *alpha androstenol*, which smells in concentrated form like sandalwood, may do just that. When the Royal Shakespeare Company in London doused certain theater seats with the substance, women gravitated to those seats. Both men and women dallied longer in phone booths sprayed with alpha androstenol.

Perfume manufacturers were not long in taking advantage of these studies. In 1981, Jovan introduced Andron, a fragrance available for both men and women that contains a tiny amount of the substance. Alpha androstenol costs an astronomical $44,000 per pound, but according to Jovan's president, "as little as 6 parts per million produces a response." Andron sold moderately well, and no one really knows whether fragrances with alpha androstenol work any better than musk, civet, and other fragrances.

Laboratory studies have uncovered other possible human pheromones called *copulins*. Copulins are estrogen-dependent (only found where estrogen is found) fatty acids found in the vaginal secretions of some women. These secretions are chemically similar to those of an ovulating female rhesus monkey. In one study, smears from a human vagina applied to the vagina of a female monkey attracted male monkeys. In another study, University of North Carolina researchers found that both males and females engaged in sex more often when they smelled a synthetic vaginal pheromone. A male synthetic pheromone would elicit a similar response, the scientists said.

It's also known that young animals who are exposed to odors from the opposite sex reach puberty more quickly than those who don't have that exposure. The animals are being primed for reproduction. Researchers are investigating whether or not the same phenomenon occurs in humans.

The G-Spot

Like the existence of human pheromones, the G-spot, an alleged female pleasure point found along the anterior (front) vaginal wall, has not been proven or disproven. First described in 1944 as "a zone of erogenous feeling" by a German gynecologist, Dr. Ernst Grafenberg (hence the "G"), the G-spot was resurrected in a bestselling book called The G-Spot and Other Recent Discoveries about Human Sexuality, published in 1982.

The authors contend that physicians and nurses trained by them found the spot in 400 women tested in Florida, Vermont, and New Jersey in 1981. Pressing the G-spot purportedly causes sexual arousal. But Dr. Kermit Krantz, chairman of obstetrics and gynecology at the University of Kansas Medical Center and world expert on sexual anatomy, does not believe the G-spot exists. "I am not a woman, obviously, and have not read the book," he says, "but in all the tissue specimens I have studied, I never found any specific nerve endings in the vagina that can be associated with sexual satisfaction."

Many agree with Dr. Krantz, including Daniel Goldberg, who briefly collaborated with the authors of The G-Spot. Goldberg, a psychologist at Jefferson Medical College in Philadelphia, tried unsuccessfully to duplicate the studies covered in The G-Spot. In one study, he found that four out of eleven women had sensitive spots in their vaginas, five did not, and two were uncertain.

In another study, Goldberg also questioned the belief that women ejaculate in so-called "uterine orgasms." In a test of six women, he found that the female ejaculate was actually urine, and not a secretion similar to semen without the sperm, as a 1981 study published in the Journal of Sex Research claimed. The JSR study is one of only two documented scientific studies cited in the The G-Spot.

Just as the publicity over the G-spot's existence was beginning to die down, sexologist Dr. Theresa Crenshaw announced in 1983 that the G-spot indeed existed and was really a female prostate gland. The prostate is a glandular body found in men that secretes a fluid that is a principal constituent of ejaculatory fluid. "There is another special erotic zone in women that some find sexually pleasurable and capable of producing orgasms," she says. "While we can't say for sure, because we don't have a large number of studies, I think it's fair to conclude all women have a prostate."

Dr. Crenshaw's hypothesis has yet to be proven.

High on Love

Some people seem to shy away from becoming attached to another person, either physically or emotionally. Either they've had too many blind dates, or they're suffering from too much of a good thing. Not too much sex, but too much of the brain's own drugs.

Studies suggest that *phenylethylamine* (PEA), the brain's naturally occurring amphetamine-like substance, seems to quell the longings for romantic love. Similarly, endorphins, the brain's version of opiates, apparently dull desire for the more permanent pair bond that comes after that initial romantic high has worn off.

Research psychiatrists Michael R. Liebowitz and Donald F. Klein of the New York State Psychiatric Institute discovered the importance of PEA while working with what Klein calls hysteroid dysphorics. Based on whether or not they are in love, these patients, like manic depressives, suffer severe mood shifts.

According to Liebowitz, "When in love they are giddy, energetic, optimistic, and totally unable to view their partners realistically. They also eat and sleep less and are very sociable; their state is like an amphetamine high. When the romance ends, however, they crash into real slumps; at these times they overeat, oversleep, feel very sluggish, and don't want to see anyone. Interestingly, the symptoms are similiar to amphetamine withdrawal."

Klein wondered whether these people, who seem to rush recklessly into affairs simply to feel the giddy elation of new love, were craving PEA.

Liebowitz tested his associate's hypothesis with help from colleagues at Columbia University. He treated several dozen hysteroid dysphorics with a monoamine oxidase (MAO) inhibitor, an antidepressant drug that prevents PEA from breaking down. Nearly all the "love addicts" calmed down.

Like amphetamines, Liebowitz believes, PEA increases the levels of the neurotransmitters norepinephrine and dopamine (and, somehow, our spirits). Liebowitz recalled one of his patients whose usually short-lived "highs" were extended when she fell in love.

"Joanne was a 24-year-old writer whose moods tended to alternate between very high and very low. Unfortunately, while the depression periods tended to last as long as a a month, the hypomanic [high] periods never lasted more than a week. Except when Joanne met someone during that week who really attracted her. 'I frequently fall in love when I'm high,' Joanne told me. 'Then I may stay high for as long as 3 or 4 weeks.' Falling in love extended the length of Joanne's hypomanic periods, by providing extra juice for her synapses. Presumably it was the same stuff she was already burning, which meant the naturally produced chemicals norepinephrine or dopamine."

Therefore, the higher the level of our brain's amphetamine-like substance, PEA, the lower our desire for the romantic love that would trigger the release of insufficiently supplied PEA. Similarly, researchers at Bowling Green State University in Ohio have found that a high level of endorphins, our body's natural opiates, seems to quell the longing for a strong pair bond (which, in humans, usually comes after that initial romantic high).

Psychologist Jaak Panksepp and his colleagues at Bowling Green studied the responses of puppies, young guinea pigs, and baby chicks separated from their companions. Only two types of drugs were found to alleviate the animals' distress without also sedating them: narcotics, particularly beta-endorphins; and *clonidine*, a drug used to reduce withdrawal symptoms in heroin addicts quitting "cold turkey." The animals not only stopped whimpering, they avoided contact with their parents and actively sought isolation.

Hence, overproduction of the brain's own "uppers" and "downers" may reduce the desire for contact with the opposite sex. Using PET scanners Liebowitz believes that soon we will be able to visualize the workings of our neurochemical systems and adjust any abnormalities with yet to be determined techniques.

Impotence

Sam Wilson, 58 years old, is chronically impotent. He is incapable of sustaining an erection firm enough for sexual intercourse. The problem came on gradually, but got worse and worse. Understandably, he became extremely depressed.

Finally his wife, Beth, convinced him to seek help. They went first to the family doctor, who suggested Sam see a psychiatrist. Sam began going to a psychiatrist once a week, but 8 months passed with no change in his condition.

Then followed 2 frustrating years as Sam and Beth approached a series of psychiatrists, psychologists, marriage counselors and sex therapists—all to no avail. Finally, a sex therapist mentioned that diabetes, which Sam had had all his life, could cause impotence.

A urologist was consulted, and the couple finally got an answer: Sam's impotence was directly caused by his diabetes. After a series of tests, the urologist determined that there was little chance of repairing the years of nerve damage wreaked by the disease. A penile implant was recommended and Sam went ahead with the operation.

"It has made me feel like a whole man again," Sam said several months after receiving the implant.

Sam is one of an estimated 10 million chronically impotent men in the United States. Chronic impotence—as opposed to temporary impotence, which all men suffer at one time or another—is commonly defined as penile dysfunction that persists for at least six weeks. Many impotent men (and their partners) are too ashamed to seek help for this disorder, and too many physicians rashly suggest the afflicted man see a psychiatrist. As a result impotent men are, as one urologist has put it, the "lepers of medicine."

Bruce and Eileen MacKenzie, of Chevy Chase, Maryland, realized the seriousness of the impotent man's dilemma. Bruce had also received an implant for impotence caused by diabetes. So in 1982, they formed Impotents Anonymous and its companion group, called I-ANON, for partners of impotent men. At least 13 chapters now exist nationwide. Modeled after Alcoholics Anonymous and

Alanon (for partners), this national self-help organization offers impotent men the opportunity to talk about their problem with others. A similar organization helps impotent men and their partners adjust to life after a prosthesis has been implanted. Called Potency Restored, the group was founded by Dr. Guilio I. Scarzella, senior attending urologist at Holy Cross Hospital in Silver Spring, Maryland.

Impotence can be caused by physiological or psychological factors, or a combination of both. An erection is a complicated phenomenon involving neurological, nervous, and circulatory systems. When the physical and the emotional factors are in synch, blood engorges two long tubes of spongy tissue in the penis called the corpora cavernosa. Almost ten times the amount of blood normally in the penis is used to generate an erection.

Until recently doctors believed 90 percent of all impotence was due to psychological disorders. If a man couldn't have an erection there was something psychologically wrong. Many doctors now think that as much as 60 percent of all impotence results from physiological problems—disorders that can be relieved or cured in more than 75 percent of the cases.

Diabetes mellitus is the principal cause of organic impotence. Between 40 and 60 percent of diabetic men suffer from erectile dysfunction. Other physical causes of impotence include arteriosclerosis (hardening of the arteries), kidney disease, pelvic and spinal surgery, Peyronie's disease (buildup of scarlike tissue in the penis), and neurological disorders such as multiple sclerosis and Parkinson's disease.

Impotence can also be a side effect of drugs, such as antihypertensives and antidepressants. A 1981 study of the most frequently prescribed drugs found that at least 15 percent of these were associated with male sexual dysfunction. Many cases of drug-provoked impotence can therefore be remedied simply by taking a patient off a particular drug or prescribing a different, but equivalent, medication.

Psychological causes of impotence are a bit harder to pinpoint, but stress (due to depression, marital discord, and fatigue), fear of hurting the partner, and fear of inadequate performance are the primary psychological factors. Virtually all researchers agree that fear of failure can actually cause erectile dysfunction.

"A mild organic problem can precipitate a more serious psychogenic problem," says Dr. Marc Goldstein, director of the male reproduction and urologic microsurgery unit at New York Hospital-Cornell Medical Center. "It's not uncommon to see a man with a little physical problem, which then causes a serious emotional problem that prevents him from reaching his potential." *All* men suffer from temporary or "situational" impotence at some point in their lives, due to the above factors as well as the deadening effects of alcohol and drugs. So men should not panic if they occasionally have trouble sustaining an erection.

Tests

If a patient feels his impotence is permanent, he should see the family physician and get a complete psychophysical checkup. Often diagnoses can be made on the basis of a thorough medical history and a complete physical examination. Physicians should do tests of the patient's neurologic and vascular systems, and evaluate blood hormone and sugar levels. Previous illnesses and medications, and factors contributing to a possible psychological etiology of the impotence, should also be scrutinized.

If this doesn't provide an answer, an array of specialized diagnostic tests can often determine whether impotence is attributable to the mind or the body.

Perhaps the most revealing test now performed is called the *nocturnal penile tumescence (NPT)* test. Impotent patients spend several nights in a special sleep center, where they are monitored by technicians for nocturnal erections. Men generally have three to six erections each night during rapid eye movement (REM) sleep. As the factors causing psychological impotence are believed to be at rest during sleep, a patient who does not achieve a firm erection at least once during the night most likely suffers from a physiologic disorder.

NPT laboratory testing is expensive—up to $1,500 per person.

As a result, many men opt for the Snap Guide, a new $15 take-home version developed by Dacomed of Minneapolis. At bedtime, the patient attaches the device, which has a Velcro band, around the base of the penis. The band has three pressure-sensitive snaps that break as penile circumference increases during an erection. If all three are broken by morning, at least one full erection is presumed to have occurred. The one drawback of the Snap Guide is that it does not indicate duration of the erection or how many took place, factors which could have important bearing on a patient's diagnosis.

Another testing device, called the *Biosonics Interface Digital Diagnostic System* (*BIDDS*), stimulates the nerves that cause erections. If no response occurs, the problem is probably neurological.

Specialists also use Doppler ultrasound to test for impeded blood flow to the penis, another common cause of erectile dysfunction. In some cases, revascularization, in which specialists surgically bypass an area of obstructed blood flow in penile arteries, can restore potency. Unfortunately, however, the problem often recurs after a few years. The arteriogram also tests the blood flow to the penis. Doctors inject a dye into the penis' blood vessels and then x-ray the organ for blockages.

Finally, doctors can x-ray the skull to search for chemical abnormalities in the hypothalamic-pituitary-gonadal axis that could also affect performance.

Psychodysfunction

If a patient fails the NPT test and if his impotence has persisted for at least 6 weeks, then he might want to consider sex therapy. This section describes a few well-known psychotherapeutic methods now in use at major psychiatric centers throughout the country.

Masters and Johnson's *behavior-oriented therapy* is based on the belief that fear of failure is at the root of all psychological impotence. During a 14-day session at the Masters and Johnson Institute in St. Louis, couples learn to become more sexually aware through a technique called "sensate focus." Patients perform specific sexual exercises that teach them to become more relaxed sexually with their partners.

One problem, according to Dr. William H. Masters, is that men often don't realize that it is natural for the penis to engorge and deflate during foreplay. "To give you some idea of how important this information is, I'll make the blanket statement that last night, thousands of men watched themselves into impotence," he said at an American Psychiatric Association meeting in 1984. "They saw this natural physiologic ebb and flow of engorgement, said 'What's wrong with me?' and then lost the rest of the erection."

A school of cognitive therapy similar to that of Masters and Johnson is *rational emotive therapy* (*RET*), developed by Albert Ellis in the 1950s. RET holds that psychological impotence results primarily from an irrational belief system, particularly the fear of failure. Like the Masters and Johnson model, RET encourages participants to make more sexual advances and be more open with their partners about sexual matters.

Ellis claims a 75 to 80 percent recovery rate of erectile potency using RET. The first controlled study was undertaken by research psychiatrists at Los Angeles County-University of Southern California Medical Center. The 6-week study of 16 men with secondary impotence resulted in increased (and successful) sexual intercourse and decreased sexual anxiety in most of the participants.

Dr. Helen Singer Kaplan of Cornell Medical Center in New York City teaches a more psychodynamic approach, which takes into account a patient's complete psychosexual history. Factors such as early sexual traumas, feelings of inferiority and troubled interpersonal relationships are carefully scrutinized.

Interestingly, more and more men with long-standing psychological impotence are getting penile implants. If months of sex therapy prove useless, getting a device that produces at least an artificial erection may give them the psychological edge they need to overcome the problem. Doctors are quick to warn, however, that there is no guarantee that a prosthesis will clear up deep-rooted fear, and many urologists will perform an implant operation only after extensive sex therapy has failed.

Hormone Shots

Men with hormone imbalances can get intramuscular shots of testosterone, gonadotropin, and other male sex hormones. Shots of testosterone usually elicit an immediate sexual response that lasts 2 to 3 hours, and men can receive up to 10 shots per month.

In a study conducted at Beth Israel Hospital in Boston, 105 impotent men between the ages of 18 and 75 were tested for endocrine disorders. Dr. Richard Spark, director of the steroid laboratory at the hospital, found abnormalities in the hypothalamic-pituitary-gonadal axes of 37 of these men. After hormonal treatment, 90 percent of the 37 returned to potency.

One patient had become impotent after radiotherapy for a pituitary tumor and had remained so for 12 years, despite repeated visits to internists and psychotherapists. Following hormone treatment at Beth Israel, the man regained potency in less than 48 hours.

But studies have shown that androgen treatment is effective only in the few men with low serum testosterone levels. Hormones are necessary for normal male sexuality, but many endocrinologists believe a threshold exists beyond which added amounts of androgens will have no effect.

Prolactin inhibitors are also being tested as a cure for hormone-related impotence. Prolactin is a milk-stimulating hormone released by the pituitary gland. When released in high quantities (a condition called hyperprolactinemia), prolactin seems to block the stimulating effects of testosterone. A prescription drug now available called *Bromocriptine* inhibits prolactin production in the pituitary. In a Masters and Johnson study, 11 men with high prolactin levels found improvement in sexual desire with shots of Bromocriptine.

New Arteries

For men with chronic blockage of the penile arteries, commonly caused by diabetes, several experimental techniques are now in clinical trials.

Revascularization, a technique developed by French and Czech surgeons, surgically bypasses blocked arteries so blood can engorge each corpus cavernosum of the penis. Vascular operations have low success rates and remain experimental, primarily because the problem often recurs several years after the operation. Moreover, the technique has caused a permanent erection in some cases.

Other techniques for restoring blood flow have been successful, in curbing impotence but they remain even more experimental. Microsurgeons at Baylor College of Medicine have restored potency (in some cases) by replacing blocked or damaged vessels with synthetic arteries. And soon Dr. Ismet Karacan, an impotence specialist at Baylor, will attempt to transfer arteries from the foot to the penis of an impotent patient.

Mechanical Aids

Presently under development by the same people who produced BIDDS (see Tests) is a device that will shock a patient into excitement. The *Male Electronic Genital Stimulator* (*MEGS*) is a plastic-coated mechanism about 3 inches long and just under an inch in diameter that's implanted in the rectum. MEGS is remote controlled by an electronic component that can be hidden in a watch or other piece of jewelry. The device causes a natural erection by electrically stimulating the nerves leading to the penis. "Each unit will be custom-made," says Dr. Henry S. Brenman, Biosonic's research director, "so that the man doesn't end up accidentally opening someone's garage door."

Another device very similar to MEGS may supplant penile prostheses in the future. Called the erection pacemaker by its inventor, Dr. Tom F. Lue, the device is now undergoing animal tests at the University of California at San Francisco. The pacemaker stimulates penile nerves to cause a natural erection. As with MEGS, a remote radio transmitter activates the device. The pacemaker has been successfully implanted in five monkeys, one of which has had it for over 2 years, according to Dr. Lue, an assistant professor of urology.

Blood Catcher

Soon impotent men may just need a good pair of rubber bands to maintain an erection. Urologist Perry W. Nadig, of the University of Texas Medical School in San Antonio, has developed a revolutionary device that creates a normal erection by drawing and capturing the patient's own blood in the corpora cavernosa of the penis. A vacuum constriction device engorges the penis and then ordinary rubber bands worn during coitus keep the blood where it belongs.

Nadig's invention consists of a clear acrylic cylinder that fits over the penis. The top end of the cylinder is closed off by a piston syringe that creates the vacuum needed to draw the blood into the penis. The device is pressed tightly against the body, creating an airtight seal, and the vacuum is activated. Blood fills the penis, making it erect.

Two rubber bands attached to the device are then wrapped around the base of the penis to constrict it, and the cylinder is removed. The penis will remain erect until the rubber bands are removed and the blood flows back into the body.

Although problems such as numbness and minor hemorrhaging have occurred, patients have been generally satisfied. In a 2-year study, Nadig found that 75 percent of 130 patients continue to use the device regularly, and at least 15 urologists in the San Antonio area now recommend it to their patients.

Potency Drugs

Yohimbine and other pharmacologic agents are being studied in hopes of combating impotence. In a test at Queen's University in Kingston, Ontario, researchers gave yohimbine to twenty-three physically impotent men for 10 weeks. Six achieved a complete return of potency, including orgasm, and four improved to a lesser degree. *Papaverine*, an opium derivative chiefly used as an antispasmodic, also has great potential for reversing impotence. When injected, it prompts erections. Dr. Adrian W. Zorgniotti of New York University treated 31 physiologically impotent men with 30 milligrams of the drug along with 0.5 mg of the alpha blocker phentolamine. Twenty-nine of these men had intercourse within one half hour after injection. "I have seen some patients for more than 6 months now, and all are happy with the results," said Dr. Zorgniotti at a meeting of the American Urological Association.

Vasodilators, drugs that will increase blood flow to the penis, are also being studied. Perhaps the best-known vasodilator is *amyl nitrite*, or "poppers," which gives those who inhale it a euphoric "headrush," in addition to producing a vasodilation. Other vasodilators that don't dilate the mind should be in drugstores soon.

Prostheses

If all else fails, a penile implant is usually recommended. Over 100,000 men have received implants and the industry (if urologists will permit the term) now boasts a 90 percent success rate.

The most widely used type of implant is the semi rigid or "malleable" version, first developed in 1972 by Miami urologists Michael Small and Hernan Carrion. Two silicone rods are inserted into each corpus cavernosum of the penis. The *Small-Carrion prosthesis* forms a permanent semierection that, unfortunately, can often be visible under clothing.

A newer version, called the *Jonas implant*, is cosmetically more appealing. It features paired silicone cylinders, each containing a length of coiled silver wire that can be bent down when an erection is not wanted. University of Iowa urologists reported a 96 percent success rate with the Jonas implant in a study of 57 patients receiving the implant over a 2-year period.

The luxury model is the *inflatable prosthesis*. It was developed in 1973 by urologist F. Brantley Scott of Baylor University, and neurologist William Bradley and bioengineer Gerald Timm of the University of Minnesota. It consists of two balloonlike tubes placed in the copora cavernosa, a pump housed in the scrotum, and a fluid reservoir hidden in the abdomen. By squeezing the pump, the patient releases a saline solution from the reservoir that fills up the tubes in the penis. This prompts an erection. When flipped, a release valve attached to the pump in the scrotum will send the solution back to the reservoir in the abdomen, and the penis will become flaccid.

Semirigid prostheses cost about $1,500, plus the cost of surgery, which usually takes less than an hour and can often be done on an outpatient basis. The inflatable implants, on the other hand, cost about $2,500 and require at least a 4-day stay in the hospital.

The principal advantage of the semirigid—besides its low cost— is that it contains no mechanical parts that can break or wear out. By contrast, the inflatable prosthesis has been known to spring leaks in as many as 40 percent of the cases. But improved surgical techniques and more sophisticated implants will bring this figure down.

Many doctors and their patients prefer the inflatable prosthesis because it produces a more natural erection than the semirigid, and offers greater penetration. Early models of the semis sometimes buckled and made treatment of urinary and prostate problems difficult.

The latest penile implant to hit the market is a combination of the semirigid and the inflatable prostheses. Called the *Hydroflex*, the prosthesis is a self-contained device that, in many cases, can be implanted on an outpatient basis. The Hydroflex consists of two expandable cylinders implanted in the corpora cavernosa. Each device has a tiny inflation pump that shunts fluid from a rear reservoir to a small inflation chamber in the front of the cylinder. Small release valves located side by side in the head of the cylinder inflate and deflate the device. The Hydroflex costs about $3,500 for the prosthesis or approximately $9,000 for the entire implant procedure.

One doctor has estimated that by the year 2002, 1 million men will have received penile implants. Such devices have restored the sex lives (and confidence) of hundreds of thousands of impotent men already—from young men to men in their eighties. Dr. F. Brantley Scott, an inventor of the inflatable prosthesis, reported recently that of the more than 1,400 inflatables he and his associates have implanted, 132 were in men over 70 years of age. As one elderly man put it: "I feel 30 years younger."

Timeline

1988 • Surgical implantation of inflatable prosthesis for the penis now performed on an outpatient basis.

1989 • Yohimbine available without a prescription.

1990 • Human pheromones found in most fragrances.

1993 • Shots of luteinizing hormone-releasing hormone (LHRH) available for men and women with flagging sexual desire.

1995 • Arteries from animals (such as a baboon) implanted successfully in the penises of men whose own arteries are blocked by arteriosclerosis.
• Twenty clinics devoted strictly to impotence now in operation around the country.
• Nonaddictive drugs to lift libido used as widely as aspirin.

1997 • Drugs to control levels of dopamine, serotonin, and other neurotransmitters in the brain used in the home and in hospitals.
• Revascularization, the surgical shunting of arteries around a blocked area in a penile artery is now successful 80 percent of the time because of advanced diagnostic and surgical techniques.

2000 • Electrical stimulator of nerves to the penis activated by thought.

2002 • One million men have received penile prostheses.

2005 • Family doctor can administer electrical stimulation of the pleasure centers of the brain to increase sexual desire. Self-stimulators also available at low cost from the local drugstore, with or without a prescription, depending on the sophistication of the device.

2010 • Techniques and drug treatments perfected whereby humans can learn to regulate at will the release of sex hormones from the pituitary and sex glands.

2020 • Ten-minute diagnostic test available that uses a PET scanner to determine abnormalities in the hypothalamic-pituitary-gonadal axis.

2050 • First successful penile transplant.

2100 • First completely robotic penis fashioned out of real human flesh and electronic components.

=Access Guide=

Here is a list of the top impotence clinics in the country. Some treat only psychological impotence, some treat only physical dysfunction. All have pamphlets describing the diagnostic and treatment services they provide. Costs for initial consultation (IC) and treatments are provided in only a few cases. At most centers, cost is determined by type and length of diagnosis and treatment.

Impotence Clinics

Anacapa Potency Center
2438 Ponderosa Drive North
Suite C217
Camarillo, CA 93010
(805) 484-7960

Full diagnosis and treatment of impotence. In-house treatments include hormone therapy and penile implants. Regular referrals for psychotherapy. Closely allied with Pleasant Valley Hospital, which runs a ROMP center (see below).

The Association for Male Sexual Dysfunction
520 East 72nd Street
New York, NY 10021
(212) 794-1616

Complete psychosexual and medical evaluation, basic and specialized lab tests; medical (medication) and surgical (penile implants) treatment, though the latter done in hospital; psychiatric services, including relationship therapy, marital-family therapy, sex therapy, individual psychotherapy, and psychopharmacology.

Atlanta Center for Male Sexual Dysfunction
3280 Howell Mill Road
Suite 125
Atlanta, GA 30327
(404) 352-8220

IC: $70. Take-home NPT testing. Treatments include hormone treatments, revascularization and semirigid and inflatable penile implants. Private impotence support group in-house.

Baylor University College of Medicine
One Baylor Plaza
Houston, TX 77030
(713) 791-3835

Known for semirigid and inflatable penile implant operations (F. Brantley Scott here; inventor of inflatable prosthesis). Also, hormonal injections and psychotherapy available. Custom-designed programs for each individual.

Center for Male Sexuality
1575 Hillside Avenue
New Hyde Park, NY 11040
(516) 354-1638

Sleep Center and other diagnostic tests. Treatments include hormone treatments, sex therapy, and all types of penile implants.

Cleveland Clinic
9500 Euclid Avenue
Cleveland, OH 44106
(216) 444-5590

Full diagnostic assessment, including NPT and real-time tumescence testing, arteriograms, and even injections of papaverine, an opium derivative sometimes used to unblock clogged arteries. Treatment includes revascularization and implants: malleable, inflatable, and new Hydroflex. Psychotherapy and sex therapy available.

Colorado Men's Clinic
2005 E. 18th Avenue
Denver, CO 80206
(303) 321-4212

IC: $45. Blood flow studies ($90), hormone testing, psychological screening. Treatments include papaverine injections; 6-week hormone treatment plan (commonly two shots per week, $8.50 per shot); and all types of penile implants. Sex therapist and psychologist on staff.

Impotence Clinic of East Tennessee
1907 N. Roan Street
Suite 404
Johnson City, TN 37601
(615) 926-2969

Initial diagnosis includes blood flow testing, NPT monitoring, and psychological evaluation. Procedures include hormone and papaverine treatments and all types of penile implants.

Impotence Institute of Eastern Oklahoma
1725 East 19th Street
Suite 80
Tulsa, OK 74104
(918) 743-8765

Initial evaluation includes blood pressure, NPT, Doppler, and hormonal tests and a psychological evaluation. Treatments include pharmacologic treatments (mostly papaverine), hormone treatments, psychotherapy, revascularization, and all penile implants. Also has Impotents Anonymous chapter.

Masters and Johnson Institute
24 South Kings Highway
St. Louis, MO 63108
(314) 361-2377

Three basic options in psychotherapy for sexual problems offered: (1) Two-week intensive therapy in which partners are seen daily; (2) 16-session progression, in which couples are seen for appointments on three successive days the first week, twice a week for 3 weeks and finally, once a week for 7 weeks; (3) program tailored to individual needs and circumstances, possibly including treament of single individuals; number of therapists, and length of treatment are other variables. Follow-up sessions also.

Mayo Clinic
Department of Urology
Rochester, MN 55901
(507 284-3722)

Initial evaluation includes psychological testing, sleep study, and vascular studies. Treatment includes psychotherapy and sex therapy, hormone treatments, and malleable and inflatable penile implants.

The Men's Clinic
c/o Penrose Hospital
2215 North Cascade
Colorado Springs, CO 80907
(303) 632-5944

Two-hour in-depth IC, including most tests: $294. Diagnostic procedures include blood and hormonal testing and psychological screening. Treatments include hormonal, yohimbine, and papaverine injections; sex therapy; and all types of penile implants.

Morrow Impotence Center
77 West Grenada
Ormond Beach, FL 32074
(904) 673-5100

Evaluation includes sleep laboratory and vascular testing. Treatment includes hormone and yohimbine injections and semirigid and inflatable implants.

New England Male Reproductive Center
720 Harrison Avenue
Suite 606
Boston, MA 02118
(617) 638-8485

Diagnosis includes NPT testing, arteriograms, and hormone tests. Treatments include hormone and papaverine treatments and all types of penile implants.

New York Hospital-Cornell Medical Center
525 East 68th Street
New York, NY 10021
(212) 472-5454

Evaluation includes blood tests, NPT testing, ultrasound, and penile arteriograms. Optional therapy and counseling include discussions with sexual counselors, psychologists, nurses, psychiatrists, and other physicians. Physical treatments include revascularization and all types of penile implants.

Northwest Center for Impotence
1231 116th Avenue Northeast
Suite 202
Bellevue, WA 98004
(206) 454-9049

Initial psychological and physical screening, including vascular testing, costs $200–$300. Tumescence testing, psychological and sex therapy, minor revascularization procedures, and penile implantation (all three types). All diagnostic and surgical procedures tailored to individual.

Potency Plus
Beverly Hills Medical Tower
1125 South Beverly Drive
Suite 410
Los Angeles, CA 90035
(213) 277-1444

First clinic strictly for impotence in the world. Complete physical and psychological evaluation, blood tests, and sleep center for NPT testing. Semirigid, inflatable, and Hydroflex penile implants. No overnight stay required, and all tests and surgery done in-house.

Sexual Impotence Center of San Diego
1662 East Main Street
El Cajon, CA 92021
(619) 574-6477

Diagnosis includes NPT, hormone, and blood testing. Treatment devoted strictly to all types of penile implants.

Self-Help Impotence Organizations

Impotents Anonymous/I-ANON
National Headquarters
5119 Bradley Boulevard
Chevy Chase, MD 20815
(301) 656-3649

Run by the Impotence Institute of America, also headquartered here. Like Alcoholics Anonymous and Alanon (for partners), these two groups help impotent men and their partners come to terms with their problem. Information and advice on impotence available.

Impotence Information Center
P.O. Box 9
Minneapolis, MN 55440

Sponsored by American Medical Systems, this center provides free literature on impotence, including "Impotence: Causes and Treatments"; "Impotence: A Guide for the Diabetic Man"; and "Impotence: A Guide for Men with Cardiovascular Difficulties." Also provides lists of physicians around the country who diagnose and treat impotent men.

Potency Restored
c/o Dr. Giulio L. Scarzella
8630 Fenton Street
Suite 218
Silver Spring, MD 20910
(301) 588-5777

First support group for impotent men and their partners in the country. Support for penile implantees and their partners before, during, and after surgery. Dues are $5.00 per family per month and those joining receive a regular newsletter.

Recovery of Male Impotence (ROMP)
Grace Hospital
18700 Meyers Road
Detroit, MI 48235
(800) TEL-ROMP

Hospital-based, multidisciplinary educational and self-help group. Fourteen ROMPs in existence. Informational (rather than psychotherapeutic) services for physically impotent men and their partners. Free and totally confidential. ROMP also puts out a brochure: "Solving the Problem of Impotence."

7

An End to Pain

Matt Payton, a 31-year-old Chicago electrician, had a spinal fusion after a motorcycle accident in 1972. The doctors said he would have no problems with his back after that. But he did. Every few months, his back would suddenly go out, leaving him prostrated on the floor in excruciating pain. Matt's wife Eileen could do nothing but comfort him until the episode passed.

Matt had a second spinal fusion operation in 1975, but after a hiatus of several months, the pain returned with a vengeance. Over the next 5 years, Matt and Eileen saw a series of orthopedists, chiropractors, physical therapists, even a psychiatrist—to no avail. Finally, in 1980, Matt received a hand-held electrical stimulation device that he could place directly over the painful area in his lower back. Doctors believe such devices, which are very successful in relieving pain, cause the release of our body's natural painkillers or somehow block transmission of pain signals to the brain. After 8 years of agony, Matt finally found relief.

Pain is our species' most relentless enemy. From that first scraped knee, every child knows that pain must be checked—at whatever cost. That cost is estimated by some pain experts to be $70 *billion* a year in the United States in medical fees, lost working days, and legal fees. Chronic pain—pain like arthritis and lower back pain that lasts for at least 6 months—affects some 40 million Americans and is the single most common reason for seeing a doctor. Another 50 million people suffer from intermittent chronic pain, such as a pinched nerve or a sudden migraine headache. Often persistent pain, even if it is minor, can lead to anxiety, depression, insomnia and extreme irritability, literally taking over the lives of its victims. In the words of Albert Schweitzer, pain "is a more terrible lord of mankind than even death himself."

From the earliest times, humans have sought to relieve pain, and many of the treatments discovered thousands of years ago are still used today in modified form. Opium, administered the world over as a potent painkiller, was recommended as an analgesic in a medical work called the *Ebers Papyrus* used in Egypt in the fifteenth century B.C., during the reign of the Pharoah Amenhotep. For centuries, chronic pain sufferers have been "tricked" into feeling better by primitive shamans and modern day physicians alike. These doctors take advantage of "the placebo effect," whereby a patient who thinks he or she has been given a potent painkiller—but has actually been given an inert substance such as a sugar pill—gets better.

Though we have gone to enormous lengths to find a pain panacea, even to the extent of drilling holes in the skulls of headache sufferers (a practice of prehistoric surgeons in Stone Age Europe and Peru), pain in its many guises still plagues the lives of millions of Americans. In the last 15 years, a veritable explosion of research into the causes and cures of all forms of pain has taken place. Pain specialists are learning how to block the passage of pain signals from a wound site to the brain, where pain is perceived; and they are figuring out why the quality of pain differs from person to person and from circumstance to circumstance. Doctors now understand that just because a specific mechanical cause for pain cannot be found, the pain is not necessarily imagined.

Back pain afflicts more people than any other type of chronic pain. Everything from common drug treatments and back exercises to less-known techniques like nerve blocks are used to treat the problem. In addition, some 200,000 Americans undergo back surgery each year. In 80 percent of those cases, the pain returns sometime in the future. Scar tissue left behind after some back operations— such as the laminectomy, in which a part of a vertebra is removed—will actually cause the patient more pain.

Next to backache, migraines and other headaches send more Americans scurrying to the family doctor than any other type of pain. Muscular headaches, also known as tension headaches, are caused by excessive contraction of the muscles in the head and neck, while vascular headaches, which include migraines, arise from irregular blood flow in the head.

Arthritis, a painful disease of muscle joints, afflicts over 30 million people in this country. The two major types—osteoarthritis and rheumatoid arthritis—account for $4 billion a year in lost income and health care costs. Osteoarthritis is a degenerative arthritis appearing most often in people over 50; it attacks the fingers and occasionally the hips and spine. Rheumatoid arthritis commonly afflicts people from ages 25 to 50, and causes inflammation, swelling, and sometimes disintegration of joints.

The most feared and often the most painful chronic pain syndrome, one which torments nearly a million, mostly elderly, people in this country, is the pain of terminal cancer. Often a cancer patient's perception of the pain will be exacerbated by the belief that cancer kills—a kind of reverse placebo effect. Cancer pain is caused by the growth of tumors that compress and destroy sensitive nerves and tissue surrounding major organs and bones. Ironically, chemotherapy and other cancer treatments can also exacerbate pain.

With dying cancer patients, stopping the pain is the important thing. Very often, however, patients suffering from severe pain are not getting the relief they so desperately seek. In a study conducted by psychiatrists Richard Marks and Edward Sachar of Montefiore Hospital in New York City, 75 percent of patients given analgesics for minor to severe pain felt no relief. The researchers discovered that physicians prescribing the drugs and nurses administering them often gave substantially less than the dosage required to quell the patient's pain, apparently because they overestimated the power of the drugs. As a result, patients often received less than 50 percent of the dosage necessary to kill the pain.

Part of the problem is that chronic pain was, until recently, so little understood. The study of pain does not fit neatly into any one medical discipline, which seems to be the reason it is seriously neglected in medical schools. Dr. John Bonica, founder of the International Association for the Study of Pain and a world leader in pain research, found in a study of 17 standard textbooks that only 54 pages out of a total of 22,000 furnished information about pain.

"We have the necessary tools to treat [chronic] pain successfully," says Dr. Steven Rothenberg of the Walker Pain Institute, "but most physicians in the United States are unaware of them and are sorely lacking in education. It's not necessarily their own fault, but the fact is that the whole system right now isn't set up for chronic pain."

But over the last few years, specialists of all sorts have started to band together at specialized pain clinics and at major hospitals in the fight to understand and treat pain. Sophisticated new diagnostic techniques like *thermography* and *bioelectric function diagnosis* are helping pain experts with this formidable task. The new field of *algology* (from *algo*, the Greek word for pain) reflects this new blending of specialties, as does a host of new professional titles: neurophysiologist, psychobiologist, neuropsychiatrist. The explosion in pain research is "one of the most dramatic things happening in medicine," says Dr. Donlin M. Long, codirector of the Pain Treatment Center at Johns Hopkins in Baltimore.

Pain's Genesis

During World War II, pioneer pain researcher Henry Beecher discovered that soldiers critically wounded at the bloody battle of Anzio felt less pain than civilians back home who were suffering from severe injuries. This circumstantial lessening of pain has since become known as the "Anzio effect": To the soldiers, serious injury meant going home, and therefore the pain was superseded by the knowledge that, for them, the war was over.

Pain experts have long known that people's perception of pain differs. People of northern European extraction, who consider stoicism a virtue, tend to have higher pain "thresholds" than more emotional people like those of Italian and Jewish heritage. And each individual human being seems to have a personal pain threshold that is dependent on a mix of physical, psychological, neurochemical, and social factors.

What, then, is pain and where does it originate? Pain experts have long wondered whether the body contains specific pain sensors, or whether cells sensitive to touch and temperature relay messages of pain to the brain. Edward R. Perl of the University of North Carolina School of Medicine found the answer when he identified nerve endings deep within the seven layers of the skin and in the internal organs that are activated only when a stimulus is of sufficient intensity to be painful.

If you smashed your big toe against a solid wall or accidentally placed your hand on a hot stove, chances are the nerve endings in the affected area would consider the stimulus intense enough to alert the brain to what doctors call "noxious stimuli." In other words, you'd hurt like hell. When activated, the nerve endings cause the release of chemicals associated with inflammation, such as prostaglandin and bradykinin, that in turn dispatch neurochemical messengers to the brain. Within milliseconds, these "neurotransmitters" work their way up the spinal column to the thalamic and limbic systems of the brain.

Once in the brain, the pain impulse is passed from neuron to neuron—like passing the baton in a road race—to its destination in the cerebral cortex, the "gray matter" covering the brain's surface, where pain is perceived. Brain experts have estimated that the brain contains anywhere from 10 billion to 1 trillion neurons, each of which may be only a neuron or two away from being connected to every other neuron in the brain.

What is being developed today in pharmaceutical think tanks, medical colleges, and high-tech hospitals to combat cancer pain, migraine headache, backaches? The business of pain relief is an extremely competitive segment of the economy, with pharmaceutical houses continually touting a new, nonaddictive, side-effect-free opiate mimic or *the* one and only pill to alleviate the nauseating throb of migraines. We will tell you which of these drugs, techniques, operations, and tests are available now, and which will soon be available.

Natural Painkillers

By far the most exciting development in the history of pain research was the discovery in the mid-seventies that the human brain contains its own painkillers. Soon each one of us may be able to unleash these nonaddicting opiate-like pain relievers with little more than a deep thought.

The beginning of the revolution in pain research came in 1965, when neuroanatomist Patrick D. Wall of the University of London and psychologist Ronald Melzack of McGill University in Montreal announced a "gate control" theory of pain. The researchers theorized that the nervous system can only process a certain amount of sensory information at one time. Cells located in the dorsal horn—a neurochemical switchboard through which signals from all parts of the body pass on their way to the brain—block any overload. Pleasure signals, they postulated, such as those generated by rubbing a sore knee, tend to get preference over pain impulses, and hence the victim of an injury tends to feel less pain than if he didn't rub it.

Wall and Melzack's theory dovetails nicely with what are unquestionably the two most important breakthroughs in the history of pain research—the discovery of opiate receptors and the discovery of the natural opiates that fit those receptors.

In 1973 Candace Pert, then a graduate student working at the National Institute of Mental Health (NIMH), and Solomon Snyder of the Johns Hopkins School of Medicine, discovered that nerve cells in the brain have receptors that "attract" narcotics like morphine. They reasoned that the body would only have developed an opiate receptor if the body itself produced its own form of opiate to fit those receptors.

Scientists launched a massive search for the theorized natural opiates, and within 2 years, two pharmacologists at the University of Aberdeen in Scotland succeeded in isolating a powerful chemical in a pig's brain that binds to the receptors just as an artificial narcotic would. They termed these naturally produced opiates "enkephalins," from the Greek "in the head." Several other natural painkillers were subsequently found and are now collectively labeled endorphins.

Interestingly, the endorphins seem to be concentrated in just those areas in the brain and spinal cord where Wall and Melzack believed the hypothetical pain control "gate" to be. "Our team at NIMH has proposed that the endorphins, our natural opiates, are a filtering mechanism in the brain," says Pert. "The opiate system selectively filters incoming information from every sense—sight, hearing, smell, taste, and touch—and blocks some of it from percolating up to higher levels of consciousness."

One of the naturally occurring, morphine-like substances that has especially intrigued pharmacologists and neuroscientists is *beta-endorphin*, a hormone-like chemical produced by the pituitary gland. Because it is released at the same time as adrenocorticotropic hormone (ACTH), a hormone involved in stress, researchers believe the systems that control pain and emotional stress in the body may be closely linked.

Another opiate-like substance in the brain that has pharmaceutical houses buzzing is *neurotensin*, which, like beta-endorphin, seems to be manufactured in the regions of the brain that synthesize pain and stress signals. A study by the Merck pharmaceuticals company showed neurotensin to be at least 1,000 times as effective as enkephalin in relieving pain.

Serotonin, a brain chemical thought to be involved in the regulation of sleep, may be a painkiller as well. Dr. Samuel Seltzer and his colleagues at Temple University's Maxillofacial Pain Control Center, in Philadelphia, administered 3 grams daily of tryptophan, an amino acid that is found in milk and that stimulates the brain's production of serotonin, to 15 patients suffering from migraines, arthritis, and several types of neuralgia. Another 15 patients received placebos. Patients receiving tryptophan reported up to a 100 percent decrease in pain intensity, while those administered placebos felt about 50 percent relief.

Tricyclic antidepressants, drugs that elevate moods, may also be added to the painkiller arsenal. Scientists believe these drugs stop serotonin from being reabsorbed by nerve cells once its message has been transmitted, so that it continues to provide pain relief signals. Researchers at the National Institutes of Health in Bethesda, Maryland, have shown that one of these drugs, called *amytryptoline*, has a pain-relieving effect that is distinct from its mood-elevating action.

Endorphin Mimes

The initial excitement over the natural opiates was somewhat dampened when researchers discovered that endorphins seem to be as addicting as artificial narcotics. Rats treated with enkephalin and beta-endorphin have been found to acquire many of the symptoms of morphine addiction. Endorphins are also broken down rapidly by enzymes in the brain, making their efficacy short-lived.

So pharmaceutical researchers are working day and night to produce analogues to endorphins that both resist the brain's enzymes and relieve pain without producing the serious side effects of narcotics. Making the job tougher is the fact that these analogues must also be able to cross the "blood-brain barrier" from the bloodstream into the brain. The power of a drug is often determined by how quickly it crosses this barrier into the brain.

Hope lies with a drug called *d-phenylalanine* (DPA), developed by Seymour Ehrenpreis of the Chicago Medical School. Like enkephalin, DPA is a string of amino acids (amino acids are the building blocks of our proteins), and so the brain is equipped to deal with the drug metabolically. DPA seems to inhibit the action of the destructive enzymes, thereby raising enkephalin levels (which, in chronic pain sufferers, are often low) and producing pain relief naturally.

Laboratory tests with rats and a small number of humans have shown that DPA is nonaddicting and does not sedate, and that there are no withdrawal symptoms after it is stopped. Furthermore, the patients who responded to DPA treatment generally needed only 2 days of treatment in order to obtain a month's relief. Ehrenpreis believes that a long-term buildup of enkephalin levels in the brain is the reason for such long-lasting pain relief.

Researchers are also developing analogues to natural painkillers that bind to receptors in the spinal column rather than the brain. Some researchers believe that such drugs would not have the debilitating side effects—like sedation and addiction—that plague users of narcotic drugs.

An analogue was recently discovered for dynorphin, a natural painkiller that binds to a specific kind of opiate receptor called a kappa receptor. Scientists believe that kappa receptors may be highly concentrated in the spinal column. Hence, this medication would block pain signals as they travel up the spinal column, and the well-known side effects of narcotics would be avoided. Pharmacologists testing the drug and other endorphin analogues remain cautious, however, as such analogues may have their own cache of side effects.

Will we someday be able to unleash our body's natural painkillers at will? "I don't think it takes too much scientific license to say that we will discover mental activities that can produce specific analgesia," University of Washington's Dr. Bonica says. "In 10 or 15 years, perhaps we can begin to teach people to control their own pain."

Pains and Needles

For centuries the Chinese have been controlling pain without using drugs. Their prescription: acupuncture. Interestingly, it took the discovery of opiate receptors and endorphins to open the eyes of Western physicians to natural pain relief. Western researchers now know that stimulating nerve endings with needles releases endorphins, thereby activating our body's own pain suppression system.

When Li Xujen entered the acupuncture unit at Peking's Guananmen Hospital, doubled over, unable to move and barely able to speak, she was surprised to find an American doctor ready to treat her. But Mrs. Xujen, 53 years old, sat quietly while the doctor placed long metal needles into her skin at various strategic locations. After a few minutes, she felt movement coming back into her arms and legs. She exclaimed "*Xie, xie* (thanks)," gave the doctor a thumbs-up sign, and strolled out of the hospital.

The American was one of a group of 25 foreign doctors taking a 3-month acupuncture course that was sponsored by Peking's Academy of Traditional Chinese Medicine in late 1984. The technique, which has been used in China for centuries as a general anesthesia for medical procedures ranging from pulling teeth to delivery of babies, has been gaining respect in this country ever since Richard Nixon's historic trip to China in 1972. Today, thousands of licensed acupuncturists, as well as physicians, dentists, and chiropractors, regularly employ the technique to relieve all kinds of pain. Medical colleges offer courses in acupuncture, and insurance companies cover acupuncture treatment as long as it is performed by a doctor.

The practice of acupuncture is based on the traditional Chinese belief that disease is caused by imbalances in the flow of T'chi, the "life energy" that runs through our bodies along 14 vertical "meridians." Along those meridians are nearly 800 points that correspond to specific body organs. For instance, a point between the thumb and forefinger is the "window" to the large intestine. Twisting and turning very fine metal needles in such spots, acupuncturists believe, directs energy to corresponding organs, thereby stabilizing the flow of T'chi.

The link between acupuncture and endorphins has been demonstrated in several experiments. In one experiment, neurobiologist Bruce Pomeranz of the University of Toronto reduced sensitivity to pain in two groups of mice by using acupuncture. In one group, Pomeranz first administered naloxone, a drug that blocks the action of enkephalin. These mice remained sensitive to pain even after acupuncture was used, which suggests that, because of the naloxone, the endorphin system was not being activated by acupuncture, as it apparently was in the second group of mice.

Studies with human subjects have produced similar results. David Mayer of the Medical College of Virginia administered slight electric shocks to the teeth of volunteers, thereby producing mild pain. Acupuncture was found to raise the pain threshold. Mayer then administered naloxone, which significantly reduced the painkilling effects of the acupuncture. Once again, naloxone seems to have kept the endorphin system from being activated.

Noninvasive Needling

Traditional acupuncture is now practiced around the country. But for people who would rather not have dozens of needles stuck into their bodies, several alternatives are available.

One of these is *laser acupuncture*, in which low-power laser beams are fired in short bursts at traditional acupuncture points. During the treatment, a patient's pulse is monitored. A stronger pulse indicates that the laser has hit the acupuncture point. The treatment, which is now being used to relieve arthritis, migraines, whiplash, and back pain, is inexpensive and cannot damage nerves or blood vessels. Dr. Wolfgang Bauermeister, director of the Pain Control Center at Parkwood Hospital in New Bedford, Massachusetts, claims an 80 to 85 percent success rate with laser acupuncture.

The ways of stimulating acupuncture points might be more numerous than anyone would have thought. Ronald Melzack, the McGill University psychologist who, with Patrick Wall, first described the "gate control" theory of pain, has found that ordinary ice, when applied to an acupuncture point between the thumb and forefinger called the Hoku point, can relieve the pain of toothaches. Eighty percent of the patients Melzack tested felt that the pain had been reduced by as much as fifty percent after ice was applied to the Hoku point.

Another needle-less form of acupuncture now employed by many specialists is *electrical acupuncture*. In electrical acupuncture, electrodes placed on the surface of the skin direct a mild electric current at acupuncture points and relieve pain by causing the release of endorphins.

One new device that is used by some electroacutherapists is the *Electro-Acuscope*. About the size of a stereo component, this $7,000 device sends mild electrical bursts directly through the body between two designated acupuncture points. The Acuscope, say its designers, restores electrical activity to cells that have been damaged in an injury, thereby returning equilibrium to the flow of T'chi.

Electrical Aspirin

Despite the fact that it is linked to acupuncture, the Acuscope was approved by the Food and Drug Administration (FDA) as a *Transcutaneous Electrical Nerve Stimulation (TENS)* device (transcutaneous means "through the skin"). Experts believe TENS devices do not work at the pain site itself, but rather somewhere along the pain pathway, either by blocking the transmission of pain signals to the brain or by stimulating the release of endorphins. Patients can rent or buy portable TENS generators at costs ranging from $60 to $400.

With TENS, electrodes are attached to the skin surface above a painful area. A mild current is generated to compete with the pain signals, just as rubbing a stubbed toe generates pleasurable signals that compete with pain messengers. Doctors also use electrical stimulation in areas of the brain and spinal cord where the natural opiates are known to be concentrated, in order to trigger the release of endorphins.

Ruth Faulk had severe, intractable pain in her hand and arm which affected virtually everything she did, even driving. In late 1984, Dr. Ronald Young, a neurosurgeon at the University of Southern California, implanted a permanent electrical stimulation device into the limbic system of her brain. At a meeting at the National Institutes of Health several months later, Faulk said she felt great relief after her operation and had even resumed working on one of her favorite hobbies—needlework.

Electrical stimulation of nerves under the skin (subcutaneous nerves) has been practiced since the early 1950s, and may be the best way to prompt production of the natural opiates. Dr. Robert Heath of Tulane University was the first researcher to implant electrical stimulation devices in the brains of patients with severe chronic pain and psychotic disorders. These "brain pacemakers," placed directly on the cerebellum, the part of the brain that originates pain signals, produced mild electric shocks that brought significant pain relief in many of the chronic pain patients.

In a way, those seminal studies presaged the discovery of receptors and endorphins. "In those studies it turned out that the pain/pleasure systems were in inverse relationship," Heath says. "Stimulating the pleasure sites automatically inhibited the pain sites, and vice versa. If we stimulated the pleasure system, violent psychotics stopped having rage attacks. All of this makes sense: When you're feeling pleasure, you don't feel angry; and when you're in a rage, you certainly can't feel pleasure."

One of the most comprehensive studies was undertaken at the University of California at San Francisco. One-third of 141 chronic pain patients who had had deep-brain electrical stimulation devices for an average of 4 years—and as long as 12 years in a few patients—felt pain relief from the devices. This figure is low, but these are patients who have failed to find relief from painkillers, psychotherapy, TENS devices, and other treatments.

Do It Yourself Relief

For chronic pain sufferers who would like to take as much of their treatment as possible into their own hands, techniques like bio-feedback and hypnosis, which require strong commitment from the patient and can often be practiced at home, are gaining in popularity. These techniques can be as involved and sophisticated as the patient wishes, but their "do it yourself" nature is appealing to the many people who have failed to find long-term relief after many high tech (and high cost) treatments.

Biofeedback is one facet of a new discipline called behavioral medicine in which the patient learns to control certain body states—such as muscle contraction and blood pressure—that were previously thought to be autonomic, or involuntary. In biofeedback training, a patient uses information "fed back" by electronic sensing devices attached to the surface of the skin to learn how to change certain body processes voluntarily.

For instance, doctors have found that the hands and feet of migraine headache sufferers often become extremely cold just before an attack. With the help of biofeedback, a patient can learn to rapidly increase the temperature of these extremities and thereby offset or substantially reduce the severity of the migraine. (This body-warming technique has been used for centuries by Tibetan monks living high in the Himalayas, who have long been known by Western physicians to be able to consciously raise the temperatures of cold hands and feet by several degrees.)

A migraine sufferer can learn pain-relieving techniques at a biofeedback clinic. During a typical session, the patient lies down and electrodes covered with a conducting fluid are attached to his or her forehead. The electrodes are connected to an *electromyograph (EMG) machine*, which monitors muscle tension. The patient hears a high-pitched tone that indicates tension. The biofeedback trainer will then begin describing a series of pleasant scenes to help the patient relax. Soon the tone begins to drop as the muscles relax and tension ebbs away. The process is very simple and, usually after initial training, can be done at home with simple, temperature-sensing devices that cost as little as a quarter.

Soon, the first thing a person may do in the morning after turning off the alarm clock will be to check the condition of his or her body using biofeedback. According to Tom Budzynski, clinical director of the Biofeedback Institute in Denver, Colorado, "You'd wake up in the morning and plug yourself into a device that would tell you what in your body needs to be adjusted to maintain optimal health. You could wear the device like a wristwatch. It would sound a warning whenever a physiological system went out of a 'normal' range."

Besides chronic lower back pain and migraine headaches, biofeedback has been used successfully in the treatment of stroke paralysis, epileptic seizures, hyperkinetic behavior in children, and even the zero-g motion sickness experienced by astronauts. And biofeedback training has helped sufferers of phantom limb pain, the most bizarre chronic pain syndrome of all, in which an amputee will "feel" intense pain in the missing appendage. As many as 80 percent of amputees suffer at some time from the disorder, which doctors believe may be due to muscle spasms in the stump.

Like biofeedback, hypnosis induces a state of profound relaxation, and the technique is also beginning to gain wide repute in the orthodox medical establishment. Skeptics have denounced hypnotism ever since the days of Franz Mesmer, the eighteenth-century German physician who was expelled from Vienna and Paris for practicing the hypnotic treatment later called mesmerism. Today, numerous physicians practice hypnosis, with much success.

Hypnosis has been used in treating severe burns, chronic lower back pain, migraine headaches, and cancer pain. As it has no side effects, it can be a good substitute for anesthesia, and has controlled pain during orthopedic, cosmetic, and eye surgery.

Most often a hypnotist or a doctor trained in hypnosis will talk to a patient in order to induce a trancelike state. "We don't put people under," claims Dr. David Colvin, a psychiatrist at West Virginia University. "Hypnosis is a natural phenomenon which people already do. They just don't realize they do it. For example, riding down the highway and not remembering the last 2 miles. It's a state of focused awareness, increased relaxation."

For those who would rather put themselves under, self-hypnosis can be just as effective as hypnosis by a specialist. In 1984, an 8-

year-old boy from Pueblo, Colorado, suffered burns over 35 percent of his body when hot grease spilled on him. Doctors taught him how to hypnotize himself during the painful skin graft procedures.

"What leads to the greatest damage and pain for these patients is not the burn itself but the body's reaction to the burn—the inflammation and swelling," says Dr. Martin Orne, director of the Unit for Experimental Psychiatry at the Institute of Pennsylvania Hospital. "Research now underway suggests that it may be possible to hold back the body's response to burns through hypnosis, and thereby reduce the painful swelling."

Healing Touch

Various modern forms of "the laying on of hands" have been experimented with during the past few years. Perhaps the most controversial of these is *therapeutic touch*, a pain-relief technique that relies on the electromagnetic energy given off by the human body.

According to Dolores Krieger, the nursing Ph.D. who developed the technique in 1968 and has taught the process to thousands of health professionals, therapeutic touch helps postoperative patients heal themselves. A trained therapist moves his or her hands up and down the patient's body about 4 to 6 inches above the skin surface, searching for aberrations in the "energy fields." Once these abnormalities are located, the practitioner can then redirect energy away from or toward the affected spot. The therapist does this by concentrating intensely and using specialized hand movements, thereby stabilizing the flow of energy and accelerating the healing process.

The theory that the laying on of hands involves some sort of energy transfer gained support after a series of carefully controlled studies at McGill University in Montreal. These experiments, undertaken by biochemist Bernard Grad, showed that the rate of healing in mice and the rate of growth of plants could be accelerated through a therapeutic touch technique in which, again, no actual physical contact was made. In the mouse experiments, the actual touching was done to the container in which the animals lived. In the plant studies, the treatment was applied to the flask of salt water

used to water the seedlings. Dr. Grad concluded that because the
healer never actually touched the mice or the plants, "it must be
assumed that some physical agent, an energy, was responsible for
the effects."

Whether an energy transfer or some as yet unexplained phenomenon takes place, "We should not ignore the technique just
because we don't know exactly how it works," insists Dr. Janet
Quinn of the University of South Carolina at Columbia, the first
recipient of a federal grant to study the technique. "Perhaps it's
just ritual. But much of mainstream medicine is probably ritual
that focuses the patient's attention on what is needed to get well.
Maybe now we need to find rituals—like therapeutic touch—that
are less invasive than the usual treatments used in medical care."

Acupressure

The appellation "therapeutic touch" is a bit of a misnomer, as the
practitioner does not touch the patient. Two pain-relief techniques
that involve actual physical manipulation of the body and that can
be particularly effective in treating chronic low-back pain are *acupressure* and *massage*. Acupressure is acupuncture with fingers
instead of needles. While acupressure uses the points of acupuncture to relieve pain, massage goes directly to the external pain area
itself to get at the root of the pain. By rubbing, stroking, kneading,
and creating friction, a masseur or masseuse can invigorate tired
skin tissues and muscles and improve circulation.

Two other hands-on techniques to relieve pain are *chiropractic*
and *osteopathy*. Chiropractic is the second largest system of health
care in the world; only allopathic (the name given to standard
Western medical practice) health care is larger. Chiropractors believe that pain results primarily from abnormal functioning of the
nervous system. By repositioning the nerves around the spinal column, often by a vigorous wrenching of various parts of the body,
they believe that the pain can be alleviated or eliminated. Chiropractors occasionally use other chronic pain treatments, such as
electrical nerve stimulation. People should be aware that chiropractors are not M.D.s.

Similarly, osteopaths hold that most pain is caused by a poorly aligned skeletal arrangement, and that an adjustment of the bones will alleviate the pain. As osteopaths rely mostly on manipulation and drugs, pain relief is often short-lived, but many people with lower back pain find that the treatments allow them to resume a normal life.

Music Medicine

As a boy of 10, Charles Lanning had to fight a fierce battle against Hodgkin's disease. On the eve of his twenty-eighth birthday, he was told that he would have to fight cancer again, this time another, unrelated form of lymphoma even harder to treat. He returned to New York's Memorial Sloan-Kettering Cancer Center, hardly able to believe it was happening a second time. He became depressed as the pain worsened, feeling that he had no control over his life or his disease.

Lucanne Bailey came to the rescue. A full-time music therapist at Sloan-Kettering, Bailey, like a growing number of pain therapists around the country, plays music to divert the minds of cancer patients from their pain. She sang and played guitar, and for Lanning, it was the best medicine. "In spite of all the medication, you have to be able to take your mind off pain and onto other things," he says. "I can lose myself in the music." After returning home, Lanning bought a guitar and began singing with his wife, Tammy.

Music therapy does not have to be live to be effective. In a study at the Dusznikachzdroju Medical Center in Poland, 408 patients suffering from severe headaches and painful neurological diseases were split into two groups. The first group listened periodically to symphonic music, while the other group did not. After 6 months, the first group required far fewer painkillers than the control group.

Some music therapists are so skilled at diagnosing exactly what a patient needs that some patients—from post-op patients to terminally ill cancer patients—can stop taking painkillers. Researchers believe that painkilling endorphins may be released when the brain's pleasure center is titillated by the aesthetic sensations of the music.

"I Shall Please"

It has long been known that a patient's expectations of relief from pain aid in that relief substantially. Faith healing still takes place in many parts of the world, with witch doctors holding the most respected place in the social hierarchy.

Modern researchers know the effects of faith healing as the placebo effect. "Placebo" is Latin for "I shall please." Research has shown that 33 of 100 patients suffering severe post-operative pain feel marked relief when given a placebo—usually an inert substance such as a sugar pill—which they think is a true analgesic.

Pain researchers at the University of California at San Francisco suggest that placebo pills may have a physical as well as a psychological effect. They may, in some cases, trigger the release of endorphins. Why would placebos produce a natural opiate response in some people and not in others? Pain experts believe stress may be the key, because patients under extreme stress react best to placebos and because the natural opiate beta-endorphin and the stress hormone ACTH are released simultaneously by the pituitary gland. Regardless of why, the one-third who respond to placebos can continue to reap the rewards of ardent, if misplaced, faith.

Reliable Relief

Painkillers have been the number one method of relieving pain since the fifth century B.C., when the Greek physician Hippocrates—"the Father of Medicine"—first told women in labor to chew willow leaves to relieve the pain. The leaves contain salicilin, the naturally occurring form of salicylic acid, the principal pain-relieving ingredient in aspirin.

Today, Americans spend $1.4 billion a year on mild analgesics such as aspirin, acetaminophen, and ibuprofen—the latter only recently available without a prescription. Aspirin has been tried and proven in over 100 years of continuous use (one estimate holds that Americans swallow 90 million aspirin tablets daily). But researchers have only recently begun to understand how the substance works.

Aspirin is believed to block the synthesis of prostaglandins, hormone-like substances released at the site of an injury. Prostaglandins perform a number of duties. They induce inflammation, as well as prompting nerve fibers to release chemicals that activate electrical messengers. These messengers then travel to the brain in the form of pain signals. Aspirin may also block synthesis of pain signals once they have reached the spinal cord.

Acetominophen has the same safe, effective pain relief action as aspirin, but does not curb inflammation, so experts believe that it does not operate at the wound site by inhibiting the action of prostaglandins. Instead, it orchestrates the blockage of pain signals in the spinal cord.

Ibuprofen is the first new analgesic for nonprescription use to be approved by the FDA in 30 years. It is sold over the counter as Advil or Nuprin. Tests have shown that it is at least as effective as aspirin in relieving pain and reducing inflammation, but it has been implicated in several side effects, some of them severe. Like aspirin, it seems to block the action of prostaglandins. But prostaglandins help the kidneys work effectively and if people with diabetes and hypertension take two or more ibuprofen tablets per day, says Dr. Leslie Dornfeld of the University of California at Los Angeles, they could have acute kidney failure. People who can take aspirin may be allergic to ibuprofen and should check with their physician before taking the medication.

Super Drugs

The seventeenth-century British physician Sir Thomas Sydenham once stated that "of all the remedies which the almighty God has seen fit to bestow upon mankind, none is so universal or so efficacious a remedy as opium." Indeed, if it were not for dangerous side effects like sedation, buildup of tolerance, and addiction, no drug or pain-relief method would ever replace narcotics like morphine for the relief of severe pain.

For many chronic pain sufferers, such side effects can be far worse than the pain itself, and so other treatments are preferred. But for terminal cancer patients with intractable pain, morphine and opium are often the only hope for relief. When a person has such a short time to live, side effects such as addiction are unimportant; the pain must be stopped.

New techniques for applying these high-powered drugs have been introduced in recent years. Physicians at Houston's M.D. Anderson Hospital and Tumor Institute are injecting opiates directly into the brain, where pain is felt. A tiny hole is drilled in the skull above the forehead to create a reservoir for the painkilling substance. Once a day, the drug is injected. The hole is then covered by a flap of skin and a wig.

Other medical centers, including the Mayo Clinic in Rochester, Minnesota, inject opiates directly into the cerebrospinal fluid surrounding the spinal cord, through which pain signals pass on their way to the brain. The technique yields great pain relief with no apparent effect on motor function or consciousness.

Another new technique for relieving terminal cancer pain that is gaining wide support is *patient-controlled analgesia* (PCA), in which patients suffering from severe pain administer their own doses of morphine and other opiates. Studies have shown that patients using PCA can control their pain more effectively using lower doses of medication, because they can treat the pain at the onset rather than when it has become unbearable.

Killer Drugs

Warnings about controversial new drugs like ibuprofen are justified. In August, 1982, a rheumatoid arthritis drug called *Oraflex* (*benoxaprofen*), which had been heralded by its manufacturers prior to release as a "miracle drug," was suddenly withdrawn from the market after reports linked it with 61 deaths in England and 33 deaths in America. The miracle drug had become a killer drug, causing acute kidney and liver failure in some of its elderly users.

In the 1970s *Butazolidin* (*phenylbutazone*) and *Tandearil* (*oxyphenbutazone*) were considered miracle drugs for pains ranging from arthritis to sprains. But the Public Citizen's Health Research Group estimates these two drugs have killed 3,000 Americans—a death rate of approximately 120 per million users. According to the

Drug and Therapeutics Bulletin, a British publication for physicians, "Ample data incriminate both drugs in fatal bone marrow depression and other serious hazards. Between them they have caused well over 1,000 deaths in Britain."

Fears about the side effects of painkilling drugs have kept many supposed miracle workers off the market. Perhaps the most well known sure-cure drug in this country to get a bad rap from the FDA is *dimethyl sulfoxide (DMSO),* an industrial solvent. Dr. Stanley W. Jacob, associate professor of surgery at the University of Oregon, first used the oily, colorless liquid—a cheap by-product of the wood and pulp industry—in 1962 to prevent cellular damage while deep-freezing kidneys for storage. Jacob and others soon found that the substance could be used to treat headaches, sinusitis, arthritis, and mild burns. When rubbed into the skin, DMSO appeared to do away with severe bruises literally overnight.

More than 100,000 people had used DMSO for chronic pain and other disorders—with great apparent success—when it was banned by the FDA in 1965 because test animals given large doses of DMSO had suffered irreversible eye damage. In humans, the worst side effects so far have been itchy skin and occasional nausea, but many people swear by it.

Even so, the FDA still holds out against DMSO, and two decades after its therapeutic use was first discovered by Dr. Jacobs, the drug remains illegal for use in musculoskeletal injuries or arthritis.

Pain Clinics

Martha was a 51-year-old Los Angeles homemaker and mother of five when she began suffering from severe pain in her neck, back, and abdomen following two automobile accidents. She lost 34 pounds and took large doses of antidepressants before enrolling at the pain clinic program at the University of California at Los Angeles.

She participated in group therapy sessions and acupuncture classes and learned relaxation techniques. Afterward, her weight returned to normal and she stopped taking so many drugs. She realized that household responsibilities were adding to her pain, and she began using the relaxation procedures taught at the clinic to help her cope with those responsibilities. "I am cutting down on the amount of input I get from other people," Martha says. "I realize that adds pressure and causes some of my pain. I'm feeling much better."

Pain clinics have been helping people solve physical and psychological problems ever since 1960, when Dr. John Bonica opened the first multidisciplinary chronic pain clinic in the United States in Seattle. Now there are approximately 150 around the world, mostly connected with large hospitals or medical colleges. Specialty clinics, which treat one type of chronic pain, such as backache, also exist throughout the country.

Treatment at a chronic pain clinic usually begins with a thorough psychological, physical, neurologic, and orthopedic checkup by specialists in the field. If a physical cause of pain such as a slipped disc is diagnosed, the patient is usually referred to a surgeon or other specialist. Otherwise, treatment proceeds in-house, often beginning with weaning the patient off painkilling drugs.

The staffs of chronic pain clinics may include neurophysiologists, psychiatrists, physical therapists, neurosurgeons—and the clinics may offer treatments ranging from biofeedback to electrical stimulation. A comprehensive list of these clinics can be found in this chapter's Access Guide.

=Timeline=

1987 to 1990
- DMSO approved by FDA for general use.
- Heroin cleared by Congress for use in treatment of severe pain.
- Direct link between stress and pain systems in the brain found.
- Most hospitals and all pain clinics use hypnosis regularly.
- Therapeutic touch gains new respect as electromagnetic link between healer and the healed proven.

1991 to 1995
- At-home acupuncture kit introduced.
- Every major hospital now has a pain clinic.
- Biofeedback devices to check the body's systems in every home.
- D-phenylalanine (DPA) pill introduced.
- Dynorphin drug synthesized that stops pain in spinal column before it's "felt" in the brain.
- Computer that designs optimal music therapy program for each chronic pain sufferer is now used in pain clinics.
- Tricyclic antidepressants, used for minor pain, available over the counter.

1996 to 2000
- Deep-brain electrode implants widely used.
- Robot massager developed for lower back pain.
- Hand-held, low-power laser available by prescription for migraine sufferers.
- Nonaddicting endorphin pill introduced.

2001 to 2010
- Home-med robot marketed that uses biofeedback, hypnosis, and electrical stimulation to treat mild aches and pains.
- Imaging techniques release endorphins at will.

2100
- Chronic pain eradicated?

Access Guide

Here is a list of the top pain clinics in the country—both multidisciplinary and specialized. All patients must be referred by a physician, and complete medical histories must be provided. As diagnosis and treatment differ with each individual, costs must be discussed prior to treatment in most cases. Some initial consultation (IC) fees are listed, as are estimated costs of some of the more-structured programs.

Top Pain Clinics

Boston Pain Center
Spaulding Rehabilitation Hospital
125 Nashua Street
Boston, MA 02114
(617) 720-6669

Twenty-one bed inpatient program lasts 4–6 weeks. Outpatient program meets 3 nights per week. Treatments include detoxification, body mechanics, physical therapy, massage, electrical stimulation, biofeedback and relaxation techniques. Also individual, group, family, and vocational therapy.

Diamond Headache Clinic, Ltd.
Foster-Western Medical Building III
5252 N. Western Avenue
Chicago, IL 60625
(312) 878-5558

Treats mostly headache sufferers. Initial visit includes neurological examination, laboratory tests (blood chemistries, urinalysis, EKG, and thyroid testing). Inpatient treatment unit at Louis A. Weiss Memorial Hospital includes detoxification, psychological analysis, biofeedback, physical and recreation therapy.

Emory University Pain Control Center
Center for Rehabilitation Medicine
1441 Clifton Road, Northeast
Atlanta, GA 30322
(404) 329-5492

Drug detoxification, nerve blocks, transcutaneous electrical stimulation, biofeedback, physical and occupational therapy, relaxation exercises. Two types of programs: a compact 2-week program for patients outside driving distance from Atlanta and a 6-week program for those within driving distance of the center.

Johns Hopkins University School of Medicine
Pain Clinic
600 N. Wolfe Street
Baltimore, MD 21205
(301) 955-3270

Usually 3-week sessions, though custom-designed per individual. Treatment includes group therapy, drug awareness classes, relaxation and stress management, biofeedback, assertiveness training, exercise, and occupational therapy. Also nerve blocks and nerve stimulation.

Mayo Clinic
Rochester, MN 55905
(507) 284-8311

Treatments include nerve blocks, nerve stimulation, cryoanalgesia (freezing of nerve fibers), and drug prescription. Above usually combined with physical therapy and exercise program, social service and occupational therapy, drug detoxification program, and psychotherapy and behavioral modification.

Memorial Sloan-Kettering Cancer Center Pain Clinic
1275 York Avenue
New York, NY 10021
(212) 794-6594

Center for the study of cancer and neurologic pain. Concerned primarily with diagnosis of chronic pain, but also offer outpatient treatments. Treatments include nerve blocks and other drug treatments, electrical stimulation, and psychotherapy. Also inpatient consultation service.

Mount Sinai Medical Center
Pain Center
4300 Alton Road
Miami Beach, FL 33140
(305) 674-2070

Specializes in treatment of shingles (herpetic neuralgia), myofascial pain, lower back pain, and headaches. Treatment includes drugs (painkillers, tranquilizers, and antidepressants), physical exercise, hypnosis, massage, transcutaneous electrical stimulation, biofeedback, psychotherapy, acupuncture, and nerve blocks.

Mount Sinai Medical Center
Headache Clinic
1 Gustave Levy Place
New York, NY 10019
(212) 650-7691

Meets only Mondays and Wednesdays from 1-4 pm, but expert treatment for headaches. Neurological consultation, followed most often by pharmacological treatment.

New Hope Pain Centers, Inc.
55 E. California Boulevard
Pasadena, CA 91105
(818) 405-9944

Divided into three branches: individual outpatient pain clinic, inpatient services, and outpatient pain unit. Programs include medication management, psychotherapy, physical therapy, nervous system coordination training, skeletal muscle autonomic balance training, neuromuscular tone education, occupational therapy, recreation therapy, discharge planning, and follow-up.

New York University Medical Center
Pain Consultation Service
530 First Avenue
New York, NY 10016
(212) 340-7316

Specializes in nerve blocks: 25 to 30 different types available. Also nerve stimulation, minor and major analgesics, and physical therapy.

North Texas Back Institute
3801 W. 15th, Suite 100
Plano, TX 75075
(214) 867-2720

Multidisciplinary spine injury rehabilitation. Programs include psychological counseling, biofeedback, physical therapy, occupational therapy, hydrotherapy, extended exercise, industrial injury prevention programs, and hospital inpatient care.

Northwest Pain Center Associates
10615 S.E. Cherry Blossom Drive
Suite 170
Portland, OR 97216
(503) 256-1930

Fifteen-day session includes lecture and discussion groups, therapeutic exercises, posture classes, functional application, relaxation exercises, biofeedback, transcutaneous electrical stimulation, and vocational counseling.

Pain Treatment Center
Hotel Dieu Hospital
Dr. Donald E. Richardson
1415 Tulane Avenue
New Orleans, LA 70112
(504) 588-5561

Ten-bed inpatient facility. Treatments include drug detoxification, behavior modification, physical and occupational therapy, family counseling, diagnostic studies. Pain inhibiting procedures include transcutaneous nerve stimulation, spinal cord stimulation, and stimulation of pain inhibiting areas in the central nervous system.

The Rehabilitation Institute of Chicago
Pain Manangement Program
345 E. Superior Street
Chicago, IL 60611
(312) 649-6011

Four-week chronic pain inpatient treatment. Procedures include exercise, physical and occupational therapies. Also biofeedback and relaxation training, psychological counseling, vocational counseling, and other services.

UCLA Pain Management Center
Department of Anesthesiology
UCLA School of Medicine
Los Angeles, CA 90024
(213) 825-4292

Treatments include nerve blocks, transcutaneous electrical stimulation, acupuncture, physical therapy, detoxification, individual psychotherapy, and behavior modification, relaxation and self-hypnosis training, biofeedback, pain management classes, and limited inpatient services.

University of Nebraska Medical Center
Pain Management Center
42nd and Dewey Avenue
Omaha, NE 68105
(402) 559-4364

Ten-hour per day outpatient/day clinic. Treats people with brain injuries, brain dysfunction, and chronic pain syndromes. Treatments include drug detoxification, physical therapy programs, biofeedback, and relaxation techniques. Program usually lasts 4 weeks, though may be longer.

University of Washington RC-76
Pain Clinic
Seattle, WA 98195
(206) 548-4284

Outpatient clinic (5 days per week) and inpatient 10-day service in the University Hospital. "Screening evaluation" includes psychological tests, interviews and diagnosis. Three-week inpatient behaviorally-based pain management program includes didactic sessions, group and individual therapy, physical therapy, occupational therapy, vocational counseling, and assessment.

Walker Institute
1964 Westwood Boulevard
Los Angeles, CA 90025
(213) 475-6766

Neurological rehabilitation clinic for people with spinal cord injuries and other neurological disorders, including chronic pain and multiple sclerosis. Complete diagnostic facilities. Outpatient physical therapy program (soon to be inpatient) is 8 hours per day for 3 to 6 months, tailored to each individual. Laser stimulation also available.

Washington Pain Center
2026 R Street Northwest
Washington, D.C. 20009
(202) 387-4735

Outpatient treatments include detoxification, nerve blocks, electrical acupuncture, biofeedback, and hypnosis. Individual, group, family, and occupational therapy also available.

Washington Pain Assessment Group
5530 Wisconsin Avenue
Suite 806
Chevy Chase, MD 20815
(301) 951-4466

Full service outpatient pain management program, but inpatient services also available. Treatment includes biofeedback; physical and occupational therapy; individual, group, and family therapy; electrical stimulation; selective injections; acupressure; and individualized home exercise regimen.

Pain Associations

International Association for the Study of Pain
c/o Louise E. Jones, BS
Executive Officer
909 NE 43rd Street, Rm. 204
Seattle, WA 98105
(206) 547-6409

International nonprofit organization to foster research of pain mechanisms
and pain syndromes. For scientists, physicians, and other health professionals interested in pain research and management. Membership is $20
plus suggested dues on basis of income. Monthly journal *Pain* and periodic
IASP newsletter included with membership.

8

Off the Disabled List: Medicine for Tomorrow's Athlete

"There's nothin' wrong with muscles," quipped Mae West. "And they're useful for bein' able to open cans and beat the men back from the door." They're also useful for winning an olympic medal or breaking a world record. But as the drive for perfection in sport has evolved, so has our understanding of what it takes to be an elite athlete. Muscles alone do not a champion make.

The Russians were the first to delve into the uncharted territory of the physiology and psychology of athletic achievement, the explorations were part of their space program in the 1950s. Natural talent, they learned, was only one component in a circuit board of skills that pushed an athlete from competence to greatness. Drawing on the tradition of the martial arts, Soviets trained their athletes' minds as well as their bodies. They experimented with drugs to increase muscle strength, and developed methods for matching young athletic performers with the sport that best suited their builds. The Soviets, in other words, learned how to make superior athletes. The world of sport had entered a new age.

It didn't take long before Western countries followed suit, putting more time and research dollars into sports medicine, a field that had once been concerned solely with the treatment of sports injuries. Today, sports medicine encompasses the whole spectrum of athletic endeavor—training regimens, mind calisthenics, reconstructive surgery, and rehabilitative techniques. Once the territory of orthopedic surgeons, sports medicine is now populated with general practitioners, podiatrists, physiologists, and psychologists. With the fitness boom, the field has grown to meet the demands of countless joggers, bikers, tennis players, and other amateur athletes who find that a regular physical workout adds to their sense of well-being. Today there's even a sports medicine hotline that provides general information and referrals to sports enthusiasts across the country.

In this chapter we'll take a look at some of the more innovative facets of sports medicine, everything from the biomechanics of throwing a baseball to the physiology of running, from the brain wave activity of an Olympic archer to the mental imagining techniques of an amateur golfer. We'll also show you what's in store for the twenty-first century.

Back in the Race

She looked calm, almost serene, as she pulled ahead of the pack. Her dark hair was wet with sweat and with the water she had sprayed on it along the way. But her stride was steady. That was the main thing. The ease with which Joan Benoit won the marathon at the 1984 Olympic games masked the rough, at times seemingly endless, road she had run to get there.

Just two months before the Olympic trials, Benoit was plagued with a debilitating pain in her right knee. She was given cortisone shots and another anti-inflammatory drug which provided only temporary relief. Repeatedly, she broke into tears during her training runs. She was ready to go home and forget about the Olympics. But Stan James, an orthopedic surgeon Benoit consulted, thought her condition could be reversed. On April 17, just 25 days before the qualifying run, James performed arthroscopic surgery on Benoit's knee, removing a small section of collagen fibers that appeared to be the source of her pain.

Since its development in the 1970s, the *arthroscope*, a small fiber-optical device that's inserted through a pencil-size opening made in the knee, has helped countless athletes return to their sports. By attaching a miniature television camera to the arthroscope, doctors are able to see the inside of the knee on a monitor and can perform delicate operations without cutting open the entire joint, thus minimizing swelling and reducing recovery time. Benoit was able to return to her training after only 5 days.

Perhaps she returned too soon. On a training run, Benoit strained
her left hamstring. "I overcompensated with the other leg," she
explains. Before she could pack her bags and head back home to
Maine, Benoit heard about an unusual treatment that might give
her yet another chance. The treatment utilized an electro-acuscope,
an instrument that speeds the healing process bv administering
low levels of electricity to the ailing muscle. Knowing she had
nothing to lose, Benoit underwent treatment. Four days before the
olympic trials she ran 17 miles without any problem. She went on
to qualify for the Olympics and on the hot, sunny day of August 5,
1984—the day of the first Olympic marathon for women—it was
hard to believe that Joan Benoit had ever had a problem running
at all.

Ten years ago, Joan Benoit's injuries would have prevented her
from winning the gold medal, but today her story is just another
account of a sports medicine success. All of the liabilities of competitive sports—runner's knee, volleyball necks, pitching shoulders, tennis elbows—stand a good chance of being put back in
order quickly thanks to advances in medical treatment.

The most common and generally debilitating injuries among athletes involve ligaments, the connective tissues that link bones to
one another. Knee ligaments suffer the hardest knocks in competitive athletics and are often the cause of early retirement. Fifteen
years ago, a serious knee injury usually meant the end of an athletic
career.

But athletes' chances for recovery from a knee injury have increased dramatically in the past few years, primarily because physicians have learned to diagnose problems with greater accuracy.

Three-dimensional computer analysis of the joint has made the
difference. Historically the knee was thought to operate like a hinge
with just one motion, backwards and forwards. Now doctors think
of it more as an airplane in flight: It can go up and down, or move
sideways. It can also roll and pitch. A new machine called the
Genucom can track the motions of the knee in those three dimen-
sions, giving doctors the equivalent of an electrocardiogram
(EKG)—actually called a Knee-K-G—of the joint. Because ligaments control the knee's movements, this new analytical tool, along

with manual examination of the joint, can reveal exactly which ligament has been injured.

Left alone, ligaments can take years to repair themselves and will never be as sturdy as they were before the trauma. If the ligament has been torn from the bone, however, it must be reattached surgically. "I tell my patients," says Dr. Frank Noyes, director of Cincinnati Sportsmedicine/The Midwest Institute for Orthopaedics, "that tearing one of these major ligaments is just like pulling a tree out of the ground. If we can reimplant it right on the spot from which it was pulled, we can heal it 80 to 95 percent of the time."

Unfortunately, athletes sometimes tear a ligament repeatedly. "Trying to suture it then is like trying to suture spaghetti," Dr. Noyes explains. Instead, he and other surgeons use a graft made of tissue from the patient or a cadaver. Called a "stint," this type of graft supports and adds strength to the damaged ligament. With it, surgeons hope to eventually be able to build ligaments that have at least 70 percent of their original strength.

Another major breakthrough in ligament repair came 3 years ago when surgeons first began implanting ligaments made from synthetics. As with the grafts, artificial ligaments are attached inside the knee using the arthroscope. The damaged ligament is first removed and then its artificial replacement is attached to the bones with tiny screws. If the synthetic substitute is attached even slightly out of place, however, normal stresses can tear it loose. To guard against this, surgeons use a special computer image that indicates within 2 or 3 millimeters where the ligament must be placed.

Although the short-term success of the artificial ligament has been good, surgeons use it only as a last resort. In part this is because artificial ligaments are made of fabric, and surgeons feel that the material may not wear well over time. "The big problem is with the people who have an artificial ligament implant and want to go skiing again," Noyes says. "Will the ligament survive that kind of stress? We don't yet know."

In the next 10 years, however, researchers will create ligament material capable of withstanding the stress of athletic competition. The same synthetic ligaments will be implanted in other joints, including the shoulder. Also on the horizon for improved knee care is the demise of the cast. Doctors are finding that moving a joint and putting some weight on it after surgery actually speeds the healing process. But the most important breakthrough in ligament repair will come 25 to 50 years from now, when researchers learn to accelerate healing by injecting a chemical directly into a cell which instructs the cell to produce collagen, a protein that helps build cartilage, bone, tendons, and ligaments.

Similarly, researchers have made headway in repairing soft tissue injuries, such as ruptured tendons. Experimental work at the Nova Scotia Sport Medicine Clinic indicates that damaged tendons respond favorably to electrical stimulation. Doctors at Nova Scotia Clinic wrap damaged tendons with a wire that's connected to a small electrical stimulator outside the body. Then they pulse a steady current to the injured site. Not only does this speed the healing of the tendon, but it also allows the patient to regain mobility more quickly (no cast is used). And a tendon treated in this fashion regains more of its original strength than one repaired surgically —without the benefit of electrical stimulation.

The next 10 to 20 years will see the perfection of these techniques. Athletes once benched because of a strained or ruptured tendon will find themselves back in the competition in world record time.

Biomechanics

Along with new medical treatments has come an emphasis on prevention. Specialists have found that by paying attention to an athlete's biomechanics (the way his or her body moves during athletic performance), they can help the athletes avoid many injuries entirely. Athletes who apply the principles of engineering to the human body can tailor their movements for increased efficiency and power. As Gideon Ariel, a pioneer in the field of biomechanics put it, "People are subject to the same physical laws as bridges."

The roots of biomechanical analysis go back to the 1930s when coaches started filming sports events and then "reviewing" an athlete's performance to help improve the person's game. Today, high-seed film and video analysis has a place in almost every sport and, in tandem with computer analysis, is useful in keeping numerous athletes off the operating table. A professional baseball pitcher, for instance, is less likely today than ever before to have an injury treated surgically.

Dr. Paul Bower, an orthopedic surgeon and consultant to the San Diego Padres, has led a personal crusade for the past 5 years to improve pitchers' biomechanics. "If a pitcher had a real bad problem with his elbow," Bower explains, "we can give him a cortisone shot to relieve the pain. But what good will that do if we don't also check his biomechanics? If it's the way he delivers the ball that's causing the pain, a cortisone shot won't help in the long run."

The process Bower and others use to check a pitcher's biomechanics involves a film or tape of the player in action and a complicated computer analysis of the motion. The computer, in a process called digitizing, translates the athlete's movements into stick figures on a computer screen. The figures reveal details impossible to see on ordinary film. Every factor involved in throwing the ball is charted onto the computer, allowing the pitcher to witness his pitching motion. It shows the angle of the arm when it releases the ball, the placement of weight on each foot during the pitching motion, and the position of the body during each part of the windup. "The best pitchers know how to change their biomechanics," Bower says. "But for some, too many changes or a major alteration will throw them off psychologically. We have to be careful. Our real goal is to teach young pitchers how to throw efficiently from the beginning."

Another important tool for biomechanical analysis is the force platform, a device that measures the forces generated when the foot contacts a surface. By walking on a force platform, athletes can see whether they are walking on the inside or outside of their foot, if they are striding evenly, and how much weight is being put on each leg. Favoring one side over another or an unequal distribution of weight can cause injuries, especially among race walkers and runners. But using the platform can also improve performance. In a study conducted with archers, researchers discovered that every time an archer scored a 10, he or she was leaning into the target. When they scored lower, they were leaning on their back foot. Once aware of the subtle shifting of weight, an archer can correct the movement for improved performance. The *electrodynogram (EDG)*, which measures the forces on the foot inside the shoe, is also used in biomechanical analysis. The EDG equipment consists of 14 small discs attached to the soles of the feet; wires connect the discs to a recording device strapped around the athlete's waist. When the athlete walks or runs, the EDG measures how stress is distributed through the foot. Ideally, pressure is distributed evenly, but if the foot turns inward (pronation) or outward (suppination), this can lead to injuries. Podiatrists are using the EDG for both the athletic and nonathletic patient, often correcting problems by constructing special devices called *orthotics* to equalize the pressure on the foot. An EDG examination is already commonplace for athletes and, in the future, may become a mainstay of every orthopedic examination.

Sudden Death and the Runner's High

"Fewer and fewer people these days argue that running shortens lives, while a lot of people say that it may lengthen them," wrote author James Fixx, whose books on running made him a national celebrity. At age 36, he had taken to the road to avoid his father's fate—death from heart disease at 43. Running made him feel better, ended his cigarette habit, decreased his weight, and improved his outlook on life. But in July, 1984, during a 10-mile run along the back roads of Vermont, the 52-year-old fitness icon died of a heart attack. His sudden death caused concern, however unjustified, among the growing number of joggers who believed that exercise could only improve their health, not endanger it.

In fact, deaths from jogging are rare. For middle-aged men and women without coronary disease, the risk is small: About 1 in 5 million for men and 1 in 17 million for women. But the odds change for those with bad hearts. One study found that death rates for men and women with heart disease were much higher among those who jogged than those who engaged in sedentary activities. Other research, however, suggests that moderate activity benefits people recovering from heart attacks. It appears to be a matter of degree.

Exercise can help fight the buildup of fat in blood vessels, but for individuals whose habits and heredity place them at high risk, it may be dangerous. That's because once arteries have been clogged, heavy exercise may force the heart to work harder than it's capable of doing in order to supply enough blood. A heart attack may be the result of this increased effort.

Strenuous exercise has also been implicated in a phenomenon called post-exercise sudden death. The syndrome is believed to occur when the body misinterprets the sudden drop in blood pressure after exercise as a sign of impending shock. It immediately releases a flood of two hormones—adrenaline and norepinephrine —that stimulate the heart. In individuals with coronary problems, the flood may cause a heart attack. Harvard Medical School's Joel Dimsdale, one of the leading researchers into the phenomenon, cautions people to cool down slowly after vigorous exercise. "Walk for several minutes before sitting down," he explains. "This will lower blood pressure gradually, decreasing the hormonal response."

For healthy fitness buffs, however, the risks of heavy exercise take a backseat to its "highs," most particularly the so-called runner's high. This euphoria experienced during a workout has yet to be documented scientifically. Nevertheless, endorphins have been shown to act as analgesics and to produce a sense of euphoria, and until recently it was thought that exercise increased the body's output of the chemicals. But several new studies reveal that blocking the release of endorphins doesn't prevent the runner's high. And not every runner who shows high levels of endorphins in the bloodstream experiences the mood change. The high may occur primarily in athletes whose constant training allows circulating endorphins to penetrate the brain.

Dr. Otto Appenzeller of the University of New Mexico's School of Medicine suggests that the runner's high may result from a combination of physiological changes. "It's probably a very personal experience, unique to each individual," he observes. "It's a feeling that may depend on a number of things." Endorphins and the hormone vasopressin, which increases blood flow in the brain, may both play a role. When lactic acid is released during muscular contractions, vasopressin is also released. "Several factors that we don't understand might have to come together at the right time and in the right sequence before they produce the runner's high," Appenzeller says.

The charting of the mechanisms which produce the runner's high is expected to be complete by the end of the second decade of the twenty-first century. This investigation will have applications outside of sports medicine. Several studies have shown that runners have a much higher pain threshold after they run than before, suggesting a future treatment for sufferers of chronic pain. Because many patients who live with prolonged and unrelenting pain have no physical malady that causes their pain, they are prime candidates for the analgesic effects of exercise. An endorphin-producing exercise may one day be used for relief from pain caused by a specific athletic injury, if the exercise can be performed without further damaging the injured site. In the coming century, the harnessing of the brain's natural opiates will be a key factor in keeping patients healthy and pain-free.

Sports Psychology

"Once you reach a certain level," said Olympic gold medalist Evelyn Ashford, "sprinting is mostly psychological." She might have said the same thing about any athletic endeavor. For years sports psychology was limited to coaches pep talks and vague ideas about the importance of getting "psyched." But psychology is becoming an integral part of every sport.

Gymnasts, pole vaulters, football players, cross country skiers, and even the weekend jogger have enlisted the aid of sports counselors to teach them psychological skills. A number of professional baseball players use hypnotists to help them over a slump or to improve their attitudes. The North American Society for the Psychology of Sport and Physical Activity began in 1966 with a handful of members. It now has almost 500. And the U.S. Olympic Committee enlisted the services of numerous sports psychologists to work with athletes for the 1984 Olympics.

Sports psychologists tend to focus more on getting the mind in shape for peak performance than on helping athletes who have emotional problems. "We deal with anything from strategies used to run a race to coping with anxiety or the fear of failure," says Craig Wrisherg, a physical education professor at the University of Tennessee. Many sports psychologists, in fact, are not clinical psychologists but psychological educators trained in physical education. Others are involved in research, looking into the effect exercise and athletic competition have on the mind.

The emotional stress of competing can sometimes overwhelm a competitor and give rise to obsessive behavior. Eating disorders, for instance, are common in the athletic population. Obsessions with body fat can produce anorexic behavior. "I've even seen some teenage athletes pick their noses and let it bleed to lose weight." says Glen Johnson, an assistant professor at the Center for Youth Fitness and Sports Research at the University of Nebraska. An article in *The New England Journal of Medicine* reported that one group of runners with eating disorders also exhibited psychological problems. They had trouble expressing anger and showed a tendency toward depression. In addition, they had extraordinarily high self-expectations, especially in athletics.

One of the biggest hurdles for athletes, psychologists are finding, is realistic goal setting. Many times anxiety, poor concentration, and lack of self-confidence interfere with athletic performance. "Many athletes only goal is to win, which is an unrealistic goal when you're competing," explains Rainer Martens, a physical education professor at the University of Illinois. No one, he adds, is entirely responsible for winning. The opposition, environmental factors and luck also determine the outcome of a competition. "Athletes should set goals for their own performance and focus their attention on achieving those performance goals," Martens says. In other words, during the process of striving to win an athlete should not concentrate on winning, but on giving his or her best effort.

Martens firmly believes that the best athletes of the future will be the ones who have mastered their minds. Athletes who learn how to arouse themselves without becoming anxious, to maintain a concentrated internal state and relax into their actions, will be the ones who break the records.

But how can an athlete learn to do this? Many sports psychologists think the answer lies in making pictures in the mind. "When I'm going to sleep at night," says 60-year-old Mary Shaw, who is a weekend golfer, "I start playing the course. I tee off on the first hole, and watch to see where the ball lands. Then I putt it into the hole and move onto the second. I get such great scores, it's thrilling. The only problem is I usually fall asleep on the fourth hole."

Mary Shaw will never be a competitor in the U.S. Open, but by learning some new psychological skills, including the ability to "image" (imagine) her game, she has become a much better amateur player. In 1984, she met J. Brian Hennessey, a doctoral student in neuropsychology and education at Stanford University. Hennessey, an athlete himself, guided her through an unusual training regimen that improves sports performance by "remodeling" the mind.

"I've always played better after watching the pros," says Shaw. "But it only lasted a little while. Before I knew it I'd be right back to my old habits." Hennessey's program is designed to leave a longer-lasting imprint. At Psykon Achievement Systems, Inc. in Palo Alto, he has established what may, in the future, be a commonplace type of psychological training center. As part of the regimen, Hennessey uses flotation tanks equipped with a video screen and speakers. (A flotation tank looks like a large, enclosed bathtub and is filled with a saline solution. In it, a person can relax completely and float without sensory interference from the outside world.)

While Shaw was relaxing in the tank, she viewed a videotape of world-class golfer Al Geiberger. After she had watched different strokes for several minutes, the film was shut off and Hennessey guided her through an imaginary game. "In my mind's eye," Shaw explains, "I played the first hole at my local club. I saw myself playing, heard the ball being hit and tasted the well-hit ball. To me, it tasted like cinnamon." The imagery session helped to create a visceral memory of good golf, which Shaw contends still helps her on the links.

Hennessey sees the tank and videotape as a temporary training device. "You're meant to create your own tapes and leave the video behind," he says. The most important aspect of these mental tapes, however, is the editing. "I try to teach people how to edit their memory so that they remember the things they do right, not wrong," he says. "People have to learn how to image to achieve. Most people only know how to image to fail."

Hennessey teaches imaging to succeed with a three-step skill exercise: replay, reform, create. Athletes must learn to replay each step of their game, imagine how the plays should have been, and then envision a future game in which they play flawlessly. A skier, for example, who has just had a lousy day of skiing, should replay what he or she did correctly first, then reform the mistakes and rehearse the next day's performance. "The great athletes who are out there now tend to future image habitually," he explains. "They tend not to see failures and they tend to recall successes."

The unconscious naturals—those who have a lot of innate ability and don't think much about what they're doing—are an endangered species. The future, he says, belongs to the conscious naturals—those with raw talent and good psychological skills.

Some sports counselors, however, don't think it's necessary to use high tech videos or tanks. "Every athlete's got all the film he ever wants in his own head," says Marlin Mackenzie, a sports counselor at the Department of Movement Sciences and Education at Teachers College of Columbia University in New York. "What I try to do is make athletes aware of the pictures they're making and then help them learn which pictures to pay attention to."

Often athletes will talk to themselves so much while competing that they perform badly. Mackenzie has found that if they pay attention to one external piece of sensory data—a sight, sound, or taste—it keeps their minds from being cluttered and allows the unconscious mind to take over. After Mary Lou Retton made a vault that scored her a perfect 10 at the 1984 Olympics, she was asked about what she was thinking before the jump. "All I thought about," she said "was stick, stick, stick." In order to stick, she had to do everything else leading up to landing perfectly. She didn't talk to herself, she imaged the perfect landing. And that, to Mackenzie, was the key to her success. "Mary Lou's 'stick' was a metaphor for everything," he says. "It's the metaphorical work that really quiets the conscious mind. It puts an athlete in a trance."

For Mackenzie sports psychology is also a matter of asking the right questions. "The therapeutic and medical types ask the question 'What's the matter?' And then they try to answer it," he contends. "But why is something the matter? My question is 'What do you want and how can you get it?' Those are very different questions."

In the future, mental workouts will be an essential element in every athlete's training. Already there is a group that markets videos to teach and reinforce the images of perfect play to both the amateur and the elite athlete. As one doctor put it, "Everyone who wants to excel will have to learn how to harness the powers of the mind."

Steroid Performance

Rick DeMont won a gold medal in swimming at the 1972 Olympics. But he didn't get to keep it. A drug test detected the stimulant ephedrine in his blood, which is on the Olympic Committee's list of banned substances. Unlike athletes who use anabolic steroids, however, DeMont had not taken the stimulant to enhance his performance; it was merely an ingredient in his allergy medicine. In fact, he was unaware that his medication contained a banned substance. His doctor had filled out his medical records for the Olympic physicians, who evidently did not notice his prescription for the allergy medicine. Despite this, Olympic officials reclaimed his medal.

Rick Demont's run-in with the Olympic Committee illustrates the seriousness with which some sports organizations have been trying to curb the skyrocketing use of drugs among athletes. Drugs that promise increased muscle strength, especially anabolic steroids, are most frequently abused. A conservative estimate is that at least 1 million fitness buffs and athletes in this country regularly use steroids.

Steroids, which are synthetic derivatives of the male hormone testosterone, were first introduced during World War II by members of the Third Reich, including Hitler and his S.S. troops. Indeed, one of the steroids' major effects is an increased aggressiveness, which may result in violent outbursts in some of the men and women who use them. But anabolic steroids also increase skeletal muscle mass, the number of red blood cells, and the amount of calcium in the bones—all highly desirable effects for competition. Some athletes report that they are able to withstand much more pain while taking steroids. They also report a greater desire to maintain long and arduous training regimens. Often anabolic steroids produce a "psychological high" that may help the athlete avoid thinking about the drugs' less pleasing long-term effects, including liver tumors, heart disease, and cancer.

But steroids are detectable in preperformance urine samples. Because of this, many athletes are experimenting with more easily concealed substances, such as *human growth hormone (hGH)*. Produced naturally by the pituitary gland, human growth hormone stimulates the growth of bones and muscles, and is medically useful in treating children with growth problems. This once rare hormone can now be produced in the laboratory and will become easier to obtain.

Like steroids, hGH also carries a heavy health risk. The hormone can create a Frankenstein-like enlargement of the face, feet, and hands. Eventually, osteoarthritis can strike prematurely. Perhaps most dangerous, human growth hormone can increase the size of the heart and lead to congestive heart failure. Despite these dangers, however, more and more athletes (and younger ones) are using hGH to improve performance. "The significant height and muscular increases afforded by repetitive human growth hormone administration," says Dr. William Taylor, author of *Hormonal Manipulation: A New Era of Monstrous Athletes*, "will most likely make current sports records obsolete in a few years—and by a large margin of performance."

Taylor and an increasing number of physicians are worried that unless hGH is carefully controlled, hormonal tinkering will become an essential element of future athletic training. And hGH isn't alone on the substance abuse horizon. By 1990 two other synthetically produced growth hormones—*growth hormone releasing factor* and *somatodmedin- C*—will also be available. There's even a hormone in use in Eastern Bloc countries that stunts the growth of young gymnasts, for whom a small frame is a competitive edge. That hormone, though, has an unfortunate side effect: It delays puberty.

In the twenty-first century, however, athletes will be using a safer method of building strength. Researchers at several sports medicine centers have demonstrated that stimulating muscles with electricity while an athlete is working out produces a dramatic increase in muscle strength. "We've seen increases in strength as high as 60 percent after a 6- to 8-week training period," says Dr. Robert Mangine of Cincinnati Sportsmedicine/The Midwest Institute for Orthopaedics.

Although he had used electricity to speed healing in patients for years, Dr. Mangine began experimenting with it on healthy athletes only recently. He first attaches an electrode—about the size of the palm of a hand—to each leg; then he guides the athlete through a series of isometric and isokinetic exercises, as a current, which creates a pins and needle sensation, is pulsed through the muscle. Each session lasts about 30 minutes and the sessions are repeated three times a week.

Mangine has tested about 150 athletes so far and is planning a large-scale study in the near future. His hope is to make the technique available for athletes preparing for the 1988 Olympics. But his ultimate goal is more far-reaching.

"Our purpose in experimenting with this technique," he explains, "is to show athletes that there is an alternative to anabolic steroids or other artificial drugs. We can now say to to the athletes, 'You don't have to take anabols. We can get you a strength gain that is more significant than you could get on your own and we can do it safely.' "

Already, Mangine and other researchers have portable electrical units that athletes can use at home or at the gym. But Mangine warns athletes against the "stimulation salons" which promise strength gain as a result of simply lying still and being zapped. Although some Russian research reports increased muscle strength from electrical stimulation without exercise, American researchers have been unable to duplicate those results. "If I knew of anything in the literature that says I could burn off my body fat by getting stimulated without working at the same time, I'd be the first one on the table," says Mangine.

At the biomechanics lab of the United States Olympic Committee (USOC), another muscle-building alternative to drugs is being developed. Researchers are experimenting with implanting transducers directly into the muscles, then firing the transducer to increase the force of a muscle contraction. This in turn speeds up the rate of muscle growth. "We could do that tomorrow," says Chuck Dillman, who heads the biomechanics and sports science lab for the USOC in Colorado Springs. "But our philosophy is to help each athlete reach his or her own natural potential. We could go beyond that and get into manipulation, but then Olympic competition could become a competition among scientists, not athletes."

Heart Sounds

When 18-year-old marksman Pat Spurgin won the Olympic gold for air rifle at the Los Angeles games, more than training was responsible. True, she had spent the year and a half leading up to the games training 6 days a week. And, she had worked hard at keeping herself steady. Shooters sway back and forth slightly as they shoot, and they must learn to minimize the sway in order to consistently hit the bullseye. "I tried to keep the weight in my feet consistent," explains Spurgin. "That helped keep my body still. If your body's still, your gun's going to be still."

But Spurgin also had the right heart for her sport. She did what all topnotch air riflers do naturally: She shot the rifle between heartbeats. Several years ago, psychologist Daniel Landers tested a group of 10 world class shooters prior to a championship in Korea. He found that all but six of their shots were fired between heartbeats. "The six shots that were fired on the heartbeat itself," Landers explains, "were about a full point lower than those that were fired between heartbeats."

To see if this phenomenon occurred in other shooting events, Landers tested .22 caliber shooters. He found that only some of them shot between heartbeats. The difference, he believes, may be due in part to the muzzle velocities of the guns: The bullet comes out faster in the .22 caliber gun. It may also be due in part to the lighter weight of the air rifle. "As a shooter rests it on the shoulder, the air rifle may pick up the vibration of the beating heart," Landers says. The air rifle shooters may be unconsciously shooting between those vibrations.

Average shooters will someday be able to train themselves to shoot between heartbeats to improve their scores. Landers has already taught some athletes to do so. "But we haven't really followed them up at a later time to see if they're still doing it, so I hate to claim that we've actually taught them the skill," he adds. Landers has been successful, though, at helping shooters to control their breathing. Using biofeedback methods, shooters are trained to alter their breathing patterns so that they hold their breath till a little bit after the shot is released. This keeps the gun steadier during the exit phase of the bullet.

Landers' lab at Arizona State University contains one of the most advanced biofeedback training systems in the world. The equipment measures physiological responses such as muscle tension and heart rate, during athletic performance. Landers' goal is to learn what happens both physically and mentally when athletes perform at their peak. He can then figure out what's gone awry when an athlete falls into a slump. When archer Rick McKinney came to the lab complaining of headaches, for instance, Landers discovered that he was tensing the muscles around his eyes as he shot. By placing electrodes which were hooked to a biofeedback machine on those muscles, Landers was able to help McKinney notice when he was tensing the muscles, and learn to relax them before shooting.

It was during a session with McKinney that Landers made one of the most amazing discoveries of sports research: Athletes' brain waves change during the various phases of performance. The left side of McKinney's brain produced alpha waves just before he shot an arrow. Alpha waves are produced more frequently in states of relaxation. Without knowing it, McKinney was shutting down his analytical faculties and letting the right, intuitive, side of his brain take control. Further investigation showed similar patterns among other athletes, leading Landers to design a biofeedback machine for the future. Tiny sensors attached to the athlete's body will feed brain wave activity into a computer for analysis. A tone will be relayed back to the athlete, allowing him or her to monitor—and control—states of mind. "We're still working on it," Landers says, "but we have most of the technology."

As more and more people become engaged in some form of regular physical activity, will the human animal begin to change? Dr. Appenzeller, editor of the *Annals of Sports Medicine*, says there is no doubt about it. "What we perceive around us, not just the plants and objects, but our fellow beings, is largely determined by an inner homeostasis, a balance between the release of various hormones and the activity of the brain," he explains. "So if we change hormonal release by prolonged, frequent, or different muscle contractions, then we will change our perception of our surroundings and of our fellow beings."

His vision of the future includes a shift toward more physical activity and a change in the cultural value we place on certain behaviors. Already, he points out, friendships are being made through sports, eating habits are changing—less beef, more vegetables— smoking cessation has become a battle cry for the New Age. These are the first signs of an evolving society. "I think it's sporadic," Appenzeller said, "but a new movement is clearly there to be seen."

In the twenty-first century, athletes will be living in a society that not only applauds, but also embraces, their efforts. And the benefits—in medicine alone—that society garners from the study of athletic endeavors will be enormous. From bionic knees to exercise analgesics, from mental imaging classes to electrical salons for building muscles, advances in sports medicine will play a role in the lives of even the most sedentary individual. Sports medicine in the future will be a discipline that involves us all.

Timeline

1988 to 1990
- Force platforms are used in amateur athletic clubs to assess members' motions.
- Synthetically produced hormones become available and are used by athletes to increase strength.

1991 to 2000
- Casts are no longer used for post-surgical recovery: instead electrical healing devices are employed.
- Artificial ligaments allow elite athletes to return to their sports.
- Amateur athletes go through complete biomechanical analysis to improve their performance and protect against injury.
- Biofeedback methods to help athletes control brain waves become popular.

2001 to 2010
- Ligament grafts will give injured joints 70 percent of their original strength.
- Steroid use by athletes is replaced by electrical stimulation.
- Researchers unravel the chemistry of the ''runners' high.''
- Exercise is prescribed instead of drugs for many sufferers of chronic pain.
- Psychological training centers for the amateur athlete become commonplace.
- Transducers are implanted in athletes' muscles to build strength.

2011 to 2030
- Drugs are injected into cells to accelerate healing of athletic injuries.

Access Guide

Organizations and Practitioners

The American College of Sports Medicine
401 West Michigan Street
P.O. Box 1440
Indianapolis, IN 46206
(317) 637-9200

A membership organization for sports medicine professionals. The college publishes pamphlets and other information for the lay public and will put you in touch with a sports medicine doctor or psychologist in your area.

The American Orthopedic Society for Sports Medicine
70 West Hubbard, Suite 202
Chicago, IL 60610
(312) 644-2623

Another source for a list of sports medicine practitioners in your area.

Sybervision
Fountain Square
6066 Civic Terrace Avenue
Newark, CA 94560

Sybervision publishes a catalog of home training guides in the form of videos for a variety of sports. Like Brian Hennessey, Sybervision believes you can learn faster and better by closely observing the experts. Call (415) 790-3637 for a catalog.

Cincinnati Sportsmedicine/The Midwest Institute for Orthopaedics
1 Lytel Place
Cincinnati, OH 45202
(513) 421-5113

Contact Dr. Frank Noyes for appointments for complete knee analysis with the latest equipment; also ligament replacements. Contact Robert Mangine for inquiries about physical therapy, including electrical stimulation of the muscles.

Marlin Mackenzie
Department of Movement Sciences and Education
Teachers College
Columbia University
New York, NY 10027
(212) 678-3325

Personal training sessions for psychological skills.

Telephone Hotline

There is a national 24-hour sports medicine hotline, staffed by orthopedic surgeons and athletic trainers. They won't offer a diagnosis over the phone, but will give out general information and tell you where to go in your area for treatment. Indiana residents call toll free, 800-23-SPORT; residents of other states, dial (317) 926-1339.

Publications

The Physician and Sportsmedicine is a somewhat technical, but very readable, monthly magazine on the field. Aimed at sports medicine practitioners, the magazine publishes original research and, each September, an extensive listing of sports medicine facilities around the country. Write to the magazine at:

4530 West 77th Street
Minneapolis, MN 55435.

Sports Health: The Complete Book of Athletic Injuries, written by William Southmayd, M.D. and Marshall Hoffman, is a comprehensive medical guide for the lay public.

9

The Healing Ray: Turning the Laser's Beam against Disease

The tumor that threatened to block the child's breathing was benign, but kept growing back. In a matter of weeks it would have to be removed again. James Koufman, a surgeon at Wake Forest University's Bowman Gray School of Medicine, in Winston-Salem, realized the operation would be tricky. A tumor in the throat is hard to extract with a scalpel. Bleeding would be a problem, and healing too slow. Koufman's scalpels were not used in this operation; instead, the patient was wheeled into a special operating room next to a large apparatus that looks like a dentist's drill. Koufman reached for the arm of the machine, focused on the tumor, and zapped it with an infrared beam of light—a laser.

Lasers have become standard treatments for several diseases and medical conditions. Gynecologists, dermatologists, even podiatrists routinely use them for conditions ranging from infertility to ingrown warts. Because there's little bleeding with laser surgery, it has been used by doctors in Israel to circumcise a 12-year-old hemophiliac. Laser surgery has even been touted as a miracle cure for the chronic pain of arthritis, or a needle-less form of acupuncture.

New research labs for lasers have been built, like the $1.6 million unit at Massachusetts Institute of Technology. Tomorrow lasers may be used to repair torn nerves and blood vessels, unclog human arteries that have been packed with plaque—maybe even hunt down and destroy cancer cells. Lasers on the drawing board for the Strategic Defense Initiative, commonly known as Star Wars, may one day find themselves in hospital operating rooms.

225

Seeing Is Believing

Thanks to insulin, a diagnosis of diabetes no longer means death. But the disease can still cause blindness. The gradual obstruction of sight, called diabetic retinopathy, occurs when abnormally weak blood vessels grow on the surfaces of diabetics' retinas. These fragile vessels can block light from the retina or can leak blood into the normally clear fluid found inside the eye, blurring the victim's vision. Some diabetics go blind before they reach the age of 30.

Fortunately, argon lasers—argon is an inert gas found in the air—can be used to reach inside a diseased eye and try to fix the damage. To be treated, a patient sits in a chair at his or her ophthalmologist's office, and looks through a set of lenses as in an ordinary eye examination. The ophthalmologist looks through the other end of the lenses, takes aim, then taps a foot switch. Bursts of painless light—the brightness of the laser beam is less than a watt—strike the back of the patient's eye, destroying the abnormal blood vessels. After treatment, the patient climbs out of the chair and heads home.

This treatment, called *laser photocoagulation*, was pioneered by Francis L'Esperance, a New York City ophthalmologist. He claims a 75 to 80 percent success rate with the specialized laser he employs, of which about 10,000 are in use worldwide. Some 20 million eyes threatened by diabetic retinopathy have been put under the laser gun. The treatment can occasionally cause retinal damage, but researchers hope that use of different laser wavelengths might lessen this side effect.

A laser treatment might not always prevent blindness, but blindness can be forestalled by months or even years. In one study, ophthalmologists in the United States treated one eye of a patient with a laser, than compared vision changes in the laser-treated and untreated eye. In most cases, the laser-treated eyes fared better.

That's only one eye treatment for which lasers are used. Retinas, those thin layers of nerves that sense light in the back of the eye, are subject to tears, and when this happens they can become detached, causing loss of sight. Forty years ago a German physician, Gerd Meyer-Schwickerath, examined a number of patients who had burned their retinas by looking directly into a solar eclipse.

After studying the patients' scars, Meyer-Schwickerath had an idea. By aiming a beam of intense light into the eye of a patient with a torn retina he could cause a scar to form. By doing so he thought he might be able to stop the torn retina from ripping farther. Meyer-Schwickerath set up an elaborate apparatus, first using sunlight as a source of power, then artificial light. Neither was practical. Years later the laser was developed by a physicist, Theodore Maiman.

A small beam of single-wavelength light focused precisely on a spot on the retina will form a scar that can stop a tear from spreading. But if the tear is not caught early, the retina will continue to rip until it detaches, and the victim will lose his or her sight. Once the retina has become detached, not even lasers can reverse the damage.

Another major cause of blindness is glaucoma, which is a buildup of excess fluid inside the eyeball. The fluid exerts too much pressure and damages the eye. Glaucoma affects 2 percent of people over 40 years old, and is especially common among those who are severely nearsighted. Again, lasers come to the rescue. They can punch tiny holes into the eyeball, releasing the excess fluid, thus reducing the pressure.

Cataracts under Attack

The newest laser treatment for eyes helps patients escape a common complication of cataract surgery. Cataracts occur when the eye's lens grows cloudy or opaque. To counter cataracts, surgeons replace the diseased lens with a plastic one. When the surgeon scoops out the cloudy lens, he or she generally leaves behind the rear membrane (posterior capsule) that holds the fluid inside the eye. That membrane is transparent, but oftentimes after surgery, the membrane also becomes cloudy, like wax paper.

The solution: An ophthalmologist uses a set of optics to look into a patient's eye, focuses on the membrane, and fires a switch. A beam of laser light rifles through the optics and into the patient's eye. For billionths or trillionths of a second, the invisible laser beam has been focused to an extremely high intensity on a point just one or two thousandths of an inch across. The intensity is so great that it makes a spark and a little pop. Inside the eye, that tiny spark punctures the membrane without affecting the rest of the eye, or the plastic lens implanted next to it. In 10 minutes, an ophthalmologist can punch a series of holes in the membrane, and the cataract patient can see again.

Refractive Surgery

Fortunately, few people are threatened with blindness, but many others are hampered by more mundane eye problems like nearsightedness or farsightedness. These occur when the eye cannot focus light on the retina. The standard treatments, of course, are glasses or contact lenses, which combine with the eye to provide proper focus. Now some ophthalmologists use traditional surgical techniques to adjust the eye so it no longer needs corrective lenses. In the future lasers may do the job better and with less risk.

It will be a long time before everyone can throw away their glasses, but tens of thousands of Americans undergo refractive surgery each year. This procedure, called *radial keratotomy*, first gained popularity in the Soviet Union. A surgeon can alleviate nearsightedness by cutting a spokelike pattern in an eye's outer layer, or cornea, with a diamond knife. When the cuts heal, the cornea curves more gently and focuses light closer to the retina.

The surgery is tricky. The cuts must go through 90 to 95 percent of the cornea without piercing it. (A cornea is one-fiftieth of an inch thick). Nor can cuts be made in the center of the cornea because scars there might obstruct vision. Results are hard to control; although most patients become less nearsighted, they may still have to wear glasses. In a quarter of the cases, vision changes for 2 years after the operation as the eye stabilizes, and questions remain about long-term effects of the operation and strength of the healed cornea.

Lasers might cut the cornea more precisely. In 1982, R. Srinivasan of IBM's Thomas J. Watson Research Center in Yorktown Heights, New York, discovered that short, intense pulses of ultraviolet laser light could cut plastics cleanly and precisely. He and others quickly found that the ultraviolet pulses could do the same to tissue. In 1984, Carmen Puliafito of the Massachusetts Eye and Ear Infirmary, Boston, used laser pulses to perform radial keratotomies on rabbits and found that their corneas healed well. Each pulse would cut part way into the cornea, making the operation easier to control. The operation has yet to be done on humans.

Another experimental refractive surgical procedure involves removing the cornea, freezing it, machining it to shape, and replacing it on the eye. Eventually a laser might reshape the cornea without removing it from the eye. But that idea has yet to be demonstrated even on animals.

Laser Dermatology

A portwine stain is a dark red birthmark, that gets its color from many abnormally large blood vessels close to the skin surface. Unlike some other birthmarks, portwine stains get darker with age, and worse, are often conspicuous. Many people try to hide them with makeup. Dermatologists have tried to remove them with conventional surgery, abrade them, or tattoo over them with light-colored dyes—all with little success.

Because a dark birthmark absorbs much more light than the surrounding lighter skin, it was a logical target for laser treatment. Now dermatologists routinely turn the blue-green beam of the argon gas laser on portwine stains. The laser burns the dark skin, and as the burn heals, the blood vessels close and the stain fades in a matter of weeks. About 70 percent of portwine stains can be lightened without noticeable scarring, making the laser burn far better than any other treatment. Unfortunately the argon laser doesn't work well for the remaining 30 percent. And it often is not useful for treating children; the stain hasn't yet grown dark enough for the treatment to be effective.

The solution might be a different laser. At the Massachusetts General Hospital laser lab, Dr. Oon Tian Tan tested an organic-dye laser that can emit the yellow light most strongly absorbed by hemoglobin in the blood. Thus concentrating the laser energy in the blood vessels, Tan proved that the dye laser could bleach some light birthmarks with little risk of scarring. She uses a laser with pulses so short the energy only goes into the blood. The patient feels only a series of pinpricks, not burns, and doesn't require anesthesia. More clinical trials are needed, however.

Similar laser treatment can attack tattoos. The goal is to bleach away the tattoo by breaking down the dyes that color it. Although lasers have not been spectacularly successful, after several treatments they can bleach away most of a tattoo, leaving smaller scars than other types of treatment.

Laser Microsurgery

Why spend $20,000 or more for a surgical laser to replace an inexpensive scalpel? Indeed, knives and saws cut bone much better than lasers. But a laser's value lies not in its power but in its finesse. A laser beam can be focused in places the most nimble-fingered surgeon can't reach. It can skim away soft surface layers without causing bleeding. A laser can perform surgery literally from head to toe. Some of the greatest successes of laser surgery, however, have involved throat surgery and gynecology.

The most common surgical laser is the carbon dioxide gas laser. Types emitting thousands of watts are used in industry, but surgical lasers need generate only 100 watts of infrared light. During surgery that light is absorbed by water, which makes up about 90 percent of soft tissue. The laser light is so completely absorbed by the water and tissue that the surrounding areas hardly feel any effects. If the carbon dioxide laser can't do the job, surgeons can use a solid-state neodymium-YAG laser or an argon laser.

The carbon dioxide laser's ability to cut tissue without causing bleeding makes it invaluable in gynecology. In the case of DES daughters, women whose mothers took the drug DES (diethylstilbestrol) during pregnancy, the laser is used to remove the abnormal, often precancerous, cells that grow on the surface of their vaginas. Because the cells that are spread over the surface cutting them away would be painful and ineffective. Scanning a laser across the cells vaporizes them with little damage to the healthy underlying cells. At the same time the laser cauterizes the cells, preventing bleeding and deadening nerves.

Lasers can also be used to treat endometriosis, a condition affecting some 6 to 8 million American women. Cells that belong in the uterus grow in patches elsewhere—on the vagina, vulva, cervix, ovaries, or even the tissue lining the abdominal cavity. Those cells bleed during menstruation, as if they were in the uterus, sometimes making intercourse painful, fusing other tissues together, and, causing fertility problems for 30 to 40 percent of sufferers.

Drugs and conventional surgery can help, but are not always totally effective. Dr. Joseph Bellina, codirector of the Omega Institute, a fertility treatment and research center at Bonnabel Hospital in New Orleans, found that 65 percent of a group of 108 women who had been infertile because of endometriosis became fertile after laser treatment. The laser is also attractive because it causes little scarring and can be used on thin tissue such as bladder walls. Laser treatment also provides an alternative to surgery or prolonged drug treatment.

Carbon dioxide lasers also are ideal for surgery on the larynx. The laser beam can be passed down a tube in the throat to remove small cancers or the much more common papillomas, small wartlike growths that make the sufferer's voice perpetually hoarse. The tightly focused laser beam can vaporize growths one-twenty-fifth of an inch across, without causing bleeding or damaging the larynx.

The beams from other types of lasers can be piped deeper inside the body through optical fibers. For example, lasers can be used in this way for treatment of life-threatening bleeding ulcers. Loss of blood makes some patients too weak to survive major surgery. As an alternative, Los Angeles physician Richard Dwyer sends the beam from a solid-state neodymium-YAG laser through a bundle of optical fibers inserted down the throat. Although the laser treatment does not guarantee a cure, it can stop bleeding. Lasers and fiber-optic endoscopes also can help stop other gastrointestinal bleeding and can be used to remove tumors in those areas.

Blocked Arteries

Plumbers can unclog pipes by ramming "snakes" through the blockages. Heart surgeons, on the other hand, must avoid a clogged artery and borrow a blood vessel from another part of the body to bypass the clog. Coronary bypass surgery has become common— about 170,000 procedures were performed in 1982; however, the surgery is serious and expensive, costing $20,000 to $40,000.

Some researchers hope to combine lasers and optical fibers to make a simple, inexpensive version of a plumber's snake. If a laser beam were fired into a thin, flexible optical fiber that was inserted into an artery, the laser should open a path for blood—a much easier technique than a bypass. Or so it would seem.

In practice, a *laser angioplasty* is not that simple. One problem is guiding the fiber through the artery. Optical fibers are stiff; arteries are not. Particularly near the heart, arteries are curved and convoluted, and a poorly thrust fiber could pierce the arterial wall. Surgeons need a fluoroscope to guide the fiber through the artery. They also need a means of directing the energy to the end of the fiber to remove plaque, because most current methods also can remove the arterial wall. And too much energy can cook tissue.

While experiments on tissue samples and animals have been encouraging, the first tests on humans were not. New York City physician Dr. Daniel S. J. Choy performed the operation on five people, all of whom received bypass grafts as backups. In two cases the arteries were damaged, one perforated by the fiber, another cooked by excess heat. The three other laser-cleaned arteries clogged again soon after the operation. A second researcher, Dr. Robert Ginsburg at the Stanford Medical Center, found that laser angioplasty did not help patients as much as did a recently developed technique called *balloon angioplasty*, in which a balloon is inserted into a blocked artery, then inflated.

Some researchers are looking at ways of combining laser angioplasty with balloon angioplasty to treat peripheral arteries in arms and legs. Blockages in those arteries can cause severe pain and sometimes loss of the limbs. After a balloon angioplasty, about 40 percent of the arteries close up again, apparently because the arterial walls have been disrupted. One corrective approach is illuminating the walls with laser light to help prevent them from closing again. A better approach may be to use laser light to heat a metal tip on the end of a fiber and then to burn through the blockage with the tip. For peripheral arteries, this procedure is much less traumatic than bypass surgery. While the patient lies on an operating table, the surgeon cuts through the skin to open a hole in a large artery. Then the surgeon inserts the fiber optic probe into the artery, watching on a fluoroscope as he or she threads the probe to the blockage. When it's on target, the surgeon turns on the laser to burn through the blockage.

The metal tip is easy to see with a fluoroscope, and there is no uncertainty about where the laser energy is delivered and how much is used, which means that there is no danger of punching through the arterial wall.

The big push for the metal tip comes from Trimedyne, a small company in Santa Ana, California, which also makes fiber-optic probes (*Optiscopes*) that look inside blood vessels. Trimedyne's metal tip *Laserprobe* has been combined with balloon angioplasty in tests on patients at the Boston University Hospital and at Northern General Hospital in Sheffield, England.

Dr. Timothy A. Sanborn of Boston University Hospital reports that 39 of the 42 diseased arteries were opened. He blamed two of the three failures on inadequate balloon dilation. The third was due to a blood clot that occurred because the patient mistakenly had not been given an anticoagulant. Long-term studies of humans remain to be completed, but Sanborn considers animal results promising.

This approach eliminates the need for major surgery only in the case of peripheral arteries. The arteries surrounding the heart are too full of twists and turns to thread today's fibers through. The unclogging of coronary arteries with lasers remains a few years from practical use, and may still require open-heart surgery.

Lasers versus Cancer

Lasers have been drafted in the war against cancer. They can be used to remove tiny tumors on the vocal cords, or skim cancer cells from mucous and skin surfaces. But those techniques only use the laser as a flashy scalpel. What about using laser light as a weapon in itself?

That is the idea behind *laser photodynamic therapy*, a technique pioneered by Thomas J. Dougherty of the Roswell Park Memorial Institute in Buffalo. As with other cancer treatments, what laser researchers seek is to kill cancer cells without harming healthy cells. The key to that selectivity is a dye that concentrates in cancer cells and produces toxic byproducts when illuminated by laser light.

The dye is *hematoporphyrin derivative* (*HpD*), which stays much longer in cells that divide rapidly (i.e., cancer cells) than in normal cells. HpD strongly absorbs red light at wavelengths near 631 nanometers, while other tissue absorbs this light only weakly. After the HpD absorbs the red light, it reacts with oxygen molecules in the cancer cell to produce excited oxygen, which in high concentrations can kill cancer cells.

After an injection with HpD, the patient waits 3 days for the dye to wash out of normal cells. Then the area is treated with red laser light, enough to cause lethal reactions in cancer cells but not in healthy cells. Any light of the right wavelength and intensity can trigger the reaction. The advantage of lasers, containing organic dyes or gold vapor, is that they can be attached to optical fibers or endoscopes that can deliver the light to tumors inside the body.

The results can be impressive. In one of the trials of the technique, Francis L'Esperance and Dougherty tried photodynamic therapy on a man whose cancerous eye was going to be removed. It took four tries to reach the right dosage level, but they finally completely obliterated the tumor.

More recent results are even more encouraging. At a conference late in 1985, Dougherty reported that over 2,000 "advanced-stage" patients have been treated. Some suffered from eye and skin cancer, which the laser light can reach directly. Others suffered from cancers of the bladder, esophagus, or lungs, which laser light can reach through endoscopes. Some patients treated early have survived up to 4 years without further cancer. Tumors the size of golf balls have disappeared so completely that nothing was left for histological studies.

Humans are not the only beneficiaries. Richard E. Thoma, a veterinarian in the Buffalo suburb of Cheektowaga, found that 59 percent of 75 pets with cancer that he and Dougherty treated with photodynamic therapy went into complete remission.

HpD also can help in early diagnosis of lung cancer, vital for its successful treatment. As with photodynamic therapy, the technique relies on absorption of the dye by cancer cells. The injected dye is illuminated by a fiber-optic endoscope; the result is a red fluorescence that pinpoints cancer cells. Researchers are concentrating on finding the best match of dye, laser and fluorescence detection.

Another laser technique, developed by University of Miami, Florida, researcher Awtar Krishan, can help physicians pick the best type of chemotherapy for a patient. Many different drugs are available, but none are perfect for all patients or all cancers. With conventional methods, finding the best drug takes weeks, but Krishan's technique requires only an hour. He passes a laser beam through a biopsied tumor and watches for characteristic fluorescence of the drugs. The stronger the fluorescence, the better the cells absorb the drug.

Unorthodox Laser Medicine

Orthodox medicine does not have a monopoly on lasers. Some intriguing—and sometimes bizarre—laser treatments have been developed for uses that range from easing chronic pain and speeding wound healing to acupuncture and smoothing away wrinkles. However, caution is wise. A laser in the hands of a quack may effectively perform only a walletectomy.

Orthodox medical practitioners admit that lasers can help stop bleeding stomach ulcers and cauterize blood vessels. Can low-power lasers speed the healing of skin lesions? Some European researchers say yes, but laboratory results are mixed, and some observers remain skeptical. A milliwatt or so of laser light has, it has been claimed, alleviated chronic pain, such as pain from arthritis. Joseph A. Kleinkort, a San Antonio physical therapist, says laser treatment works best for inflammatory pain, such as arthritis. He explains that steady illumination with a milliwatt or so, usually red light from a helium-neon laser, alters cell metabolism to reduce swelling, and he has submitted documents to the FDA to demonstrate the effectiveness of the laser treatment for arthritis of the hand.

Initially skeptical about laser treatment, he says, "Of all the modalities I ever used for pain management, the laser is the most effective, the least dangerous, and has the fewest side effects." Conceding the laser's limits, notably that it only works on small areas of the body, he believes that the laser could replace ultrasound, heat, and cold therapies for alleviation of pain.

Practitioners of unorthodox laser medicine now tend to be more cautious in their claims than they were just a few years ago. The biggest flap has been over laser "facelifts," a byproduct of laser acupuncture. When acupuncture became fashionable in the U.S. in the late 1970s, some acupuncturists sought alternatives to traditional needles. They used instead a milliwatt of red beam from the helium-neon laser, with which they illuminated the traditional acupuncture points. Practitioners insist it works, even though conventional physicians don't understand how it could.

It was just a few short steps from laser acupuncture to laser "facial toning" and claims of "nonsurgical laser facelifts." Some practitioners claimed that lasers could smooth away wrinkles. Ads appeared promising facelifts, breast enlargement and other miracles. Some laser acupuncturists worried that the claims were excessive. Orthodox physicians who use lasers worried that the public would come to associate laser medicine with quackery.

In 1982 the American Society of Plastic and Reconstructive Surgeons requested that the Federal Trade Commission act against "false and misleading advertising" because no scientific evidence existed in support of laser facelifts. Patients also complained. After an investigation, the FTC enjoined two Florida practitioners from making such claims.

Frontiers of Laser Medicine

Today's research with lasers tries to answer questions about how light and tissue interact. At the Massachusetts General Hospital in Boston, John Parrish's laser group has brought in laser physicist Thomas Deutsch to help physicians understand how lasers work. Laser light directed at the body needs to be absorbed, by tissue, blood, or an additive such as a dye. Then what happens to the absorbed light? Does it heat tissue, cause chemical reactions, or interact in other ways?

By looking at the fundamental biophysics of these events, researchers hope to find the best treatments. For instance, they will learn how to select the laser wavelength so that the beam's energy does not spread beyond the target, such as a blood vessel.

The payoffs of that basic research will be many: Dermatologists will be able to bleach portwine stains now resistant to laser treatment. Ophthalmologists will find ways to treat retinal degradation earlier, and save more and more diabetic eyes from blindness. Careful control of where and how laser energy is deposited will let physicians reach inside the body without knives. Laser refractive surgery may become precise enough—and low enough in risk—for many people to throw away their glasses.

Meanwhile, other researchers are developing new medical lasers. Traditionally these lasers have been bulky, sometimes requiring plumbing for cooling. Newer models are smaller and more efficient. Coming along soon are compact semiconductor lasers that would fit in a physician's hand, yet pack enough power for many treatments. The bulky articulated arms used to deliver the beams in early surgical lasers, which look like dentist's drills, are being replaced by smaller, much more flexible bundles of optical fibers. Compact, durable, and inexpensive lasers can be used to treat conditions such as glaucoma at much lower cost than that of drugs therapy bringing the benefits of high technology medicine to people who now cannot afford it.

Medical research also may benefit from a free-electron laser, a current favorite for use in the Pentagon's Strategic Defense Initiative program, commonly referred to as Star Wars. John M. J. Madey, the Stanford University physicist who pioneered the free-electron laser, believes smaller versions of the Star Wars laser would be valuable in hospitals because its beams can be tuned over a wide range of infrared wavelengths.

Madey and interested physicians from several leading hospitals got money for their work by staging a daring daylight raid on the Star Wars budget. They convinced Congressional budget writers to divert $10 million of the 1985 Star Wars budget to work on medical free-electron lasers. (That's the only connection between laser medicine and Star Wars—and reportedly Pentagon program managers are unhappy about it.)

It will take years to turn the free-electron laser into a medical tool. Further in the future, new lasers and better understanding of light interactions offer exciting possibilities. Researchers at the University of California at Irvine and the Soviet Institute of Spectroscopy in Moscow already have focused laser beams on tiny spots to alter DNA in cells. The laser might evolve into the genetic engineer's tool for fixing defective DNA or tailoring genes in animals—and perhaps humans.

Timeline

1987 to 1990
- Lasers begin to be used for "hot tip" unclogging of peripheral arteries.
- Pale portwine stains can be bleached with dye lasers.
- Laser photodynamic therapy used for cancer treatment.
- Laser drilling of holes in eyeball gains acceptance for glaucoma treatment.

1991 to 2000
- Laser angioplasty of coronary arteries becomes alternative to coronary bypass surgery.
- Laser photodynamic therapy gains acceptance for cancer treatment in areas that can be reached through skin or by fiber optics.
- Hand-held semiconductor lasers are tested for surgery and other treatment.
- Lasers replace knives in refractive surgery.
- Lasers accepted by medical profession for pain treatment.

2001 to 2010
- Widespread use of tiny hand-held semiconductor lasers to treat many diseases.
- Researchers learn how laser light interacts with drugs and other treatments, opening up new generation of therapies.
- Laser microsurgery is used for genetic tailoring of animals on an experimental basis; research begins on treatment of genetic defects in human embryos.

2011 to 2030
- Physicians can buy laser modules to treat specific diseases, with the wavelength they desire for that purpose.
- Semiconductor lasers are packaged as cheaply as transistor radios for many kinds of medical treatment in Third World.
- Lasers are integrated with other therapies for cancer treatment and genetic therapy.

Access Guide

Too many physicians, medical centers and hospitals have lasers to list them all individually. Local physicians generally know what specialists use lasers. You may contact the American Society for Laser Medicine and Surgery, 425 Pine Ridge Boulevard, Suite 203, Wausau, Wisconsin 54401, (715) 845-9283. The society's membership includes physicians and researchers from a wide range of specialties who work with lasers, and the organization will help with referrals.

Laser eye surgery is performed by ophthalmologists, not optometrists or opticians who prescribe and fit corrective lenses. Thousands of ophthalmologists use lasers regularly in their offices. For information on the status of laser eye research, contact The Institute for Visual Sciences Inc., which is headed by Francis L'Esperance, Jr.

The Institute for Visual Sciences, Inc.
18 East 73rd Street
New York, NY 10021
(212) 628-2223

For information on all types of refractive surgery, contact:

The International Society of Refractive Keratoplasty
14935 Rinaldi Street
Mission Hills, CA 91345

Laser refractive surgery has yet to be performed on human patients; one leader in the field is:

Carmen A. Puliafito
Massachusetts Eye and Ear Infirmary
Boston, MA 02114
(617) 523-7900

The most-advanced system for laser angioplasty (artery cleaning) is the one developed by Trimedyne that uses a laser-heated tip on an optical fiber to clear blocked peripheral arteries. For further information, contact:

Michael R. Henson
President, Trimedyne, Inc.
1815 E. Carnegie Avenue
Santa Ana, CA 92705
(714) 261-9041

Laser unblocking of coronary arteries remains experimental; information on that work can be obtained through:

Dr. Thomas L. Robertson
Chief, Cardiac Diseases Branch
Division of Heart and Vascular Diseases
National Heart, Lung and Blood Institute
National Institutes of Health
Bethesda, MD 20205
(301) 496-1081

Lasers are widely used in microsurgery of the throat and larynx. Many otolaryngologists use lasers for surgery; one leader in the field is Dr. James A. Koufman, associate professor of otolaryngology at the Bowman Gray School of Medicine at Wake Forest University. Write:

James A. Koufman, M.D.
Bowman Gray School of Medicine
Wake Forest University
300 South Hawthorne Road
Winston-Salem, NC 27103
(919) 748-4161

Many gynecologists also use lasers for microsurgery on the female reproductive system. One leader in restoring fertility using lasers is Joseph H. Bellina, who can be reached at the Louisiana State University, School of Medicine, New Orleans, Louisiana 70114. (He also is at Bonnabel Hospital in New Orleans.)

The use of lasers and fiber-optic endoscopes is growing, but not yet widespread, and the physician's skill is crucial to successful treatment of conditions such as bleeding ulcers. One of the best-known developers of the technique is Richard M. Dwyer, a gastroenterologist at the University of California Medical Center at Los Angeles. He also has a private practice:

Richard M. Dwyer, M.D
Laser Endoscopy Medical Group, Inc.
1300 North Vermont Avenue, Suite 703
Los Angeles, CA 90027
(213) 668-0100

A number of medical researchers are studying how lasers can weld tissues together. One specialist is:

Douglas K. Dew
University of Miami, Department of Orthopaedics and Rehabilitation
Microsurgery Training & Research Center
PO Box 016960
Miami, FL 33101
(305) 549-6108 or
(305) 547-6202

Research in laser photodynamic therapy for cancer is centered at the Roswell Park Memorial Institute in Buffalo. Contact:

Thomas Dougherty
Division of Radiation Biology
Roswell Park Memorial Institute
Buffalo, New York
(716) 845-3054

Laser pain treatment is not widely accepted among conventional physicians, but advocate Joseph Kleinkort estimates that over a thousand practitioners in the United States treat patients. For more information, he may be contacted at his office:

Joseph A. Kleinkort
4499 Medical Drive, Suite 380
San Antonio, Texas 78229
(512) 692-0796

The availability of laser treatment depends on approval of instruments by the Food and Drug Administration, because most laser medicine requires special devices. Normally, new medical lasers (and other new medical instruments) may be sold only in limited quantities as "investigational devices" until research demonstrates they are effective. Once FDA approval is granted, the lasers tend to proliferate rapidly among specialists and hospitals. For more information on medical device regulation, contact:

Food and Drug Administration
5600 Fishers Lane
Rockville, MD 20857

Basic research on laser medicine is performed at many universities and teaching hospitals around the country. Leading institutions include the Wellman Laboratory headed by John Parrish at the Massachusetts General Hospital, Boston, MA 02114; the Laser Research Center in the George R. Harrison Spectroscopy Laboratory at the Massachusetts Institute of Technology, Cambridge, MA 02139; and a group headed by Michael W. Berns, at the University of California at Irvine, CA 92717.

10

The Heredity Factor: A Guide to Genetic Medicine

Nancy Wexler's mother died of Huntington's disease. That means there's a 50 percent chance that Wexler has inherited this fatal genetic disorder, which doesn't rear its ugly head until midlife and gradually destroys sufferers' nervous systems. " With the disease, you can't think straight," said Wexler, 40 and president of the Hereditary Disease Foundation, "yet you know you're dying."

Until now, Wexler and thousands of other potential victims of this disease were forced to live with the shattering knowledge that they could be struck down in the prime of their lives with this incurable malady. But in the not too distant future, Huntington's disease, as well as 3,500 other genetic disorders, may be conquered by gene therapy. This trailblazing medical technique entails replacing defective genes with healthy ones that have been cloned in the laboratory.

The very real possibility of correcting genetic defects at their source—the faulty gene—represents nothing less than the front lines of the genetic revolution that began in 1953 when Frances Crick and James Watson diagrammed the three-dimensional spiral staircase structure of DNA (deoxyribonucleic acid), the basic molecule of heredity.

The human species, of course, has practiced primitive methods of genetic control for centuries. The domestication of wild animals, the systematic breeding of dogs for specific behavioral characteristics, or even the more contemporary notion of establishing sperm banks for Nobel prize winners in science to breed offspring of high intelligence, are examples of rudimentary attempts to control heredity.

Hereditary maladies cause 80 percent of mental retardation and nearly half of all miscarriages and infant deaths. Thirty percent of the children and 10 percent of adults that are hospitalized annually, at a cost that runs well into the billions, are being treated for hereditary ailments. And scientists have discovered that the onset of a whole array of other ills, such as heart disease, cancer, emphysema, peptic ulcers, alcoholism, chronic depression, and other behavioral disorders have a genetically related component.

Experts predict that their efforts within the next few decades to unlock the secrets of our genetic makeup will mean eventually reducing the awesome toll of these inherited diseases. Genetic disorders that are resistant to conventional treatment—and the vast majority are—will come under attack through the use of gene therapy.

But the critical first step in this process is deciphering the particular genetic coding errors that trigger these ailments. Three startling scientific breakthroughs in the early seventies gave scientists the knowledge necessary for figuring out the precise sequences of the four nucleotides (adenine, cytosine, guanine, and thymine, more commonly indicated as A, C, G, and T—letters of the genetic alphabet) that comprise the individual genes.

Then the development of sophisticated gene-splicing techniques in the early seventies enabled scientists to insert human genes into quickly multiplying bacteria. The effects of minor changes in genetic information could be seen within hours or days rather than over several human generations, and this speeded up the pace of research. This led to the discovery of the biochemical "language" —the sequencing of nucleotides—in which genetic instructions are "written."

Moreover, techniques of gene mapping, the painstaking process by which scientists pinpoint the location of genes on specific chromosomes, are improving so rapidly that Dr. Frank Ruddle of Yale University, echoing the sentiments of other experts, has predicted that "by the turn of this century the major outline of the human gene map should be known."

On the downside, however, the potential applications of this revolutionary biotechnology have sparked a storm of controversy among religious leaders, government policymakers, and scientists themselves. They worry that the temptation to "play God" and alter the genetic pool on a scale that rivals Aldous Huxley's worst nightmares will be too much to resist. Will employers use genetic screening tests to deny a prospective employee a job, or even dismiss a worker? And what monstrous strains of bacteria could be artificially produced and escape from the laboratory as a result of experimentation with DNA?

These and other questions will probably be hotly debated for years to come. But scientists around the globe continue to push forward one of the most exciting and fertile frontiers in medical science. The dream of eradicating hereditary diseases is no longer the exclusive domain of science fiction writers contemplating a brave new world. In fact, while the study of genetics is still pretty much in its infancy, research is proceeding at such an explosive pace that the Congressional Office of Technology Assessment describes genetics as "the most rapidly progressing area of human knowledge in the world today."

Gene Mapping

One child slowly loses all muscle control, gradually becomes blind, deaf, and paralyzed, and usually dies—perhaps mercifully—before the age of 5, a victim of Tay-Sachs disease. Another will be stricken with Lesch-Nyhan syndrome, which causes severe mental retardation, palsy, and such bizarre behavior as compulsive self-mutilation—biting off fingers and lips—and dies before her twentieth birthday.

In both cases, the heartbreaking and incurable diseases are caused by a cruel trick of nature: a simple spelling error in the genetic code of a single gene. But thanks to advances in gene-mapping techniques, the process in which genes are tracked down to their chromosomal addresses, scientists can now identify who will suffer from these fatal disorders. Typically, geneticists can detect the faulty genes by testing either cells cultured from a simple blood test or fetal tissue taken from the mother's amniotic fluid during prenatal screening tests. This is just the first step toward developing strategies for replacing or repairing the defective genes.

Geneticists are on the threshold of mapping out the exact location of the more than 100,000 genes that make up our 46 chromosomes.

More than 800 genes have been tracked down to their zip codes on the chromosomes—and a handful of others already have a street address—on that microscopically thin six-foot-long strand of DNA that's coiled inside each cell. And scientists are confident that by the end of this century they'll have a blueprint of the entire human genome.

Ironically, just a few years ago, charting the vast territory of the human genome seemed like such a herculean task that even the most optimistic scientific sleuths didn't expect to complete this work for several decades. But in 1982, a team of researchers headed by James F. Gusella of Massachusetts General Hospital in Boston discovered the existence of a genetic marker that identified potential victims of Huntington's disease.

Based on intensive screening of several families afflicted with this disease, they discovered a common variant, known as *restriction fragment length polymorphisms (RFLP)*. While these RFLP markers only indicate a gene's general vicinity or zip code, they do serve as critical guideposts to the gene's actual street address, allowing scientists to walk along the markers to find a particular gene.

"The beauty of this strategy is that you don't have to know the nucleotide sequence of the defective gene," says Dr. Arno G. Motulsky, director of the Center for Inherited Diseases at the University of Washington in Seattle. "Once a marker is identified in an affected family, you should theoretically be able to diagnose the genetic disease, regardless of whether or not you understand what's gone awry in the hereditary code. That's a big leap forward."

Indeed it is. Since then, scientists have successfully isolated RFLP markers for sickle cell anemia; Duchenne's muscular dystrophy; retinitis pigmentosa (a disease of the retina); beta thalassemia, which is a severe form of anemia; cystic fibrosis; and polycystic kidney disease; and they have found a marker which strongly suggests susceptibility to cardiovascular disease. "If you have this marker," says Dr. John Baxter, head of California Biotechnology, the firm which uncovered the heart disease marker, "it's equivalent to having blood pressure of 190."

Research teams throughout the world are racing to uncover other markers that indicate the presence of the genes or combinations of genes that trigger hundreds of other genetically related disorders.

Another set of markers, *human leukocyte antigens (HLA)*, are giving scientists hints to the genetic basis of many diseases in which the body's immune system goes haywire. The HLA substances are among the key regulators of the body's natural defense system and must be considered when deciding on the compatibility of the tissue types of organ donors with recipients.

Recent findings indicate that people with specific HLA markers are much more likely to contract certain diseases. Among these are multiple sclerosis, which affects the nervous system; myasthenia gravis, in which the muscles degenerate; systemic lupus erythematosus, a chronic inflammation of the connective tissue; Grave's disease, a thyroid disorder; diabetes; hay fever; and two rare forms of arthritis, Reiter's disease and ankylosing spondylitis.

At the present time, the practical applications of this new technology are primarily diagnostic. But even the ability to spot potential health hazards long before symptoms appear can save countless lives. Results of experimental therapies being used on juvenile onset diabetes suggest that it's possible to stop the progress of this disorder if it's identified in time; this might be true of other diseases as well.

To cite another example, more than half a million Americans die each year of heart attacks. But this new biotechnology holds out the promise of cutting down these harsh statistics. By 1988, adults and children may be routinely given a blood test which could predict their likelihood of developing heart disease, so that preventative measures such as a change of diet or a daily exercise regimen can begin early on to minimize their risks.

In addition, the ability to map a gene to a specific region of the chromosome enables scientists to analyze its normal and abnormal variations and identify the protein the particular gene manufactures. This opens the door to development of therapeutics for a gene's negative effects. Potential therapies fall into two major categories: supplying the patient with the substance that's deficient or replacing the faulty genes with healthy ones.

Already, hypopituitary dwarfism is treated with genetically engineered growth hormone supplements. It won't be long before many other ailments, ranging from heart disease and diabetes to rheumatoid arthritis and peptic ulcers, come under attack using genetically engineered natural bodily substances. As yet, there have been no successful gene transplants. But several research teams across the country are on the verge of beginning the first human gene therapy trials.

"Mapping out the fine details of human genes has immediate clinical application to diagnosis," declared a recent statement by the March of Dimes Birth Defects Foundation, one of the major underwriters of gene-mapping research. "But only the most pessimistic or unimaginative student of this new branch of biology can seriously doubt that its applications will lead to new means of preventing and treating human diseases."

Cancer Genes

Cancer claims the lives of more than 450,000 Americans every year. But the recent discovery of cancer genes (oncogenes) could dramatically reduce the toll of this ravaging illness, and has been hailed by Dr. Frank J. Rausher, Jr., senior vice president of research at the American Cancer Society, as "unquestionably the single greatest breakthrough in all our years of cancer research."

There's no question that this tremendous advance has given scientists their first real handle on what prompts a healthy cell to suddenly turn malignant. It also offers significant clues as to why some families tend to be stricken with certain types of cancer. In addition, it paves the way toward development of more effective strategies of prevention and control, as well as vastly improved diagnostic tests that will detect the illness in its earliest stages when the chances for a cure are the greatest.

Close to two dozen oncogenes have been identified and experts estimate that fifty oncogenes may be the underlying culprits in virtually all forms of cancer. It is known that normal genes can be transformed into oncogenes through exposure to such carcinogens as radiation, chemicals, certain viruses, and other environmental factors that scientists have yet to identify. Studies also suggest that genes that control cell function and reproduction must be involved to trigger the growth of cancerous cells. Consequently, at least two types of genes must be changed into oncogenes and switched on for cancer to occur: One stimulates abnormal cell growth (reproduction); the other permits this unchecked growth to occur (even if the cell is not programmed to grow in this manner).

Other research indicates that some individuals are born with "brittle" DNA (fragile sites on the molecules that tend to break) that may heighten their chances of developing cancer. "In all likelihood, a combination of internal and external factors sets the stage" explains Dr. Jorge J. Yunis, a geneticist at the University of Minnesota Medical School in Minneapolis who has linked several forms of leukemia and lymphoma to brittle DNA. He points out that the chemicals in tobacco often damage one region of chromosome number three. "Anyone with an inborn weakness in this area should stay away from cigarettes if they don't want to get lung cancer," he says.

In fact, Yunis, along with other researchers around the world, is on the brink of developing tests to identify healthy individuals prone to cancer. Once scientists prove conclusively that there is a correlation between cancer and fragile sites, a simple blood test could reveal a predisposition to the disease.

What's more, Yunis's research on chromosomal aberrations in cancerous cells may eventually provide physicians with an indispensable tool for prescribing the most effective treatment regimens for cancer patients. Yunis has discovered that chromosomal changes in cancerous cells are reliable indicators of the severity of a particular cancer.

In the not too distant future, it's likely that physicians will closely monitor people with cancer genes and switch these deviant genes for "good" ones at the first sign of trouble. In addition, those individuals who've been identified as likely cancer candidates could minimize their risks by avoiding such known cancer-producing agents as certain petroleum-based chemicals and cigarette smoke. And some evidence suggests that by increasing their intake of folic acid, a B-complex vitamin, potential cancer victims might be able to protect chromosomes from the breakages that trigger the onset of cancer.

DNA Probes

Frank Spence was a heavy cigarette smoker for more than 30 years before he finally kicked the habit a decade ago. The 66-year-old Florida home builder was recently stricken with a mild case of emphysema. If he had never smoked at all, it's quite likely Spence would never have developed the disease. But if he hadn't quit smoking, he probably would have died of severe emphysema.

That's because the otherwise healthy Spence has a minor genetic quirk that made him susceptible to the disease. His body doesn't produce sufficient quantities of the enzyme that keeps a protective coating on the lung tissue—and this condition was seriously aggravated by years of smoking. Thanks to advances in DNA technology, however, it will soon be possible to obtain a complete rundown of your genetic makeup, including predispositions to a broad spectrum of ailments—like emphysema.

DNA probes are the most precise instruments to date in the biotechnological toolkit that's aiding scientists in their quest to unlock the secrets of our genetic code. DNA probes are merely fragments of DNA that are synthetically produced in the laboratory.

Because of special properties of DNA, these tiny sleuths can ferret out the precise location of a specific gene or detect the presence of a faulty gene.

The DNA molecule is composed of two microscopically thin strands that are dotted with thousands of genes and are tightly coiled inside the nucleus of each cell. The strands line up next to each other like two sides of a zipper. But scientists have discovered that the two sides of the zipper can fit together in only one way.

Consequently, even tiny bits of DNA—the probes—will only bind or attach to segments of DNA that have an identical structure.

Currently, DNA probes are used to detect the presence of several different hereditary disorders. Within the next few years, these DNA fragments will be used for cancer diagnosis, early detection of infectious diseases, and tissue typing, which will help upgrade efficiency in matching organ donors with recipients. In fact, the potential applications of this technology are so vast that, according to Betty Silverman, biotechnology analyst for Robert S. First, Inc., the 1990 worldwide market for commercial DNA probe tests may total over $1 billion.

Already, DNA probes have enhanced the scope of prenatal screening. Tests using DNA probes can yield results quickly because cells don't have to be cultured, as they do in regular tests—the DNA itself provides the information. By the end of this decade, these genetic detectives will routinely scan fetal tissue for genetic indications of Huntington's chorea, cystic fibrosis, and polycystic kidney disease.

What's more, such biotech firms as Enzo Biochemical, Integrated Genetics, and Cetus are racing to place on the market probes to diagnose viral and bacterial infections like salmonella and hepatitis. Probes that detect numerous gastrointestinal, respiratory, venereal, and other infectious diseases are also being researched.

In the immediate future, these tiny detectives will be put to work spotting genetically related health problems long before symptoms appear. Early detection means that we can modify our lifestyles or begin treatments that may delay—or even prevent—the onset of the illness. For example, probes are being developed that would examine oncogenes. "By the time we diagnose cancer today, it's often fairly far along," explains Steve Turner, president of Oncor, Inc., a biotechnology firm which sells oncogene probes to researchers. Some day these special probes will monitor genes and send out alarms if even slight changes occur.

The ramifications of these mind-boggling advances have forced scientists to grapple with dozens of ethical issues. "Right now, our diagnostic ability is outpacing our capacity to treat a whole range of conditions," says Dr. Frank Ruddle of Yale University. "So what good does it do to tell someone that he's susceptible to a serious disease that can neither be prevented nor cured? One might even argue that you were doing that individual more harm than good. Of course, [genetic] research should eventually lead to improved therapy, but until such time there's apt to be an uncomfortable hiatus."

Prenatal Screening

Sylvia and Rupert Boynes decided not to have any more children after their daughter, Nkenge, died a slow, lingering death from sickle cell anemia, an inherited blood disorder that afflicts more than 60,000 Americans. So the New Jersey couple faced an emotionally charged dilemma when they were told they were expecting their second child.

But thanks to a prenatal screening test, which showed conclusively that the fetus did not have the defective sickle cell anemia gene, Sylvia Boynes went on to give birth to a healthy baby girl. If genetic screening hadn't been available, Mrs. Boynes said abortion would probably have been the couple's only alternative.

"In perhaps no other area of medicine can new knowledge be applied so rapidly and readily for the benefit of patients," says Dr. Harold M. Nitowsky of New York's Albert Einstein College of Medicine. The rapid advances in DNA research have transformed genetic screening from a hit or miss proposition in which high risk groups were simply told the odds of having an afflicted child, to a more precise tool that predicts the probability of the child's developing a specific disorder.

Since 1980, *amniocentesis*, a procedure in which cells shed by the developing fetus are extracted from the amniotic fluid and examined for abnormal genes or chemicals, has become the most widely used prenatal screening technique.

Amniocentesis, normally done in tandem with ultrasonography (in which a "picture" of the fetus is drawn by bouncing sound waves off the fetus) can detect the presence of more than 190 chromosomal defects. The conditions for which defects can be pinpointed include Down's syndrome, which results in severe mental retardation; and genetic disorders like sickle cell anemia; Tay-Sachs disease; Duchenne's muscular dystrophy; spina bifida, a severe spinal deformity; anencephaly, a condition in which the skull is not completely formed and leaves brain tissue exposed; and the life-threatening blood disease beta thalessemia.

That's just for starters. On the immediate horizon, the *chorionic villus biopsy*, a new procedure that's already been approved for use at 22 genetic counseling centers across the country, makes test results possible within the first 9 to 11 weeks of pregnancy. In the near future, more precise prenatal screening tests will make it possible to scan fetuses for even minor problems early in pregnancy.

For example, Jorge Yunis has already developed a test that can detect missing kneecaps, mild mental retardation, and possible infertility. Given these incredible technological leaps, it's no wonder Dr. Savio Woo of Houston's Baylor College of Medicine predicts that "we're going to see an explosion of information in the next 5 to 10 years that will lead to prenatal diagnosis for tens, if not hundreds, of genetic diseases."

While prenatal screening is still primarily a diagnostic tool, it has advanced from the stage of specialized research to routine medical practice at the nation's 400 genetic counseling clinics. Its function: to provide parents in high risk groups with information about fetal abnormalities. Obviously some parents then decide to abort the fetus. This is exactly why prenatal screening has become one of the most controversial areas in medicine and the target of attacks by right to life groups. "But," responds Dr. Mitchell Golbus, a geneticist at the University of California at San Francisco, "we've shown time and again that 95 percent of those screened are healthy, which means that many more babies are born—by a huge margin—than would have been without the tests."

The ethical dilemmas inherent in genetic counseling are further complicated by the fact that it's virtually impossible to predict how debilitating a particular disorder will be. For example, some children may only develop a mild form of cystic fibrosis that will require about the same amount of treatment as chronic bronchitis. Others, however, may be doomed to spend most of their short lives in a hospital. Unfortunately, the current diagnostic tests can only detect the presence of the abnormal gene, not the severity of the result. "Parents have to be counseled and make up their own minds on how they want to handle it," Dr. Golbus says.

At the present time only a handful of genetic disorders can be prevented or treated before birth. In utero surgery can now be done on fetuses between 18 and 28 weeks old. The most common surgical procedure is one to relieve urinary tract obstructions, which can severely damage the kidneys and retard lung development. In one case, surgery was performed on a rat fetus to correct malformations in the brain and spinal cord. In another series of experiments with rhesus monkey fetuses suffering from limb malformations, it was discovered that when the limb was removed as late as the beginning of the second trimester, a normal limb would often develop in its place.

On the immediate horizon, congenital heart defects, neural tube defects, and a whole array of neurological disorders may be corrected in the womb. In the not too distant future, physicians are confident that it will be possible to remove the fetus from the uterus, make the necessary repairs, and then replace it for normal delivery.

Vitamin Therapy

In 1968, an 8-month-old boy in a coma was rushed to Yale-New Haven Hospital in New Haven, Connecticut. Laboratory tests showed that the child's urine contained massive quantities of methylmalonic acid, the presence of which normally points to a deficiency of vitamin B_{12}. Yet blood samples showed more than adequate quantities of this vitamin.

Stymied, physicians called in a team of geneticists. Cell cultures of the child's skin provided the answer that had not been uncovered by conventional tests: His cells lacked a critical enzyme needed to carry out the body's complex chemistry and activate the B_{12} vitamin that breaks the acid into simpler chemicals. The genetic defect was unusual, but the remedy was fairly straightforward. The child needed at least 1,000 times the normal daily dosage of vitamin B_{12} to develop normally. Scientists have since identified more than two dozen other inherited disorders that respond to *megavitamin therapy*.

What's equally significant is that many of these metabolic malfunctions can be diagnosed prenatally. This means that vitamin therapy can be initiated before birth, which dramatically increases the chances that the mother will give birth to a healthy baby.

Gene Therapy

In the summer of 1980, Dr. Martin Cline of UCLA made the first attempt to cure a hereditary disease in humans at the source—by fixing the defective gene. In operations performed in Israel and Italy on two female victims of beta thalassemia, an often fatal blood disorder that's caused by a single defective hemoglobin gene, Cline removed bone marrow from both patients' thigh bones. (Bone marrow is the location in the body where blood cells form.) The marrow cells were incubated in the laboratory with quantities of the functional hemoglobin gene that was lacking, and then inserted back into patients.

The hope was that the healthy genes would function normally when injected into the cells, and would replenish the blood supply. Unfortunately, the experiment did not cure the thalassemia, and Cline was heavily censured for what was characterized as his unauthorized and premature efforts. But his approach did prove that this procedure could be carried out safely on human beings.

Since then, no other human experiments in which healthy genes were implanted in cells have been performed. But researchers have been doing extensive work with laboratory animals to lay the groundwork for the first sanctioned trials of human gene therapy, which many anticipate beginning shortly. The importance of this revolutionary approach to conquering inherited diseases cannot be overemphasized, as it offers the first real hope for the hundreds of thousands of people suffering from genetic disorders.

"Drugs and everything else we use today are palliative measures. They treat symptoms; they don't get at the basic disease," explained W. French Anderson of the National Institutes of Health and head of one of the research teams gearing up for the prospective trials. "The only way to get at the basic disease, if the disease stems from a defective gene, is to correct the genetic defect."

Right now, preliminary efforts are centered on 1,600 inherited ailments, each of which is the result of a single defective gene. Treatment of those genetic diseases triggered by a *combination* of several malfunctioning genes is beyond the scope of the currently available technology. In the initial gene therapy trials, research teams are focusing on three rare diseases for which the defective genes have been identified, and for which healthy copies have been cloned in the laboratory. The method of treatment is fairly straight-forward. Essentially, researchers plan to flood a critical pathway of the body's defensive system (the stem cells of the bone marrow) with thousands of normal genes. They hope that enough genes will land in the right place and begin functioning normally and start producing the lacking protein or enzyme.

Lesch-Nyhan syndrome, for one, a severe neurological disorder that strikes 1 in 10,000 boys, is caused by the cells' failure to manufacture hypoxanthine-guanine phosphoribosyl transferase (HPRT), an enzyme required to help regulate the complex chem-istry of the body. The lack of this enzyme causes mental retardation, palsy, kidney problems, arthritis, and such bizarre behavior as com-pulsive aggressiveness and self-mutilation.

Two other diseases which cripple the immune system—adeno-sine deaminase deficiency (ADA), which killed David, the so-called "Bubble Boy," and purine nucleoside phosphorylase deficiency—are also prime candidates for these experiments. And if the trials are successful, they will be what one expert calls "a scientific tour de force of unparalleled proportions," and will give researchers the tools to attack the more widespread but also more complicated single-gene disorders like cystic fibrosis, sickle cell anemia, mus-cular dystrophy, hemophilia, and Huntington's disease.

With the eyes of the world upon them, researchers are anxious to avoid blunders and are reluctant to proceed without sufficient preliminary data to support a human experiment. But one recent experiment, conducted in 1982 by a team of researchers led by Timothy Ley of the National Heart, Lung, and Blood Institute in Bethesda, Maryland, gave scientists their first clear signal that it was possible to manipulate genes in humans.

The experiment, involved five people—three victims of beta thal-assemia and two men stricken with sickle cell anemia. In healthy individuals each gene is ultimately responsible for production of a specific protein; if a particular part of the body doesn't require that protein, the gene may be switched off. In a developing fetus, how-ever, two genes control hemoglobin production. Once the child is born, one of these original genes is turned off and a third gene, the beta gene, takes over its chores.

Scientists wondered if there was a way to reactivate that fetal gene if the beta gene was defective, as it is in victims of sickle cell anemia. When recent research hinted that the drug 5-*azacytidine* might be able to turn on dormant genes, scientists swung into action. After they received continuous intravenous doses of the drug for a week, the fetal genes were reactivated and the anemia was dramatically reduced for up to a month afterward in all five patients. The downside is that the drug is toxic and it's possible that prolonged use could boost cancer risks. Consequently, several questions must be answered before this treatment regimen could win FDA approval.

Bolstered by this success, however, researchers in several laboratories across the country buckled down to solve some of the problems of direct gene transfer. In one experiment conducted in 1984, scientists injected a growth hormone gene into a fertilized mouse egg that was deficient in growth hormone. The mouse grew to nearly twice its normal size, which gave scientists their first clear signal that it was possible to insert foreign genes into animals and get those genes to function.

The next step, of course, was to figure out a way of transplanting genes into humans. One of the key stumbling blocks, however, has been development of an efficient delivery method. A "vector" must be found to transport the precious DNA cargo and drop the genes into a critical pathway—the immature stem cells of the bone marrow, where cells are still dividing into white and red blood cells.

But hitting the stem cells is the equivalent of finding that proverbial needle in the haystack—with your eyes closed. So scientists have begun bombarding the bone marrow cells with DNA in hopes that a few DNA strands will land on the appropriate target. To perform such a massive invasion, scientists selected a carrier (vector) with a proven track record; the virus. "The virus has solved the problem of infecting cells," says William Nyhan of the University of California at San Diego, head of the research team which identified the Lesch-Nyhan syndrome. "That's how it does business."

Other scientists—Dr. Inder Verma of the Salk Institute in San

Diego and Dr. Theodore Friedmann of the University of California, San Diego—have developed a genetic engineering technique for inserting the normal HPRT gene into a mouse leukemia virus which has been rendered benign so that it can be used as a DNA carrier.

Once this has been accomplished, millions of marrow cells from mouse bones are then removed and incubated in the laboratory with the altered mouse leukemia viruses that carry the normal HPRT gene. Once the virus deposits its DNA cargo into the nuclei of the cells, the cells are reinjected into the mouse. The final step in this experiment, which is still underway, is to determine whether the genes in the altered cells are expressed, or switched on, in the living mice.

The other scientific teams gearing up for the first gene transplants on humans have arrived at approximately the same stage in their research. But one experiment in particular should provide the first substantial evidence that gene transfer will work in humans.

Dr. Richard O'Reilly of Memorial Sloan-Kettering Cancer Center in New York City, along with the NIH team headed by W. French Anderson, recently transferred human ADA genes into four rhesus monkeys. Preliminary data indicates that this group is on the verge of overcoming the final hurdle that stands in the way of the first human gene therapy trials: determining whether the ADA gene is expressed in the animal's stem cells.

In anticipation of this revolutionary breakthrough, the Recombinant DNA Advisory Committee of the National Institutes of Health recently established strict criteria that research teams must meet to win approval for the prospective human gene therapy trials. Specifically, the directives limit experimental procedures to severe illnesses that don't respond to conventional treatment. Furthermore, the guidelines require assurances that the interests of the patients and their families will be safeguarded, perhaps in an effort to avoid a replay of the media circuses that surrounded the first recipients of an artificial heart and "Baby Fae," the infant who received a baboon heart.

What's equally significant are the committee's guidelines. These must be very carefully written to prohibit development of any experimental techniques that would implant genes that could be passed on from one generation to the next. "Gene therapy offers enormous hope for the alleviation of human suffering," says Dr. Anderson, "But we must go forward carefully as we develop greater power to alter the lottery of nature."

Genetically Engineered Natural Drugs

A panel of U.S. scientists ranked genetic engineering and the development of recombinant DNA techniques in the early seventies as "one of the four major scientific revolutions of this century, on a par with unlocking the atom, escaping the Earth's gravity, and the computer revolution." Given the current and future applications of this biotechnology, this group was not exaggerating its importance.

In late 1985, in fact, Dr. Steven A. Rosenberg, head of the National Cancer Institute research team testing a new cancer therapy that uses genetically engineered substances, gave the world an early Christmas present. Based on preliminary results on 25 patients with advanced tumors, Rosenberg announced that this experimental treatment shrunk the tumor size by 50 percent or more in 11 cases.

The promising new technique, called *adoptive immunotherapy*, relies on a genetically engineered growth factor, *interleukin-2 (IL-2)*, that mobilizes the body's own defense mechanisms to bring wayward cells under control. White blood cells from the patient are removed, cultured in the laboratory, and then incubated with IL-2, which transforms them into "killer cells." The IL-2-enhanced white cells are then reinfused into the patient's bloodstream.

These killer cells do appear to carry out their orders and attack the malignant tumors, much akin to the way that white blood cells—the foot soldiers of the body's immune system—are galvanized into action to battle against foreign invaders. While Dr. Rosenberg cautiously avoided making any extravagant claims about the significance of these early findings, he did call the research "the first new kind of approach to cancer in perhaps 20 or 30 years."

In fact, interleukin-2 is only one of a growing arsenal of genetically engineered biological weapons being developed in the battle against cancer. The opening volley of this war was fired little more than a decade ago when scientists discovered restriction enzymes, which are able to cut the DNA molecule at specific sites. At about the same time, it was found that ligase, another enzyme, could glue a gene removed from one DNA molecule into a similar region of the DNA of another organism. This technique is known as gene splicing, and the hybrid molecule formed is called recombinant DNA (recombined DNA).

The structure of bacteria makes them ideal carriers (vectors) for a snipped out gene. The gene is piggybacked on top of the bacterium molecule (it is attached to an extra chromosomal section of the bacterium's DNA known as a plasmid). Once this is done, each time the microbe reproduces, it also replicates the gene and produces more gene product, normally protein.

More recently, development of computerized gene machines has virtually eliminated the once time-consuming process of copying genes by trial and error. Consequently, when the gene responsible for the production of a particular protein is identified, scientists can very quickly produce enough altered bacteria to begin churning out prodigious quantities of previously scarce substances essential for bodily functions.

"We're looking for natural products made by the body that are deficient in diseased people," explains David V. Goeddel, a molecular biologist at Genentech and a member of the wunderkind research group that has isolated the genes for the production of human insulin, human growth hormone, and alpha and beta interferon. "If there's activity, we assume there's a gene."

Breakthroughs such as the one at Genentech have transformed the pharmaceutical end of biotechnology into a multi-billion dollar industry. In Eli Lilly's laboratories in Indianapolis, Indiana, for example, modified microbes pump out human insulin in fermentation vats (instead of removing insulin from animals). Eli Lilly's Humulin is more costly than the animal insulin currently in use. But bacterial insulin production does ensure that diabetics will have an adequate supply of the hormone, and prices should tumble as the technology advances.

Across the country at Genentech in South San Francisco, bacteria are busy at work producing human growth hormone, which allows children stricken with hypopituitary dwarfism to develop normally.

Just down the road at CooperBiomedical in Palo Alto, California, human genes growing inside yeast cells may be able to churn out ample amounts of the enzyme inhibitor *alpha-1-antitrypsin (AAT)*, a chemical that is lacking in victims of emphysema. Clinical trials are in progress, and the firm expects to place the drug on the market shortly.

Other pharmaceutical firms are racing to be the first to win FDA approval for commercial production of *Factor VIII*, the blood-clotting factor that is deficient in hemophiliacs. This is welcome news for the nation's 14,000 hemophiliacs.

Clinical tests are also underway with *plasminogen activators*, natural substances that dissolve the blood clots that cause most heart attacks. "With 700,000 heart attacks a year and a half million deaths from coronary disease, the drug could have significant impact," predicts Dr. James H. Chesebro, associate professor of medicine at the Mayo Medical School.

And this is only the beginning. On the horizon is the development of a new class of drugs which block the action of enzymes and other bodily substances that have been identified as causers of rheumatoid arthritis, blindness, kidney and nerve damage in diabetics, stress and high blood pressure and peptic ulcers.

Antigens (the foreign invaders which trigger the production of antibodies by the immune system) as well as natural body substances that may help the body battle cancer, have also come under intense scientific scrutiny. In addition to IL-2, among those arousing the most interest are *tumor necrosis factor (TNF)*—the substance that many tout as this decade's "magic bullet" because it causes tumor cells to burst while leaving healthy cells intact—and *alpha, beta,* and *gamma interferons.* Alpha, beta, and gamma interferons are proteins the body produces naturally in response to viral infections. The hope is that their virus-fighting capacity could make tumor cells more recognizable to the immune system so that the body's defenses could swing into action against the invaders.

Already, researchers at Genentech have cloned TNF, and human trials of TNF are underway at Sloan-Kettering in New York and Houston's M. D. Anderson Hospital. Clinical trials are also getting started for gamma interferon.

Scientists suspect that a combination of all of these substances may eventually eradicate this dreaded killer. "We know from chemotherapy that, with few exceptions, it took a combination of chemicals to cure childhood [cancers] like leukemia," explains Dr. Jordan U. Gutterman of the M. D. Anderson Hospital. "The same thing is going to be true of biological agents. It is going to take more than one agent to fully cure [cancer]."

Genetically Engineered Vaccines

In many parts of the Third World, 25 percent of the children born die before their first birthday, fatally afflicted with diarrhea, bacterial infections, cholera, and malaria. In Asia, 200 million people suffer from serious liver ailments triggered by the hepatitis B virus, which kills thousands of infants each year. Ironically, vaccines are available that could halt the devastating effects of these illnesses, but it's much too costly for impoverished Third World countries to institute inoculation programs.

But the development of genetically engineered vaccines will soon change this bleak picture. And this new vaccine technology may soon stop the spread of herpes, which now afflicts millions of Americans. "Mankind is now on the threshold of a new era in the technology of vaccine development and production," says a spokesperson for the World Health Organization, and other public health experts are confident that diseases like malaria and hepatitis B will be eradicted within the next decade.

Their optimism seems justified. This new class of genetically engineered vaccines are cheaper, safer, and more effective than the ones currently in use. Conventional vaccines use a weakened virus which prompts the body's immune system to swing into action, producing antibodies that would repel a stronger, disease-causing virus. But using a weakened virus that's still strong enough to stimulate a bodily reaction can be a tricky business. The upshot is that contaminated batches of some vaccines have been known to trigger the disease itself or produce disastrous side effects—most notably the brain damage in a few children caused by the whooping cough vaccine.

With genetically engineered vaccines these problems can be avoided since it's no longer necessary to use the disease-causing virus to spur the body's defense mechanisms. Scientists can now identify the antigens—proteins of the disease-producing organisms —that trigger the body's defensive reaction against foreign invaders. The gene responsible for creating a particular antigen can now be synthetically produced in the laboratory and inserted into a harmless bacterium, which starts producing the antigen so that it can be used as a safe and effective vaccine.

This technique has been employed to produce several genetically engineered vaccines, including one for hepatitis B, which is currently in the final stages of clinical testing, and others, still in development at several major laboratories across the country, for malaria and gonorrhea.

Other researchers are manipulating the cowpox virus used in the smallpox vaccine to adapt it for use as a multipurpose vaccine. Using gene-splicing techniques, a research team with the New York State Department of Health, headed by Dr. Enzo Paoletti, has successfully piggybacked the antigen-producing genetic material for three other viruses—herpes, hepatitis B, and influenza—onto the exceptionally large cowpox virus molecule.

There are several distinct advantages to this approach. Not only is there no risk of the inoculated person actually contracting these ailments (because the disease-producing virus is not present), but this vaccine is inexpensive to produce—costing about 30¢ a shot —and doesn't require refrigeration. These pluses are particularly important for Third World countries, where infectious diseases are reaching epidemic proportions.

What's equally significant is that, because the cowpox virus molecule is so large, it could be adapted as a vaccine against a whole array of other infections. "There is enough room to insert 12 to 15 different foreign genes," Dr. Paoletti says. "We could develop a polyvaccine that would render a person immune to herpes, hepatitis, malaria, and other diseases, all in one shot."

Clinical human trials of the genetically engineered combination herpes, hepatitis, and influenza vaccine are scheduled to begin next year. The vaccine itself won't be *commercially* available for several years. But the fact that it could eradicate these ailments throughout the world prompted an official at the World Health Organization to call it "a scientific achievement of the first order."

Genetic Screening in the Workplace

In the early 1960s, a group of workers at an Israeli dynamite factory were stricken with acute hemolytic anemia, a disorder which destroys the red blood cells and deprives the body of the oxygen needed to carry out metabolic functions. Plant officials were at a loss to explain what triggered this sudden outbreak of a relatively rare disease.

Several years later, researchers used a genetic screening test to solve the mystery. It turned out that what the ailing workers had in common was that they all suffered from a G-6-PD deficiency. Individuals with a pair of G-6-PD deficient genes can become ill with hemolytic anemia when exposed to certain chemicals—like the TNT present in vast quantities in the dynamite factory. The upshot: The factory gradually lowered exposures to the TNT so that workers were no longer at risk.

Recent research has revealed that minor quirks in an individual's genetic makeup can increase susceptibility to certain ills, particularly after exposure to chemicals and other harmful substances both on and off the job. This discovery has brought to the fore the idea of using genetic screening as a cost-effective tool in the effort to reduce the toll of occupational diseases.

A survey conducted by the Office of Technology Assessment (OTA) in 1982 reported that at least 59 of the Fortune 500 companies are either using or are interested in genetic testing to determine which of their employees are likely to contract particular ailments. Genetic disorders that predispose individuals to illnesses that interfere with the functioning of red blood cells—for instance, the G-6-PD deficiency or serum alpha-1-antitrypsin deficiency, which is linked to emphysema—are among the prime candidates the OTA report mentioned for these tests.

The logic behind instituting genetic screening in the workplace is obvious: Weed out those workers who are genetically predisposed to certain ailments and cut down on occupational ills. But screening can be a double-edged sword. "While on one hand genetic screening could prove to be a marvelous tool to protect workers' health," says Rep. Albert Gore, who initiated the OTA study, "it also presents us with Orwellian possibilities. It could be used to unfairly discriminate against people on the basis of their genetic heritage."

It certainly could. For example, a genetic marker has been found that helps determine who will get ankylosing spondylitis, a chronic arthritis of the lower spine, which develops mostly in young men. This debilitating condition has been linked to an antigen known as B27. Almost everybody who has ankylosing spondylitis has the B27 antigen. Yet only one out of four men who has B27 will get the ailment.

What happens to those with the B27 antigen present? Will employers use genetic screening tests for this and other inherited ills to justify denial of employment, job transfers, of even dismissal? Will insurance companies use this information as ammunition to get permission to raise the rates of those who may be susceptible to life-threatening ills? In short, will these medical advances create a class of unemployables?

Indeed, what spurred Congress to commission the 1982 OTA report was a series of articles in the *New York Times* about a program at a Dupont plant in which black employees were tested for the sickle cell trait. The *Times* stories suggested that the Delaware-based chemical corporation had been using the test to exclude those who might be susceptible to the chemicals used at the factory. Dupont denied the charges, but the story did stir up a storm of controversy.

Organized labor, for instance, contends that employers may use genetic testing merely as a smoke screen for layoffs rather than cleaning up the job sites and compensating those who become ill. "There's a tendency to concentrate on who is susceptible," says Dr. Rafael Moure, industrial hygienist for the Union of Oil, Chemical, and Atomic Workers, "rather than controlling exposure in the workplace. We see that as very dangerous."

These are legitimate issues that need to be ironed out before genetic screening in the workplace becomes an accepted practice. At the present time, only six of the the firms OTA surveyed were actually involved in some type of genetic testing, but all that can change in the near future.

General Molecular Applications Inc., a biotechnology firm in Columbus, Ohio, for instance, is in the process of testing a genetic screening system that should be commercially available within the next few years. As Thomas H. Murray, an associate professor of ethics and policy at the University of Texas, noted, "Given the enormous potential of these techniques, it may be only a matter of time before many companies embark on full-scale testing programs."

The mind-boggling medical breakthroughs outlined in this chapter only scratch the surface of the new vistas that have been opened up by genetic researchers around the world. Scientists are busy at work breeding genetically altered cattle and crops, in hopes of producing food in such abundant quantities that world hunger will become a relic of a bygone era.

Other researchers are developing high-tech machines to detect errant genes that warn of potential health hazards and inherited ills—even in the womb. In the very near future, this equipment will be as common in a doctor's office as blood-testing apparatus is today. And those with hereditary predispositions to a vast array of disorders won't have to live under the shadow of nature's lottery— methods of prevention and control will be readily available.

Imagine a world where everyone truly is created equal, a world where children are no longer victims of their heredity, a world free of hunger, mental retardation, cancer, heart disease, and the thousands of other ills that kill or cripple millions each year. For centuries, that's been the dream of medical scientists who've labored to unlock the secrets of how that amazingly complex organism known as the human body functions, in hopes of eliminating human suffering and improving the quality of life. The awe-inspiring scientific advances by geneticists, who have become Nobel laureates with almost metronomic consistency, have brought us to the brink of making these dreams a reality.

Timeline

1986	• First human gene therapy trials for ADA and purine nucleoside phosphorylase deficiency begin.

1987 to 1990	• Genetically engineered drugs to control hemophilia, emphysema, rheumatoid arthritis, diabetes, stress, heart disease, and certain cancers win FDA approval for general use.
	• Infants now routinely tested for presence of genes that trigger heart disease, emphysema, cancer, peptic ulcers, diabetes, Alzheimer's disease, Huntington's chorea, kidney disorders, multiple sclerosis, lupus, myasthenia gravis, and arthritis.
	• First human gene therapy trials for Lesch-Nyhan syndrome, cystic fibrosis, sickle-cell anemia, muscular dystrophy, hemophilia, and Huntington's chorea begin.
	• Combination herpes-hepatitis-influenza-smallpox vaccine, and vaccines for toxic shock syndrome, malaria, gonorrhea, croup, strep throat, cholera, tooth decay, and typhoid fever are approved by FDA for general use.

1991 to 1995	• Scientists map all 50 cancer genes.
	• Government approves guidelines for genetic screening in the workplace.
	• Genetically engineered vaccine for AIDS approved by FDA for general use.
	• Prenatal screening techniques for 4-week-old embryos approved by FDA for general use.

1996 to 2000	• Major outline of human gene map is known.
	• Scientists discover how to ''switch off'' cancer genes.
	• Prenatal genetic screening tests become available for home use.

2001 to 2010	• First human gene therapy trials for Alzheimer's disease and other diseases resulting from defects in more than one gene begin.

- Gene transfer therapy for 1,600 single-gene-defect diseases approved by FDA for general use.
- Genetic counseling for couples contemplating having children now required by law.

2011 to 2100
- Gene transfer therapy for all hereditary diseases becomes standard medical practice.
- All hereditary or genetically linked diseases are eradicated.

Access Guide

Here is a list of the major genetic research and diagnostic centers across the country. Unless otherwise noted, each offers genetic counseling services and prenatal diagnostic tests, and is involved in genetic research.

National Center for Education in Maternal and Child Health
3520 Prospect Street, Northwest
Washington, D.C. 20007
(202) 625-8400

University of Alabama in Birmingham
The Medical Center/Laboratory of Medical Genetics
University Station
1720 Seventh Avenue South
Birmingham, AL 35294
(205) 934-4968

Genetics Center of the Southwest Biomedical Research Institute
123 East University Drive
Tempe, AZ 85281
(602) 894-1104

City of Hope National Medical Center
1500 East Duarte Road
Duarte, CA 91010
(213) 226-3816

Los Angeles County—University of Southern California Medical Center
Department of Pediatrics
Division of Genetics
1129 North State Street
Los Angeles, CA 90033
(213) 266-3816

University of California, Los Angeles
Center for Health Sciences
760 Westwood Plaza
Los Angeles, CA 90024
(213) 825-6379

Children's Hospital Medical Center of Northern California
51st and Grove Streets
Oakland, CA 94609
(415) 654-5600

University of California, Irvine Medical Center
Department of Pediatrics
Division of Clinical Genetics and Developmental Disabilities
101 City Drive South
Orange, CA 92668
(714) 634-5791

University of California, San Francisco
Department of Pediatrics
Divsion of Medical Genetics
3rd and Parnassus Avenue
San Francisco, CA 94143
(415) 666-2981

Stanford University Medical Center
Department of Pediatrics
Genetic Counseling Center
300 Pasteur Drive
Stanford, CA 94305
(415) 497-5198

Harbor UCLA Medical Center
Division of Medical Genetics
1900 West Carson Street
Torrance, CA 90509
(213) 533-3667

University of Colorado Health
  Sciences Center
Genetics Unit
4200 East Ninth Avenue
Denver, CO 80262
(303) 394-8742 or 394-8777

Yale University School of Medicine
Department of Human Genetics
Genetic Consultation Service
333 Cedar Street
New Haven, CT 06510
(203) 436-3076

Georgetown University Medical
  Center
Department of Pediatrics
Center for Genetic Counseling and
  Birth Defects Evaluation
3800 Reservoir Road, Northwest
Washington, D.C. 20007
(202) 625-2348

Emory University School of
  Medicine
Department of Pediatrics
Division of Medical Genetics
Box AM
Atlanta, GA 30322
(404) 488-3606 or 488-3607

University of Chicago Hospital
Pritzker School of Medicine
Department of Pediatrics
950 East 59th Street
Chicago, IL 60637
(312) 947-6344

University of Illinois Medical
  Center
Abraham Lincoln School of
  Medicine
Department of Pediatrics
Division of Genetics and
  Metabolism
840 South Wood Street
Chicago, IL 60612
(312) 886-6714

Indiana University School of
  Medicine
Department of Medical Genetics
1100 West Michigan Street
Indianapolis, IN 46223
(317) 264-2241

Kansas University Hospital College
  of Health Sciences
Department of Pediatrics
Division of Medical Genetics
39th and Rainbow Boulevard
Kansas City, KN 66103
(913) 588-6043

Johns Hopkins University School
  of Medicine
Prenatal Diagnostic Center
601 North Broadway
Baltimore, MD 21205
(301) 955-3091

National Institutes of Health
Medical Genetics Clinic
Clinical Center
Building 10, Room 9C436
Bethesda, MD 20892
(301) 496-1380

Massachusetts General Hospital
Department of Children's Services
Genetics Unit
Fruit Street
Boston, MA 02114
(617) 726-3826

Peter Bent Brigham Hospital
Department of Medicine
Genetics Clinic
721 Huntington Avenue
Boston, MA 02115
(617) 732-2259

University of Michigan Medical
School
Departments of Internal Medicine
and Human Genetics
1137 East Catherine Street
Ann Arbor, MI 48109
(313) 763-2532

C.S. Mott Center for Human
Growth and Development
Wayne State University
School of Medicine
275 East Hancock
Detroit, MI
(313) 577-1066

University of Minnesota
Dight Institute for Human Genetics
400 Church Street Southeast
Minneapolis, MI 55455
(612) 376-3792

Mayo Clinic
Department of Medical Genetics
200 First Street Southwest
Rochester, MN 55901
(507) 284-8198

New York State Health
Department
Division of Laboratories and
Research
Birth Defects Institute
Empire State Plaza
Albany, NY 12201
(518) 445-5124

Albert Einstein College of
Medicine
Department of Pediatrics and
Genetics
Genetic Counseling Program
Rose F. Kennedy Center
1410 Pelham Parkway
Bronx, NY 10461
(212) 430-2510 or 430-2516

New York Hospital
Cornell University Medical Center
Department of Medicine
Division of Human Genetics
525 East 68th Street
New York, NY 10021
(212) 472-8352

University of North Carolina at
Chapel Hill
Department of Pediatrics
Genetic Counseling Program
School of Medicine
Chapel Hill, NC 27514
(919) 966-2266

University of Pennsylvania
Children's Hospital of
Philadelphia
Division of Genetics
Clinical Genetics Center
34th and Civic Center Boulevard
Philadelphia, PA 19104
(215) 596-9800

University of Pittsburgh
Children's Hospital
Department of Pediatrics
Unit of Clinical Genetics
125 DeSoto Street
Pittsburgh, PA 15213
(412) 647-5070

University of Texas Health Science
  Center at Dallas
Southwestern Medical School
Division of Clinical Genetics
5323 Harry Hines Boulevard
Dallas, TX 75235
(214) 688-2595

Baylor College of Medicine
Texas Children's Hospital
Birth Defects Genetics Clinic
6621 Fannin
Houston, TX 77030
(713) 791-3261

Center for Inherited Diseases
University of Washington
University Hospital
Prenatal Diagnosis Clinic
1959 East Pacific Street
Seattle, WA 98195
(206) 543-3370

University of Wisconsin at
  Madison
Clinical Genetics Center
328 Waisman Center
1500 Highland Avenue
Madison, WI 53706
(608) 262-2507

11

War on Fat

Americans forked over $5 billion in 1985 for diet pills, dieting books, low-calorie foods, and exercise equipment in what seems like a never-ending—and losing—war on fat. Obesity ranks as the number one form of malnutrition in this country, a country in which diseases such as scurvy, rickets, and pellagra, ailments usually associated with malnutrition, have all but disappeared. They have been replaced, however, with medical conditions that frolic among our excesses: hypertension, cardiovascular disease, arthritis, kidney stones, gall bladder disease, back pain, and gout. Obesity has been linked to cancer of the breast and uterus in women, cancer of the prostate in men, and colorectal cancer in both sexes. People with a family history of Type II diabetes could be threatened by as little as 5 extra pounds of weight. That's not to mention the many psychological and social consequences blamed on obesity.

According to the National Institutes of Health, more than 34 million Americans are overweight, and 11.5 million of those are at extreme risk. Men who are 20 percent overweight have a 20 percent decrease in life expectancy. Women who are 20 percent overweight have a 10 percent decrease. For the morbidly obese—people who carry twice their desirable body weight—the mortality rate is 1200 percent higher than normal.

At least 20 percent of our population—approximately 40 million people—are dieting. "But maintaining a normal weight in Western society is a losing battle," says Dr. Aaron Altschul, director of the Georgetown University Diet Management Program. Only 1 in 10 Americans is satisfied with his or her weight. Despite all of our renewed interest in diet and exercise, Americans are heavier today than ever. Why?

Researchers have just begun to conclude that serious obesity is not always a matter of poor diet, lack of exercise, a need for more willpower or for behavior modification. At the Physical Activity Sci-

273

ences Laboratory at Quebec's Laval University, researchers discovered that the amount and location of body fat in adopted children was more closely associated with that of their biological parents than that of their adoptive ones—a discovery that indicates that the role of heredity in producing fatness may be more important than that of environment.

Virtually no good evidence exists that proves obese people eat more than their leaner counterparts. Of course, if 40 percent of a 3300 calorie per day diet is comprised of fats, which is average for an American, this can turn a minor genetic predisposition into a full-blown problem. And it's certainly true that we become fat because we eat and drink more calories than we use. But that doesn't address the crucial question: Why do two people with similiar build who eat the same and exercise the same weigh different amounts? Researchers studying obesity in rats have wondered not only how these animals gain weight when they are put on a high-calorie ("cafeteria") diet, but also why some of the rats steadfastly refuse to gain a gram. "I think only 5 or 10 percent of our obesity can be directly blamed on environmental factors," says Dr. Rudolph Leibel, a researcher at the Obesity Research Center, at the Rockefeller University in New York.

Most researchers are aiming their efforts directly at our bodies' biochemistry in an attempt to deflate our ballooning midriffs. Perhaps in a few years, doctors will stop prescribing yet another diet or exercise routine, and instead try to manipulate an obese victim's appetite-control system, increase the efficiency of his or her body's metabolism, or inject drugs that can hunt down and destroy fat cells. If those means fail, doctors may order extensive forms of plastic surgery or call into action the most extreme of diets: human hibernation.

Fated to Be Fat

A potent appetite stimulant was recently discovered by researchers at the Rockefeller University. This stimulant, called *neuropeptide Y*, causes intense craving for carbohydrates, and may be linked to bulimia or anorexia, eating disorders that affect 5 percent of the American population. An occasional excess of this chemical could stimulate the appetite of normal people as well, causing them to overeat.

After neuropeptide Y was injected into the brains of rats, they ate twice their normal consumption within 3 days, gaining weight six times faster than normal, and tripling their amount of body fat. Dr. Glenn Stanley, a neurobiologist at Rockefeller, stresses that while neuropeptide Y causes a desire for carbohydrates, it has little or no effect on desire for proteins and fats. This jives with earlier findings that many victims of obesity crave carbohydrates, while people who suffer from anorexia are "carbohydrate phobic." By controlling the level of neuropeptide Y, researchers hope to eventually control appetite and, of course, weight.

Neuropeptide Y was discovered while researchers examined another appetite stimulant, *norepinephrine*. Both substances are found in the paraventricular nucleus, or PVN, which rests in the brain's hypothalamus. (Low levels of norepinephrine are found in people with anorexia.) The PVN controls our desire to eat and drink, and is linked to the pituitary gland, which among its other functions, controls growth and development of our bodies. Also found in the PVN were two appetite *suppressants*: *cholecystokinin* (CCK) and *serotonin*.

CCK was discovered 10 years ago at New York-Cornell Medical Center in White Plains, New York. CCK originates in the intestine and wends its way to the hypothalamus. Dr. Bart Hoebel, a professor at Princeton University, found out that CCK, when injected into the brains of rats, suppressed their feeding. Could dieters reap the same benefit from CCK in tablet form? Unfortunately, when CCK is taken orally it breaks down in the digestive tract before it can have any effect. "Besides, we don't know if CCK by itself will suppress appetite in humans," Dr. Hoebel says. "It may have to work with other chemicals found in the PVN."

One such chemical might be serotonin. As carbohydrates enter the human body, the level of serotonin rises. This suppresses neuropeptide Y and as a consequence the desire for more carbohydrates. Drs. Judith and Richard Wurtman, researchers at the Massachusetts Institute of Technology, speculate that many overeaters have inadequate levels of serotonin, and that as a result, their systems lose control of neuropeptide Y production.

If 30 percent of your diet is made up of carbohydrates, you're probably a carbohydrate craver. The Wurtmans, who advocate a diet relatively rich in carbohydrates for their patients, recently discovered that many subjects snacked on 40 percent fewer carbohydrates after taking *d-fenfluramine*, a drug that supposedly kills the desire for carbohydrates by increasing the activity of serotonin. "It's like taking an aspirin for a headache," says Judith Wurtman. "It works instantly and might be used when the need arises, like during a stressful situation, or, for women, prior to menstruation." d-Fenfluramine is sold in France and should be available to Americans in several years.

Too many stimulants, too few suppressants, or the brain's inability to react to suppressants—perhaps due to an inadequate number of receptors or receptors that malfunction—can cause overeating and eventually obesity. Also, a small imbalance could trigger weight gains over a long span of time. As few as 30 extra calories a day for 10 years could cause many people to gain 30 pounds. By suppressing these stimulants, or stimulating production of these suppressants, scientists someday hope to control abnormal cravings for some foods.

But the neuropeptide-Y research at Rockefeller has further implications. During the experiments, the lab rats that had eaten so voraciously after injections of neuropeptide Y gained weight "faster than they ate," says Dr. Stanley, further explaining that the speed and intensity of their weight gain was too great for the amount of calories they consumed. Something else was at work. The excess of neuropeptide Y may have begun a biochemical chain reaction that caused the rats' metabolism rates to collapse. They needed fewer calories than normal to gain weight. Controlling appetite may be the first step to controlling the human body's metabolism, the rate at which it consumes calories.

Fat on Ice

Tomorrow your dieting options may offer you considerably more food for thought. Now the most extreme diets, such as fasting, or outright starvation, can only be undertaken with complete medical supervision and used on morbidly obese patients who must lose weight quickly. (Oddly, the longer the fast, the easier it becomes to maintain; people on starvation diets (the most extreme fast) lose their desire to eat and drink.)

Researchers have begun playing with the notion of hibernation as a means of losing weight. What could be easier than settling down for a long winter's nap while your body whittles away its stubborn lard? Could a human being actually hibernate like a woodchuck or a mother bear, who will drop one-third of her weight during a 5-month hibernation?

Already scientists are studying these animals for clues as to how people might match the feat, not only for dieting purposes, but for suspended animation for space travel, cold climate survival, or surgery. In the early 1950s, the Air Force began hibernation research to try to find a way to keep downed fliers alive in extremely cold weather.

Dr. Wilma Spurrier, a researcher at Loyola Medical Center, Maywood, Illinois, discovered that when the blood of hibernating animals was injected into nonhibernators, these animals began exhibiting some of the behavior of hibernators. An opiate-like substance in the hibernators' blood—it was dubbed the *hibernation induction trigger (HIT)*—can also work on receptors in the brains of nonhibernators, such as monkeys, and induce a state similar to hibernation. For instance, the monkeys become quite docile. "You can pull their tails, even poke them," Dr. Spurrier says. She has injected monkeys with enough HIT to lower their body temperatures 3 degrees for 6 to 8 hours and cause their pulse to drop 40 to 50 percent. They also lost their appetites, perhaps because low body temperatures act similarly to high ones, turning off the desire for food. The monkeys ate less than half their usual amount of food for up to 3 weeks.

Many problems lie ahead, but a purified form of HIT is in the offing and will make research much easier. It will be several years—perhaps decades—before hibernation experiments can be performed on humans. Researchers could find that our tissues simply are not suited for hibernation, or they might discover that we are capable only of a state of partial hibernation, which still might help dieters. Spurrier remains optimistic. "I've been a fatty all my life and believe me, I want this to work," she says.

Brown Fat

As hibernators begin to warm up, their body cells burn a substance known as brown fat, a substance we humans also possess, although not in as great a proportion as other animals. A brown fat cell looks tan—hence its name—but more importantly it has about half as much triglyceride as a white fat cell. What also makes a brown fat cell unique, according to Dr. Barbara Horwitz, a professor of animal physiology at the University of California at Davis, is the cell's metabolic machinery; the cell contains a special protein that feeds off the triglycerides stored inside the cell. While white fat collects calories, brown fat eats them up.

This fat is turned into carbon dioxide and water, releasing energy as heat. British scientists discovered in an experiment that certain rats consumed 50 percent more calories than they needed to gain weight but remained lean. Autopsies revealed that they had a higher than average amount of brown fat. Unfortunately, the larger the mammal, the smaller the percentage of brown fat in its body. While 5 percent of the total amount of fat in a rat may be brown, perhaps only 1 percent in a human is brown. However, this statistic might not be as important as the efficiency at which the brown fat cells operate. Researchers wonder if people who are only 10 to 20 percent overweight might have brown fat cells that don't burn calories as well as those of people of normal weight. A small percentage of inefficiency, says Dr. Horwitz, could over a number of years cause gradual but noticeable weight gain.

Can brown fat cell efficiency be improved? Rats placed in a cold environment (5 to 7 degrees Centigrade) adapted to the low temperature by adjusting the metabolic machinery inside their brown fat cells, burning more calories to stay warm. Brown fat efficiency has also improved in lab rats when they ate foods that, ironically, had high fat content. Also, a category of drugs, *beta adrenergic agents*, can stimulate the growth of brown fat cells, but cause a number of side effects. "If the side effects can be licked, this treatment could probably help a lot of people with slight weight problems, so we're certainly hoping it someday can be applied," Horwitz says.

Cellular Warfare

Every dieter has woven fantasies about a miracle drug, a magic pill that could simply be popped into his or her mouth and would dissolve as much fat as needed. Many naysayers argue that our weight control system is too complicated for a single treatment to work. But a discovery made in Scotland might prove them wrong.

After working 8 years, biochemists at the Hannah Research Institute found a serum that can seek out and destroy fat cells in animals. These researchers have focused on the use of so-called biologicals, which lie inside the body and protect us against viruses, germs, and other foreign substances. (The approach is similar to the one used by cancer researchers experimenting with interleukins and protein interferons.)

At Hannah, researchers removed fat cells from rats and injected the cells into sheep. These alien fat cells bind themselves to the membranes of the normal fat cells of the sheep. The binding makes the normal fat cells seem foreign to the animals' defenses. "It's really very natural," says Dr. David Flint, a researcher at Hannah. These defenses, or antibodies, puncture the membranes of the fat cells, causing them to leak the triglycerides that had been stored inside. The stricken cells either become incapable of storing fats, or they store the fats less efficiently. Two months after the animals had been treated with the serum, they lost 30 percent of their body fat—with no other changes in diet or exercise.

The technique is being developed to rid livestock of fat, which is essential now that European consumers demand leaner meats. In theory, it could be used on humans, says Dr. Flint, although many problems loom. Chief among these: What happens to the triglycerides after they have been freed from their fat cells? They may simply float around the bloodstream until they clog arteries and veins, causing high blood pressure and increasing an individual's chance of heart disease.

This is not a concern with livestock, which of course will be slaughtered before they could be threatened by a heart attack. Commercial trials for the serum are slated to begin in 3 years, and if all goes well, the serum could be available to livestock growers in another 2 years.

Many pharmaceutical companies have contacted Hannah expressing interest in research focused on humans. Flint is hopeful about the serum's prospects. A fat-killing serum may come to the rescue, saving us from more diets and exercise routines that don't work well enough.

Why Diets Don't Work

What is obesity, anyway? The answer can't always be found spinning on our bathroom scales. Obesity means fatness, and it's possible—albeit rarely—to be overweight without being overly fat. For instance, football players are far heavier than other men of the same size and height, but these athletes weigh more because they have more muscle. These overweight men are actually underfat. Conversely, sedentary men of normal weight can have too much body fat.

Thus, obesity is defined as a body fat content over 25 percent in men, 35 percent in women. (Women probably have more fat because they need it for childbearing.) And as we grow older, we get more fatty—even if we maintain the same weight. One explanation for this development: As our ancestors competed for scarce food, the older, weaker ones could only survive if, as they aged, they needed less food to convert into fat.

We can find out what percentage of our body weight is fat with noninvasive techniques that include skinfold measurements, densitometry (weighing patient under water), whole potassium counting, or total body electrical conductivity. The old "pinch an inch" or skinfold technique is simple and can be easily performed by most doctors. About half our body fat can be observed and measured; true skin is only 1 millimeter thick, so most of the tissue we can pinch is fat.

Not everyone suffers from the same kind of obesity or for the same reasons. We may either have fat cells that have become enlarged (hypertrophic) or have grown too many fat cells (hyperplastic-hypertrophic). If we began gaining weight only as adults, our cells have probably just enlarged. If we have been overweight since childhood we usually have an excess of cells.

If we suffer from adult-onset obesity we have a good chance of controlling it with traditional techniques: diet, exercise, drugs, and behavioral therapy. But for people who have been overweight since childhood, traditional techniques fail even though these people may have nearly starved themselves.

Why? The first law of thermodynamics states that energy cannot be created or destroyed. Unfortunately we have very law-abiding bodies, so whatever we eat must be accounted for somehow. We either burn it up or store it away. Once our fat cells have stored this excess energy and swelled, we usually try to shrink the cells by dieting.

Dieters are essentially waging war against their bodies' own survival mechanism. During the evolution of the human species, people faced far more famines than they did feasts; to have a body that was very efficient at storing fat was a virtue. (One of the advantages of obesity in earlier times was that it increases resistance to tuberculosis, which may help explain why corpulence was held in high esteem by many earlier cultures. King Henry VIII was elated when he learned that one of his wives to be had a healthy double chin.) Only recently have researchers discovered how this memory of starvation haunts us today, and in turn, why diets fail.

The loss-gain–loss-gain phenomenon that is part of almost all dieting is often called the "yo-yo syndrome," but it can also be tagged with an even more ominous-sounding metaphorical title— the "rachet effect." How does the rachet effect work? Our bodies have a sort of self-regulating function that warns us to maintain a certain stable weight, called a "set point." This weight is not really set in cement; it can be moved up or down somewhat by healthy diet and exercise or the lack thereof.

We dutifully start our diets. Water, glycogen—which provides us with energy—and protein make up the couple of pounds a week we drop during the first weeks of dieting. After we have lost this "easy" weight, we plateau, which happens not only because fat is harder to shrink than muscle, but also because our bodies' metabolism rates drop, sometimes as much as 45 percent. In other words, the less we eat, the less we need to eat.

To make matters worse, the moment we stop dieting, we'll regain weight much faster than we lost it. Our fat cells lay first claim to any renewed nourishment, and we'll end up with a higher percentage of body fat than we had at the start of our diets.

Also, as we diet, our appetite heightens. Rockefeller's Dr. Leibel explains that as our cells shrink, triglycerides, which make up 99 percent of the fat in fat cells, break down into free fatty acid and glycerol. During a diet, only 35 to 40 percent of the free fatty acids remain in the cells, leaving a lot to float around in our bloodstream. And the researchers at Rockefeller speculate that this excess of fatty acid stimulates appetite. Some weight control specialists argue that we must ignore internal pressure to break a diet, and that in the future nearly everyone will be forced to *vieller sec*, a French expression that means "to age dry," by starting to diet at age 25— and never stopping.

Overweight people can never have the luxury of eating normally. They face a lifetime of staying hungry. The American Society of Bariatric Physicians (ASBP) use three criteria to judge the effectiveness of diets: safety, short-term weight loss, and long-term weight loss. The Weight Watchers diet program was ranked safest and most effective. Novelty diets that allow us to eat up to 1200 calories worth of certain foods, like grapefruits or plant juices, were criticized. Often these diets advertise that certain food combinations will target body fat for destruction by increasing metabolic rates, destroying the will to eat, or removing toxins that cause weight gain. If these diets do indeed work, they work for the same reason any diet works—because dieters ingest fewer calories per day than their bodies need to maintain their weight—reports the ASBP. Conceivably, we could lose weight on a chocolate mousse diet.

Working It Off

Why do we suffer from such wretched rebounds after a diet?

Lying in wait inside our fat cells is an enzyme: *low-density lip-oprotein lipase (LDL)*. LDL acts on certain substances that float in our bloodstream and changes them into glycerol and free fatty acids, which are transported across our cells' membranes and stored as lipid. LDL becomes very active during a diet, especially when our bodies fall below their set points. LDL not only stimulates our appetite control system, but it also makes it easier for our fat cells to suck up the lipids they need to swell, sometimes up to three to five times their normal size. As a cell swells, it can burst, splitting into more cells with their own ravenous cravings for lipids. The bad news: Once we gain a fat cell, we can shrink it but never lose it. Every time our fat cells split our weight problem grows accordingly.

Can anything arrest our insatiable LDL? Dr. Peter Herbert, a researcher at Rhode Island Miriam Hospital, has theorized that cigarette smoking may inhibit LDL, which might explain why people who stop smoking often start gaining weight. He discovered that smokers have low levels of LDL until they quit. That doesn't mean we should start smoking to lose weight, but it does pose some interesting questions. More importantly, exercise lowers the ratio of low-to-high-density lipoprotein lipase.

Most weight control specialists now stress a program of exercise combined with dieting. Exercise alters the behavior of lipoprotein lipase. While LDL stimulates the accumulation of fat in our cells, *high-density lipoprotein lipase (HDL)* counters this effect, helping to remove fatty tissue deposited by LDL in our arteries, according to Dr. Herbert. Thus, the ratio of HDL to LDL in our bloodstream has a direct correlation to our chance of having a heart attack. Long distance runners, for example, have an HDL-LDL ratio that's about 50-50. Sedentary people have HDL levels as low as 29 percent. Less HDL is broken down by our bodies if we exercise, which leaves more of it available to attack the fatty substances, such as choles-terol, that clog our arteries.

Unfortunately, exercise doesn't help everyone equally. People who suffer from an excess of fat cells (unlike those who are fat because their fat cells are enlarged) don't respond well to exercise. Usually if we have fatty thighs or buttocks, we suffer from too many fat cells. Even if those cells are shrunk to the maximum, they are so numerous that we still look fat. People who have upper body obesity usually respond better to exercise because upper-body fat cells tend to be merely enlarged, and need only to be shrunk. (The good news for victims of lower body obesity is that they are less prone to weight-related diseases.) Remember: Although exercise can shrink our fat cells, it cannot obliterate them or hamper their efficiency. That's why exercise will probably play a smaller role in weight reduction in the future.

Trimming the Fat

Unlike dieting or exercise, surgery can actually rid our bodies of fat cells, and offer clues as to how we may someday be able to slice away more of our flab. Surgical remedies were until recently thought of only as extreme measures to use in cases of morbid obesity. One procedure, the *jejunoileal bypass*, which eliminates the use of the stomach in digestion, has been all but abandoned because of its side effects, such as growth of bacteria and diarrhea. This technique, however, inspired development of other gastric procedures that merely make the stomach smaller.

Only patients who are 200 percent over normal body weight will be considered for this surgery. Those who have it are usually pleased with the results, although one out of four patients need the operation again. If the patient overeats, his or her stomach can be stretched to its original size. If the patient sticks to a diet, he or she can lose as much as two-thirds of the excess weight. The success rate for morbidly obese patients underscores another point: how badly current programs of diet, exercise, drugs, and behavioral therapy have failed in serious cases.

Is surgery an option only for victims of morbid obesity? No. For people who are as little as 20 percent overweight, a technique in which a balloon is inserted into the stomach and later inflated has been approved by the FDA. The technique, developed by Drs. Mary and Lloyd Garren, gastroneurologists at Union Hospital in Elkton, Maryland, makes eating uncomfortable for the patient, but like other gastric procedures, can be foiled by constant snacking or by intake of high-calorie liquids.

For those who are less than 20 percent overweight, another technique called fat suctioning, or *suction lipectomy*, can remove stubborn fat from parts of the body that are particularly resistant to dieting and exercise, such as hips, thighs, buttocks, and abdomens. Lipectomies can also eliminate fat from double chins and—a popular request by men—breasts.

Developed in Switzerland in the 1970s, lipectomy is really a form of plastic surgery and is used only to remove small, local deposits of fat. Doctors caution that it is not a cure for obesity; the most fat removed from a patient thus far has been only 3 pounds. Also, for best results a patient should have fairly young skin, although a 78-year-old woman has been treated successfully.

Dr. Norman Martin, of Beverly Hills Medical Center has performed over 4,000 lipectomies. Eighty percent of his patients are women. Martin explains that after an injection of saline solution and adrenaline, a one-half-inch incision is made above the pubic area, the knee, or inside the crease of the buttocks, through which a long, hollow rod is inserted. A surgeon steers the rod in a radial pattern from the point of the incision, suctioning out tunnels of fat with each thrust. The more thrusts made, the more fat removed. Although general anethesia is usually used, small areas can be treated under local anesthesia, requiring only one day in the hospital. After the surgeon finishes tunneling, an elastic dressing is applied over the treated area to support the skin until it contracts to its new, thinner shape. The dressing stays in place at least a week, and the patient must wear a girdle or other support for 1 to 2 months.

Although no research yet supports his observation, Martin has noticed that many of his patients have found it easier to lose weight after surgery. "A lot of them have told me that they lost another 10 pounds or so without really trying," he says.

Many people who exceed the 20 percent overweight limit have requested the surgery, but Martin can't perform it on them. If too much fat is removed, a patient could suffer shock, he explains, although he did break his rule for one woman who had such large fat deposits on her inner thighs she could barely walk, or even sit comfortably.

Tomorrow, techniques similar to lipectomies will become more refined, and perhaps will even be used to remove larger chunks of fat. And one service they will certainly offer is the delicate fine-tuning that will be needed by all people who have lost weight, but who still wear many of the lumps and bumps of stubborn fat that have evaded other weight loss stratagems.

Thin Pills

Americans spend more than $200 million a year on appetite suppressants. Nonprescription suppressants are generally made up of one of two drugs: *benzocaine*, a local anesthetic found in diet gums, candies, and lozenges that purport to numb the taste buds, blunting our desire to eat; and *phenylpropanolamine (PPA)*, which is similar to an amphetamine, and is sold as pills or capsules. No serious side effects have been reported by users of benzocaine. In a few cases, people who swallowed PPA may have suffered from high blood pressure, kidney failure, stroke, psychotic reactions, and other complications. Some physicians and consumer groups have lobbied the FDA to have PPA removed from the list of nonprescription drugs.

"PPA has to be taken as directed," says Princeton's Dr. Bart Hoebel, who did early research on the drug. "There might be that one in a million person who is hypertensive, drinks six cups of coffee a day, and takes too many PPA pills who has a reaction." The FDA, thus far, has refused to make PPA available as a prescription drug.

More effective than these over-the-counter drugs are *amphetamines*, but many doctors hesitate to prescribe them because of the adverse publicity that clouds their use. Amphetamines were the first appetite suppressants ever used, and their effectiveness as suppressants was discovered accidentally. They were first prescribed in the 1930s for people who suffered from narcolepsy—a condition during which the victim periodically falls into deep sleeps. These patients noticed that they lost their appetites when taking the drug, and amphetamines were soon after prescribed for weight disorders. Many specialists still consider amphetamines the drugs of choice for obese patients, depending on their medical history, family history, and occupation.

Drug therapy often undermines the confidence dieters have in their own ability to lose weight. They feel once the medication stops, they can no longer withstand the forces that compelled them to gain weight in the first place. Most patients gain 5 or 10 pounds the month after they stop taking drugs. "I only prescribe them in an emergency, or when someone has to lose weight quickly for health reasons," says Dr. Thomas Wadden, clinical director for the Obesity Research Group at the University of Pennsylvania.

Others do not agree that these drugs affect dieters' confidence. "Drug therapy doesn't sap dieters' willpower," says MIT's Dr. Judith Wurtman. "They have no willpower in the first place or they wouldn't be in the shape they're in." While weight control specialists argue over the virtues of today's medications, the outcome of the debate will probably depend upon the effectiveness of future diet drugs. If they can help a dieter lose weight and keep the weight off with no side effects, these drugs could become a staple of many diets.

Another drug therapy failure involves an unusual and initially promising tactic: impairing the absorption of food in the intestines. One drug that does this, *cholestyramine*, also impairs the absorption of fat-soluble vitamins. *Perfluorooctyl bromide*, a fluorocarbon, is taken orally and makes its way to the intestines, coating their walls like paint, thus blocking absorption of food. Like cholestyramine, the chemical inhibits the absorption of all nutrients, including fats.

Starch Blockers were removed from the over-the-counter market in 1983 by the FDA. The chemical supposedly neutralized an enzyme, alpha amylase, which is secreted by the pancreas and is needed to digest starch. One million starch blocker tablets were being consumed daily in the U.S. at the time. Some users suffered from severe constipation, nausea, and vomiting. Side effects notwithstanding, users didn't lose weight. Researchers speculated that the starch blockers failed because the dosage was too small to handle the amounts of alpha amylase present in the body.

This type of setback often casts entire drug therapy programs into an unfavorable light, and it's not surprising that many weight control specialists reject drugs outright for their patients. But there is little doubt that if obesity can be conquered, drugs will play a role. How, when, and to what extent remains open to debate.

How We Eat, How We Think

When we look at a fat person, what do we see? Someone who is lazy? Sloppy? Weak-willed? Self-indulgent? Stupid? Not only do lean people look at their fatter peers this way, so do fat people. Emotional problems have often been cited as the source of obesity, but, several studies have failed to uncover any common underlying personality trait that can be linked with obesity.

We are not fat because of a problem with our personality, but we can develop problems like anxiety, depression, and low self-esteem because we are fat. Dieting causes hunger and hunger causes irritability, hostility, and depression. Children who are forced to diet often become resentful and scheme to undermine their weight control programs. On the other hand, weight loss can work wonders on a patient's psyche, allowing him or her to become more confident, assertive, and independent.

Psychologists tell their obese patients that they must monitor their eating habits. As a short-term technique for weight loss, self-monitoring works. After awhile, other behavioral treatments are needed. Dieters are also shown how to manage their environments. For example, if they eat in front of the TV, they must turn it off.

Therapists often urge an obese patient's spouse or other family members to acknowledge the patient's progress, and generally to be supportive and helpful. Sometimes a patient and therapist will draw up a contract that specifies changes in eating habits that must be made. Success is rewarded, failure punished.

Behavior-modification programs do help, but not a lot. Average weight loss for dieters who use this therapy is 10 pounds, much of which is regained within a year after therapy has ended. To keep weight off, patients must combine behavioral therapy with exercise and diet. Georgetown's Dr. Aaron Altschul speculates that more such therapy will be used in the future. Dr. Thomas Wadden of the University of Pennsylvania agrees, adding that while specialists wait for miracle drugs to appear, behavior therapy is one of the few techniques tht can be used today with some success—even though its success rate is modest.

We Are Not What We Eat

The citizens of ancient Sparta used to drive overweight people in shame beyond the walls of the city. Today our means of expresssing disapproval might not be as cruel, but victims of obesity continue to live in shame. A fear not only of obesity, but of any odd lump or bump, has driven 80 percent of the fourth grade girls in San Francisco to dieting, according to one study by the University of California. Perhaps what many obese people will need is not another grapefruit diet or dancercise routine, but a public relations agent or a civil rights lawyer.

Part of the problem lies with the position taken by the National Institutes of Health. NIH sees obesity as a disease, and this increases the pressure on the obese to lose weight even though mounting evidence shows that most are unable to. People who would claim they never discriminate against anyone on the basis of appearance feel quite justified when they object to someone's weight because it's supposedly a health problem.

The extent to which obesity is a health problem is debatable. Despite the NIH's findings, the world's largest epidemiological study on the effects of weight and mortality presents conflicting data. Sponsored by Norway's National Institute of Public Health, the Norway Study shows one glaring exception to the general rule that obesity is harmful to your health: Among women who are five foot seven, aged 25 to 29, the risk of dying over the next 10 years (which is 1 percent) remains the same whether they weigh 198 or 115 pounds.

Researchers from Rockefeller University followed a group of women and one man, all of whom weighed more than 200 pounds but dieted until they got their weights down to normal—at least they looked normal. But their body chemistries were anything but average. Every woman had stopped menstruating. Other symptoms included abnormally small fat cells, low levels of thyroid hormone, low white blood cell counts, low pulse rates of about 50 to 60 beats per minute, and low blood pressure of about 100/60. They always felt depressed; thoughts of food harassed them constantly, yet sadly they needed 25 percent fewer calories to maintain their weight than would have been expected of others who are the same height and weight. To become "normal," these people became anorectic. And if they regained their lost weight, they felt fine. "Fat people may not be in an abnormal state when they are obese," says Dr. Rudolph Leibel.

In the immediate future, the real problem for overweight people will be to confront obesity not as a health issue, but also as a moral one. Not long ago in Pennsylvania, a convicted drug dealer who weighed 350-plus pounds had his jail sentence set to a sliding scale: 1 to 3 years, with parole to be granted if he lost 150 pounds.

To help overweight people become more aware of their plight and their options, the National Association to Aid Fat Americans was formed. The organization publishes a newsletter and supports its members with health and legal information while it tries to educate the American public about obesity. "Everybody on Madison Avenue is doing all they can to get people to eat fat-rich, processed foods that help make them obese," says Dr. Wadden. "At some point society must become supportive of the problems these people face and must understand that just as people vary in height, they vary in weight."

Timeline

1987 to 2000
- Suppressants will act on the brain's hypothalmus to curb appetite.
- Doctors will no longer prescribe amphetamines for weight control.
- More-refined surgical techniques will allow removal of larger fat deposits and restructuring of features.
- Use of the appetite suppressant PPA will substantially decrease.
- New gastric procedures developed that will section off or otherwise make stomachs smaller.

2001 to 2025
- Serums that will injure or destroy human fat cells available.
- Diet and exercise will play smaller roles in weight control.
- Treatment available that will increase the rate at which the human body burns calories without side effect.

2026 to 2050
- Technology available that will allow humans to hibernate at least partially.

Access Guide

For more information about health implications of obesity contact:

U.S. Department of Health and Human Services
Public Health Service
National Institutes of Health
Office of Medical Applications of Research
Building 1, Room 216
Bethesda, MD 20205
(301) 496-1143

For more information about current techniques in weight control contact:

Georgetown University Diet
  Management Program
Lower Level, Gorman Building
3800 Reservoir Road, Northwest
Washington, DC 20007
(202) 625-3674

Dr. Peter Miller
Hilton Head Health Institute
P.O. Box 7138
Hilton Head Island, SC 29938
(803) 785-7292

Dr. Gerard Musante
Structure House
707 Morehead Avenue
Durham, NC 27707
(919) 689-9846

Dr. Thomas Wadden
University of Pennsylvania
  Obesity Research Group
113 South 36th Street Suite 507
Philadelphia, PA 19104
(215) 898-7314

Dr. Janet Grommet
St. Luke's-Roosevelt Hospital
  Center Weight Control Unit
411 West 114th Street
New York, NY 10025
(212) 870-1743

Dr. Michael Hamilton
Duke University Diet and Fitness
  Center
804 West Trinity Avenue
Durham, NC 27701
(919) 684-6331

Beth Israel Hospital Weight Loss
  Clinic
Psychiatric Department
330 Brookline Avenue
Boston, MA 02115
(617) 735-4735

For information regarding health, civil rights, and counseling contact:

National Association to Aid Fat Americans (NAAFA)
P.O. Box 43
Bellrose, NY 11426
(516) 352-3120

12
Super Foods, Megavitamins

"Let thy food be thy medicine, and thy medicine be thy food," said Hippocrates, the father of medicine, 2500 years ago. And Maimonides, in the thirteenth century, said: "Let nothing that can be treated by diet be cured by any other means." The idea that disease can be treated by diet is one of the oldest in medicine. Indeed, from prehistoric times, people have often attributed seemingly mystical qualities to food. It was not until the twentieth century, however, that scientists began isolating and identifying the microscopic compounds in food that substantiated some folk myths. And today, as researchers learn more about the chemical roots of disease, mainstream doctors and scientists are beginning to recognize the importance of nutrition—particularly vitamins—not only in the prevention of chronic illness, but also in the treatment of such degenerative killers as cancer and heart disease.

The increased interest in nutrition began in the late 1960s when a growing body of scientific evidence prompted public health experts, such as researchers at the American Heart Association, to admonish Americans against diets rich in fat and cholesterol that were linked to the high incidence of heart disease. More recently, such foodstuffs have also been implicated in the development of many types of cancers. And in 1980, the Departments of Agriculture and Health and Human Services jointly published dietary guidelines encouraging a decreased consumption of fat, cholesterol, salt, and sugar, and increased intake of complex carbohydrates and fiber.

Today, physicians, medical centers, and health organizations have begun working with restaurants to develop health-oriented menus. The American Heart Association, for example, implemented its nationwide Creative Cuisine program with the help of numerous companies that provide food service nationwide, including Arby's, Marriott Hotels, and American Airlines, while local chapters worked with individual establishments. And the Pritikin Longevity Center has likewise established an affiliation with restaurants across the country. Meanwhile, in Texas, Methodist Hospital's Sid W. Richardson Institute for Preventive Medicine opened its four star restaurant Chez Eddy within the medical center itself, and they plan to open another in Houston's shopping district. Even the Culinary Institute of America in Hyde Park, New York, sought the help of New York Medical College in setting up nutrition guidelines for both its courses and its kitchen.

Employers are advocating healthy nutrition in the workplace. Recognizing that better nutrition leads to better health, and therefore, fewer sick days and optimal performance, employers from multinational corporations such as Xerox and municipal governments like that of Birmingham, Alabama, to small, family-operated companies, are emphasizing nutritional education and dietary counseling. Further, as computers have aided physicians in analyzing patients' nutritional needs, software programs have been flooding the market so that individuals can carefully critique their own dietary practices at home.

The renewed interest in nutrition is also causing many researchers and physicians to reexamine the applicability of the recommended dietary allowances (RDAs) published by the National Academy of Sciences (NAS). Instituted during World War II when concern over the adequacy of the national food supply turned the government's attention to Americans' nutritional needs, the RDAs defined the minimum requirements for mass-feeding whole populations. Requirements were established to prevent nutrient deficiency diseases, such as pellagra, beriberi, and scurvy.

Reviewing the latest scientific literature every 5 years, the Academy's Food and Nutrition Board touts the RDAs as the necessary requirements to maintain good health, "health" implying an absence of disease. Despite the fact that there are more than 40 nutrients identified as essential to good health, many of those are not included among the RDAs. The argument against including these: There's no indication that lack of some vitamins and minerals causes *deficiency* diseases. But research shows that inadequate amounts of some vitamins and minerals can cause physiological damage long before deficiency symptoms appear.

In 1985, committee members who produced the latest updated

RDA report found themselves in conflict with other academy panels. Among its proposed changes, the report suggested a decrease in the RDAs for vitamins A and C. Yet in 1982, another academy group had reported that foods rich in these two vitamins appeared to reduce the risk of some types of cancer. Because of the conflict over the new RDA proposals, the NAS decided not to officially issue the latest report. In effect, NAS officials chose to not accept the new guidelines.

In 1968, when Nobel Prize-winning chemist Linus Pauling presented evidence that vitamin C prevented and cured diseases other than scurvy, he was scorned and ridiculed not only by many of his peers, some of whom decided that he had become senile, but also by physicians untrained in nutrition. Pauling pointed out that for vitamin C effect to combat the common cold, a daily intake of at least 1,000 milligrams of the vitamin was apparently necessary. But the significance of his studies goes beyond the controversy over vitamin C. If traditionalists were wrong in their belief that large-dosage vitamin C supplementation is ineffective, then similar assumptions about other vitamins might also be incorrect. Moreover, as the vitamin C experience shows, vitamins may have more than one action, and amounts in excess of the RDAs may indeed be beneficial.

Nutritional Medicine

For the last 5 months, the patient has complained of insomnia, fatigue, and depression. He has had one cold after another. Long past adolescence, he has also suddenly developed adult acne. At the doctor's office, the nurse collects the standard urine and blood samples, and clips a lock of pubic hair. "It's exposed to less environmental pollution and other external chemicals," she says. "The hair analysis for mineral content will be more accurate." Then the doctor examines the patient, including tongue and fingernails. He inquires about past illnesses, exercise routine, and eating habits, and he runs all the data through the computer.

The diagnosis: Stress has increased this man's nutrient requirements. He reports that the patient is deficient in zinc, magnesium, and B vitamins. And stress has been sapping all available vitamin C. Toxic levels of lead are present; the zinc and B deficiencies have caused the acne. The prescription: the physician's own multiple vitamin formula prepared according to the needs of the individual patient, a mineral preparation, and megadoses of vitamin C. He suggests pumpkin seeds to increase the intake of zinc. And eggs and applesauce every day to remove the excess lead.

"Nutrition is the key to good medicine," San Francisco physician Richard Kunin says. "And ideally, orthomolecular medicine should become mainstream medicine.

Orthomolecular medicine is the preservation of good health and the treatment of disease through manipulation of the body's chemistry. "Disease is often a chemical imbalance," explains San Francisco's Dr. Michael Lesser, a founder of the Orthomolecular Medical Society. "We don't say drugs and surgery are bad, just that the doctor should first try correcting the problem nutritionally. We work to strengthen the body's defenses, often using vitamins, minerals, and other nutrients to do the job." But even as this growing low technology alternative to more conventional health care attracts increasing numbers of patients, orthomolecular medicine remains at the center of one of traditional medicine's most heated controversies.

Modern nutritional therapy began in 1949, when Dr. Fred Klenner, chief of staff at Memorial Hospital in Reidsville, North Carolina, told of successfully treating viral disease with enormous doses of vitamin C—up to 100 grams a day given intravenously.

Several years later, two Canadian psychiatrists tested a nutritional therapy for schizophrenia. Doctors Abrams Hoffer and Humphrey Osmond reported that the then standard treatment— psychotherapy and electric shock—were 80 percent more effective when backed up by a high-protein, low-carbohydrate diet, with megadoses of niacin, B vitamins, and vitamin C. They produced equivalent results in studies that varied in sample size from 17 patients to more than 120.

Nobel Prize-winning chemist Linus Pauling finally coined the term "orthomolecular medicine" in 1968—from *orthos*, Greek for "corrective," and "molecular," for the body's chemical makeup.

But the body's chemistry cannot be corrected unless we know what is needed. And it was Roger Williams, former director of the Clayton Foundation Biochemical Institute at the University of Texas in Austin, who proposed vitamins and minerals for nutritional insurance. Williams reported that there are vast differences in the biochemical requirements of different individuals. No one prescription of nutrients can work in every case; the recommendations must be tailored to each patient's need. This may often mean prescribing by trial and error, working to determine what dosage works, while maintaining all the nutrients in synergistic balance.

Unlike many orthomolecular theorists, Williams had a bushel of professional credits. A member of the National Academy of Sciences, he is the discoverer of pantothenic acid, a B vitamin found in all living tissue, especially in the liver, and essential for metabolism and hormone synthesis. His idea that people are as different in their biochemistry as they are in appearance gave the practice of tailoring the diet to the individual validity. In a less controversial field, his new approach might have won backing.

Traditional physicians, however, charge that orthomolecular theorists don't do proper research. Their results, they say, vary so widely that they cannot be duplicated. But this *may* say more about the way orthodox medicine conducts research than about orthomolecular practices. "Most researchers vary only one nutrient at a time, for example, administering niacin without a low-carbohydrate diet," Lesser said, in testimony before the Senate's Select Committee on Nutrition and Human Needs. "It's the classic way drugs are tested in medicine, but it's oversimplified."

Adherents to orthomolecular medicine—which includes nutritional medicine, orthomolecular psychiatry, and clinical ecology (or ecological medicine)—remain a small band of persistent pioneers. Nevertheless, they are attracting a growing number of believers, both physicians and patients. In the future, there may be individual biochemistry laboratories and an even larger number of nutrition specialists to whom people will go for regular tune-ups as easily— and as often—as they go to the dentist. And for those people who do not, there will be nutritional physicians who can correct the body's chemical imbalances and cure many diseases.

Super Fish

For generations, mothers have told their children that fish is good for them. Now everyone seems to be saying "Eat more fish," because it's nutrient-dense, supplying a wealth of vitamins and minerals. We know that fish, long referred to as "brain food," is also rich in omega-3 fatty acids, polyunsaturated oils, one of which is docosahexanoic acid (DHA). And nearly 70 percent of the brain's gray matter is made of fats, with DHA being one of the most important. Researchers at the University of Toronto have found that rats fed a diet high in polyunsaturated fats learn more quickly than those consuming saturated fat.

Though there is currently no proof that omega-3's are essential for human development, a number of studies suggest their importance. Some researchers believe that nursing mothers in America may be ingesting too few omega-3's, possibly affecting brain development in their infants, according to University of Oregon nutritional researcher William Harris. Studies have shown that depriving young animals of omega-3 while their brains are developing can impair mental function.

Seafood, however, is more than just brain food. Studies of Greenland Eskimos and Japanese fishermen, who rely on fish as a dietary staple, showed a surprisingly low incidence of heart attacks. And a 20-year study of more than 800 middle-aged Dutch males found that those who ate just 3 ounces of fish a week had a 36 percent lower risk of heart disease than those who ate no fish. Those who ate 7 to 11 ounces a week, moreover, had a 64 percent lower risk.

Ironically, physicians once warned heart patients to stay away from seafood—especially shellfish—because they believed it contained excessive cholesterol. But even shellfish, with the highest cholesterol content, contains less in a single serving than one egg. As interest grows in the use of dietary measures to prevent and treat diseases, researchers are finding that omega-3 fats can actually reduce cholesterol levels; prevent blood clots, often a major cause of heart attacks; possibly retard the development of atherosclerosis; the buildup of material, mostly cholesterol, along arterial walls, and perhaps lower blood pressure.

Other studies, moreover, indicate that polyunsaturated oils from cold water fish may have an impact on the pain and swelling associated with arthritis. Brandeis University biologist K. C. Hayes reports, for instance, that fish oil fed to arthritic mice and monkeys reduced the inflammation. It acts by altering prostaglandins, hormones that trigger cell response to infection and allergies, causing inflammation.

Long-term effects, if any, of megadosing on fish are still not known. But doctors *are* suggesting more fish in our diet. The prescriptions may vary from two, three, or more servings a week to a half pound a day. For patients who really despise the taste of fish, doctors will prescribe fish oil tablets.

Garlic Power

For millennia, practitioners of folk medicine have credited garlic with astounding attributes. The Codex Ebers, an Egyptian medical papyrus dating from about 1550 B.C., makes 22 references to garlic as an effective remedy for ailments including heart problems, headaches, bites, worms, and tumors. In India, garlic has served as an antiseptic lotion for washing wounds and ulcers.

Recently, studies in India and West Germany have indicated that garlic may help break up cholesterol in blood vessels, preventing atherosclerosis and heart disease. In an epidemiological study of three Indian populations that consumed differing amounts of garlic and onions, those who consumed the most garlic and onions had the longest blood coagulation time. Their blood was thinner and more fluid, and thus less sticky and less likely to form clots and block arteries.

And in a 1983 study at California's Loma Linda University School of Medicine, researchers reported that garlic may hold a promising position as a broad-spectrum therapeutic agent, and warrants further investigation. In a controlled study, volunteers consumed garlic oil in amounts equivalent to 10 cloves a day. In 6 months, the total blood level of low-density lipoprotein (LDL) cholesterol decreased by 14 percent. Moreover, the level of *high*-density lipoprotein (HDL) cholesterol increased by 41 percent. Both LDL and HDL transport cholesterol and other lipids, fat-like substances stored in the body as energy reserves, but HDL contains more protein and less fat, and a high level of HDL cholesterol is associated with a low incidence of heart disease.

However, consuming 10 cloves of garlic a day can have unpleasant side effects, such as diarrhea, nausea, vomiting, body odor, and, of course, bad breath.

The secret of garlic, and its cousin the onion, appears to be a number of selenium-containing compounds and other substances used by the plant to protect itself from bacteria and fungi, substances which may also benefit humans. But garlic seems to lose its potency when processed into powder or salt. In 1984, however, University of Minnesota chemists George Barany and Andrew Mott succeeded in synthesizing one of the plant's ingredients—allyl methyl trisulfide—in the laboratory. That success, Mott says, will now make possible further research into the magical powers of the allium family.

Once the chemical reactions are deciphered, moreover, physicians might begin prescribing garlic oil capsules—enclosing the oil will control its offensive odor—for a variety of ills. Or isolating garlic's magical formula will allow doctors to prescribe the chemicals in tablet form. After all, two or three cloves of garlic a day may be beneficial, but it won't encourage friendships or intimate relationships.

Mind Food

The brain, like the rest of the body, is highly sensitive to what we eat, and research is showing that food directly affects brain function. From high-carbohydrate diets that dull chronic pain to high-protein foods as a treatment for depression, scientists are looking at a range of therapies using a variety of different foods. In other words, our thoughts, feelings, and sensations can be altered by the simple components of breakfast.

Certain nutrients in our diet, it now appears, can have a direct effect on the production of brain neurotransmitters, the chemical messengers that carry signals from one nerve to the next. About 40 neurotransmitters have already been identified—some of them amino acids or derivatives of these protein building blocks—and these need vitamins B_6, B_{12}, and C for their synthesis. Neurotransmitters like norepinephrine, in fact, transmit the nerve impulses that control all emotions, perceptions, and bodily functions. They are, essentially, responsible for just about everything we do and feel.

Research at the Massachusetts Institute of Technology (MIT) and Harvard indicates that the brain's level of neurotransmitters fluctuates in direct response to the type and amount of nutrients in our blood. Tyrosine, an amino acid found in most proteins, for example, might be able to boost norepinephrine, which heightens alertness. Likewise, an increase in other everyday nutrients might enhance learning and memory, ease pain, induce sleep, or have a powerful effect on mood. Moreover, researchers say, if we can use common nutrients to manipulate neurotransmitters, we may be able to treat maladies including manic depression and high blood pressure.

MIT endocrinologist Richard Wurtman and other researchers have established that nutrients can also alter the level of such neurotransmitters as dopamine, acetylcholine, and serotonin. They frequently cite serotonin, which has a calming effect. Enzymes manufacture it from the amino acid tryptophan, abundant in high-protein foods. And Wurtman suggests whenever the brain has a shortage of serotonin, it somehow develops a craving for serotonin-increasing carbohydrates—potatoes, rice, and bread. In other words, the brain is always attuned to the body's nutrient status, and that knowledge determines what we eat. If such is the case, then doctors may begin prescribing fewer tranquilizers and sleeping pills, and suggest specific foods at specific times during the day and night.

But serotonin is not the only neurotransmitter implicated in depression. Research indicates that a deficit of norepinephrine may cause clinical depression as well. Harvard psychiatrist Alan Gelenberg has been investigating that possibility for several years. In his most widely cited experiment, he described a 30-year-old woman who took tyrosine, an amino acid from which norepinephrine is synthesized in the body, for 2 weeks: Her depression improved markedly, according to the psychological testing measures used. When a placebo was substituted for tyrosine, her depressive symptoms returned within 1 week. Although Gelenberg himself is skeptical of the results, Wurtman believes they make sense.

Depression is only one malady that nutrients may one day cure.

Their most dramatic use may be in the treatment of Alzheimer's disease, which afflicts the elderly with a progressive loss of memory and eventual full-blown dementia. In two 1976 studies, a clear biochemical abnormality was found connected with Alzheimer's disease: Virtually all victims have a severe deficit of the neurotransmitter acetylcholine.

In studies with rats, Wurtman found that an increase in dietary choline, which metabolizes and forms acetylcholine, elevated the level of acetylcholine in the brain. In experiments with human volunteers, he administered supplemental choline in the form of a naturally occurring substance called lecithin. The choline concentration in the volunteers' blood rose to levels that were high enough to stimulate brain acetylcholine in rats, he reported. In addition, Harvard doctor John Growden found that administering lecithin in combination with other drugs increased the level of choline in cerebrospinal fluid. The implication: The extra choline does have access to the human brain.

Wurtman believes that all his hypotheses must be *extensively* verified in tightly controlled human studies. Toward that end, he is busy trying to convince multinational food and pharmaceutical companies to participate in the work. Though the results are not in, Wurtman has been successful in enlisting interest from big business. Unilever, in the Netherlands, is researching the possible drug implications of lecithin, and the Thomas J. Lipton Company is producing lecithin-enriched noodles for experiments with Alzheimer's disease. Pierrel, in Italy, is testing a tyrosine intravenous solution for the treatment of traumatic shock.

The Immune System

Every day, the human body is invaded by alien bacteria, viruses, and other organisms. But with its complex, multitiered defense system—the immune system—it's able to resist such infections and fight disease. And vitamins, particularly A, C, and E, appear to stimulate and enhance the immune response.

Pauling first created a stir among the scientific community when he proposed that megadoses of vitamin C could prevent or lessen the severity of viral diseases such as the common cold and influenza.

But orthomolecular practitioners, using vitamin C in doses of 10 grams and higher, have reported even greater success in reducing the symptoms of bacterial and viral diseases. According to Dr. Robert C. Cathcart III, a Los Altos, California, physician, taking C along with eating a balanced diet speeds the recovery from mononucleosis, viral pneumonia, and viral hepatitis. But his most astounding results have been with AIDS patients, using amounts so high that vitamin C must be administered intravenously.

Cathcart believes that every infectious disease involves a severe depletion of vitamin C in the body. "It starts in the tissues directly involved by the disease, and spreads throughout the body," he says. "As the vitamin C is burned up as an antitoxin in the diseased tissues, it's slowly sapped out of other tissues. And if it's not replaced, every C-dependent function in the body is impaired."

Vitamin C spurs the body's manufacture of antibody molecules and enhances the effectiveness of the white blood cells that engulf and digest bacteria and other foreign debris. There is also evidence that vitamin C enhances the action of prostaglandin, a hormone-like substance found in blood cells that boosts the infection fighters known as T-lymphocytes. Vitamin C also increases the production of interferon, a body chemical that interferes with viral proliferation.

Cathcart classifies illnesses according to the amount of ascorbic acid needed to cure them. Hepatitis, for example, is a 60-disease. Bowel tolerance—the amount of vitamin C absorbed before it causes diarrhea—usually increases proportionately to the severity of the illness. A bad cold can increase tolerance to 100 grams a day, Cathcart explains, while severe viral infection can raise bowel tolerance to 200 grams a day. Scientific studies haven't confirmed C's effectiveness, he believes, because most researchers use too little. "Everyone is different," he stresses. "You have to take each patient right up to bowel tolerance."

But research at George Washington University in Washington, D.C., also suggests that megadoses of vitamin C may be effective in boosting the immune system's response to infection. In their study, biochemists Gary Thurman and Allan Goldstein used guinea pigs because, like humans, they cannot manufacture vitamin C. Maintaining two groups of the rodents on C-deficient diets, Thurman and Goldstein supplemented the drinking water of one group with the nutrient. Once a week for three weeks, they challenged the immune systems of both groups with harmful viruses. The results: More than twice as many C-deficient animals died as animals receiving vitamin C. In the following month, however, the scientists fed the vitamin to the deficient survivors, some receiving an amount equivalent to 100 milligrams in humans, others 1,000 milligrams. After 3 to 4 weeks, those in the 1,000-milligram group were healthy and able to resist harmful foreign substances, while those in the 100-milligram group failed to regain weight and were unable to resist immunologic attack.

Research has shown that vitamin A also has a powerful effect on specific immune system functions, stimulating both cellular and humoral immunity. The cellular immune system is made up of T and B cells derived from the thymus, the pinkish-gray mass behind the breastbone and just below the neck; the humoral system is responsible for antibody production in body fluids. Most studies of the immunological effects of vitamin A have used animals that were deficient in vitamin A. But while in England on a fellowship from Harvard University, Dr. Benjamin Cohen, a surgeon now practicing in Houston, Texas, studied humans who had had major surgery. Following surgery, patients' immune functions are often suppressed for weeks as a result of the stress related to surgery and anesthesia. Any harmful stimuli, such as physical injury or chemical poisoning, can cause stress. Usually there is a decrease in cellular immunity and in the functioning of white blood cells that fight off infections.

In the Cohen study, one group of patients received megadoses of vitamin A before and after surgery. Blood samples drawn the day before, one day after, and then one week after surgery, indicated increased T-cell activity; in the control group not receiving vitamin A supplements, immune function was diminished. And even though the megadoses were more than 30 times the RDA for vitamin A, there were no signs of toxicity.

But vitamins A and C are not the only nutrients that can stimulate the immune system. In animal studies, vitamin E supplements at levels greater that the RDA appear to have a strong influence. Having studied its effect on mice, guinea pigs, chickens, turkeys, rabbits, and sheep, animal nutritionist Cheryl Nockels, at Colorado State

University, believes that further research will show that it strengthens immune capability in humans, too.

Experimenting with mice, Nockels gave one group 60 international units of vitamin E for every kilogram of food, while giving a control group the routinely balanced diet. She then injected both groups with sheep red blood cells that cause the same reaction as bacteria in mice—their bodies produce antibodies that attack and destroy the foreign substance. In the supplemented mice, that reaction was significantly stronger: Their spleens were heavier, indicating increased antibody production, and a greater number of antibodies was found in their blood. Increased antibody activity was also found in a similar experiment with guinea pigs.

But a higher level of antibodies does not necessarily mean a greater resistance to infection. And in follow-up studies with chickens, turkeys, and sheep, Nockels wanted to determine how effective vitamin E supplements would actually be in arming the immune system. Using a variety of species, Nockels explains, makes generalizations sounder, and strengthens the argument that the findings will also apply to humans. So in later tests, she infected the animals with disease-causing bacteria and viruses. And in all three additional species, the results indicated that vitamin E significantly increased resistance to disease. The RDA level does not appear to maintain immunity at full strength; in the Colorado research, greater amounts were required to stimulate enhanced immune response.

If such results can be duplicated often enough to convince the scientific community that vitamins, such as A, C, and E, do play a major role in activating the immune system, we can expect to see vitamins prescribed on a regular basis by all doctors. We may be taking vitamin formulas, in excess of the current RDAs, to prevent or treat such seasonal ills as the flu and colds. Infections that jeopardize recovery from surgery will no longer occur. Diseases such as mononucleosis and hepatitis will be cured in weeks, or even days, instead of months. And people with AIDS-related conditions and other immune deficiency diseases will survive longer, because their bodies will be able to effectively fight off the devastating effects of the AIDS virus. Indeed, we will be sick much less often, and when we are, recuperation will be quicker.

Cancer

Cancer strikes in three out of four American families, or about 30 percent of the population. Once referred to as "the wasting disease," cancer weakens the body, disables vital organs, and diminishes immune capability. But having detected antibodies in people who may be susceptible to leukemia, many researchers believe that HTLV (human T-cell leukemia virus) is an example of viruses that cause cancer.

In his book *Origins of Human Cancer*, British cancer specialist Sir Richard Doll expressed the belief that the main advances in our knowledge of cancer will come from studying diet and nutrition. And in 1979, based on the growing literature linking diet and the possible development of cancer, the National Cancer Institute (NCI) committed itself to increase funding for nutrition research. In 1982, the Committee on Diet, Nutrition, and Cancer at the National Academy of Sciences reported to the NCI that approximately 35 percent of all cancers can be prevented by eating the right diet. The mounting laboratory and epidemiological evidence has spurred the NCI to develop and increase its research efforts in chemoprevention and dietary intervention. Chemoprevention is the use of natural and synthetic agents to halt or reverse the development of cancer, while dietary intervention involves the intake of specific nutrients and food groups.

Both the NCI and the NAS now recommend that Americans eat more foods containing vitamins A and C. Research findings have indicated that these two nutrients in particular aid in the prevention of several types of cancer, including cancers of the lung, stomach, skin, bladder, breast, and esophagus. Other studies indicate that vitamins can also increase the effectiveness of standard cancer treatments, such as chemotherapy.

Following their own controversial results with vitamin C and cancer, Pauling and surgeon Ewan Cameron concluded that supplemental ascorbate acid is "of some value to all cancer patients and can be of dramatic benefit to a fortunate few." In their initial study, the researchers supplemented 100 patients with terminal cancer with megadoses of vitamin C, and used 1,000 unsupplemented patients as a control group. Pauling and Cameron found that vitamin C, given along with chemotherapy, could at least triple life expectancy. At the Linus Pauling Institute of Science and Medicine in California, researchers continue their investigation of the seeming wonder nutrient, even though two repeat trials at the Mayo Clinic refute their original findings. Pauling and Cameron, however, insist that the Mayo methods did not precisely replicate their original study, and naturally led to different results.

In 1980, doctors told John Brooks (not his real name) that his colorectal cancer had spread to his liver, where he had developed an inoperable malignant tumor. The average life expectancy for such patients, they said, was 6 months. At Pauling's suggestion, Brooks had started taking 12 grams of vitamin C a day, and gradually increased that amount until he reached 36 grams a day. Five years after the initial diagnosis, the tumor remained, but it was no longer growing larger. Otherwise, Brooks was living well for an 81-year-old man. The most serious side effect from the vitamin C megadoses, he claims, was increased appetite. Most cancer patients experience a decline in appetite and, therefore, lose weight. As a result, they often do not eat properly, and many die from malnutrition. Not so for Brooks. "For 3 years," Brooks says, "I was trying to lose 10 pounds and couldn't."

Other research lends support to the Pauling-Cameron findings. At the University of Oregon Health Sciences Center in Portland, immunopathologist Benjamin Seigel found that vitamin C induces the body to produce interferon. This antiviral protein is produced by cells in response to a variety of viral infections, including mumps, herpes, and the common cold. According to Swiss born microbiologist Mathilde Krim and other interferon researchers, interferon can inhibit cell growth and reduce the growth of tumors. Researchers have found, moreover, that the substance is effective in the treatment of some types of cancer. But isolating the substance from human blood cells is a laborious process which makes interferon therapy prohibitively expensive. Seigel's work therefore, may prove to be a valuable alternative.

In one study by Seigel, two groups of mice were infected with a leukemia virus. The group also receiving large amounts of vitamin C not only developed milder cases of leukemia, but produced more than twice as much interferon than the unsupplemented mice. Siegel speculates that we can use vitamin C supplementation to likewise encourage interferon production in the cancerous human body.

Such Nutritional therapy would not have adverse physical effects on the patient. Unfortunately this is not the case with more conventional therapy. Patients in chemotherapy are debilitated by nausea and vomiting. Their hair falls out, and they lose weight. But doctors may be able to neutralize the side effects of cancer-fighting chemicals with *beta-carotene*—the orange substance present in such foods as carrots, yams, and cantaloupe which the human body converts to vitamin A. The effect was found in studies by biochemist Eli Seifter at Albert Einstein College of Medicine, in New York City.

Seifter wanted to learn whether beta-carotene would be a valuable dietary supplement for cancer-stricken mice already weakened by chemotherapy. During the study he found that the usual side effects of the treatment *were* markedly milder. And he was able to drastically increase the doses of anticancer drugs and increase the length of survival. When beta-carotene and chemotherapy were combined with radiation therapy, the mouse tumors completely disappeared. In follow-up tests, 92 percent of the mice were still free of cancerous cells 14 months afterward. Seifter believes the treatment works because the body converts beta-carotene to vitamin A, which restores the white blood cells necessary for immune function. And the body makes the conversion at an optimal rate.

Seifter has also found that beta-carotene appears to hinder the development of tumors. When mice are inoculated with low doses of tumor cells, normally 50 percent of the mice would develop tumors. But pretreating them with beta-carotene, Seifter reports, lowered that rate to only 10 percent. And in those mice in which tumors were allowed to grow, beta-carotene inhibited the process and, again, the lives of the mice were prolonged.

In some cases, scientists hypothesize that a nutrient deficiency can be localized, promoting the development of some types of cancer. One such case involves folic acid (folate), a B vitamin essential to cell growth, according to clinical nutritionist Charles E. Butterworth, Jr., chairman of the department of nutritional sciences at the University of Alabama in Birmingham. It's possible that such a deficiency is related to cervical dysplasia, a condition in which abnormal, and possibly precancerous, cells are found in the cervix. Butterworth tested the hypothesis in his study of 47 women who were taking oral contraceptives and who had mild to moderate cervical dysplasia. Some of the women were given daily supplements of 100 milligrams of folate, while others received a placebo. The results: Those taking therapeutic folate improved significantly; the unsupplemented subjects showed no change. Moreover, symptoms in four cases among the supplemented group appeared to regress, while four cases in the placebo group apparently *progressed*. Butterworth's conclusion is that "oral folic acid supplementation may prevent the progression of early cancer to a more severe form and, in some cases, promote reversion to normalcy."

Heart Disease

Currently, nearly 50 percent of all deaths in the United States are related to heart and blood vessel diseases, twice as high as that related to cancer. But with a 30 percent decrease in the past few years, heart disease is on the run. The decrease perhaps due, in part, to changing lifestyles—no smoking, increased exercise, and dietary changes such as decreased cholesterol intake and increased fiber consumption. There is also tantalizing evidence that certain vitamins—specifically B_6, C, and E—may aid in the prevention, or even the treatment, of heart disease.

A notable culprit in heart disease is cholesterol, a chemical naturally present in all animal fats and in the human body, including the brain and blood. In the body, it aids in the synthesis of vitamin D and some hormones, such as cortisone and estrogen. Excessive cholesterol, however, can lodge along artery walls and impede blood flow, predisposing the body to heart attacks and strokes. While there is disagreement about whether the body's cholesterol level can be effectively managed by decreasing the intake of saturated fat, this is the approach that is most common currently. Now some research indicates that vitamin C may help lower cholesterol levels by speeding its transformation to bile acids, which the body excretes.

In India, for example, nutritional researcher A. K. Bordia found that when patients with a history of heart disease took 1 gram of C twice a day, cholesterol levels dropped by 12 percent, with level of low-density lipoproteins lowered significantly while that of high-density lipoproteins rose. Bordia's research, moreover, indicated that these patients had fewer adhesive platelets and these were less likely to clot and obstruct normal blood flow.

While cholesterol, hypertension, stress, and smoking are risk factors in the development of arteriosclerosis, vitamin B_6 deficiency may, in fact, be a cause. And such a deficiency may be common, considering that this vitamin has been eliminated from most refined grains. It's also water-soluble, and often lost in cooking.

But according to a theory subscribed to by biochemist Jeffrey Bland at the University of Puget Sound in Washington, cell biologist Leonard Hayflick at the University of Texas, Austin, and others, the chemical homocysteine, a toxic substance formed in the breakdown of the amino acid called methionine, is a cause of atherosclerosis. And atherosclerosis can lead to *arterio*sclerosis, or hardening of the arteries. Conversion of homocysteine for metabolic use in the body, moreover, depends on the presence of pyridoxine, (vitamin B_6). Arteriosclerosis could be the first sign of a B_6 deficiency.

Of all nutrients, however, vitamin E has probably been the most recommended for a healthy heart—and the most controversial. The protests of the naysayers notwithstanding, vitamin E does seem to reduce the stickiness of platelets, blood particles that can clump together and block the arteries. In research by biochemist Lawrence Machlin, at the Hoffman-La Roche company's facilities in Nutley, New Jersey, E was able to reduce excessive stickiness in the blood of rats. In another study, hematologist Dr. Manfred Steiner at Brown University in Providence, Rhode Island, took blood samples from healthy volunteers and exposed them to chemical agents that stimulate stickiness. Vitamin E added to the blood, however, minimized the clumping and kept the blood more fluid. In a follow-up study, Steiner supplemented volunteers with 1,200 to 2,400 international units of vitamin E for several weeks and then exposed samples of their supplemented blood to the same agents. Again, vitamin E minimized the stickiness.

Vitamin E's effect on platelets may, in fact, be related to its protection of blood cells. Jeffrey Bland has found that circulating oxygen in the blood can weaken and damage red blood cells; vitamin E can protect the cells. Vitamin E molecules enter the cell membranes, where they become trapped in the unsaturated fatty acids and other fats. In one research study, Bland gave volunteers 600 international units of vitamin E a day for 10 days. Blood samples were then exposed to oxygen and sunlight to speed oxidation, which would normally damage most of the cells. But with the vitamin E supplements, only a small number of cells were harmed.

Vitamin E may also raise HDL levels. Nutritional pharmacologist Joseph Barboriak, at Wood Veterans Administration Medical Center in Milwaukee, gave volunteers alpha-tocopherol, a form of vitamin E. The results: higher HDL among those volunteers who initially had low levels of the lipoprotein. The only subjects whose HDL levels were not affected by vitamin E were those who already had high levels. These, it turned out, happened to be joggers or long-distance runners.

It is relatively difficult, Barboriak reports, to raise HDL levels by therapeutic means. Effective approaches often have drawbacks: Exercise may be unsuitable for some people and increased alcohol intake may lead to dependence or addiction. Barboriak is now doing a year long double blind study to further investigate vitamin E's effects.

With the help of megavitamin therapy, could we see the end of heart disease in the twenty-first century? Perhaps not. But if vitamins can increase the efficiency of the blood system, and thus the heart, early deaths from heart disease will certainly decline, if not disappear completely. Now, 45 percent of such deaths occur before the age of 65, and most of those victims are men. And there will be a decline in heart surgery and less-restrictive lifestyles prescribed to patients as cardiologists and other heart specialists promote therapeutic vitamin regimens.

Researchers are finding scientific support for many folk beliefs, and discovering even more benefits to be gained from the use of therapeutic nutrition. This chapter has highlighted only a few of the nutrients and foods that hold promise for the cure of some diseases. But with the flurry of nutritional research now going on in the United States and elsewhere, many convincing results can be expected in the near future.

As more and more studies present irrefutable evidence of the link between nutrition and disease, government agencies and medical organizations will redefine human dietary requirements. And as San Francisco's Dr. Richard Kunin hopes, orthomolecular medicine will become mainstream medicine. Rather than a two-state theory of health, where people are either sick or well, medical practitioners will focus on *optimal* health to prevent the early development of disease. They will use vitamins and other food components to correct the body's chemistry when it malfunctions, in many cases using drugs and surgery only as secondary options.

=Timeline=

1987 to 1995
- Researchers, funded by such organizations as the National Cancer Institute, begin announcing the results of major studies on the relationship of nutrition and diseases.
- Further reports on killer diseases, such as AIDS, and the effects of nutrition therapy begin to confirm orthomolecular practice.

1996 to 2000
- Nutrition education required for all medical students.
- The nutrition-disease link confirmed.
- Physicians with nutrition backgrounds begin to set up private practices.
- Vitamins A and C used in conjunction with other standard cancer therapies.
- National Academy of Sciences redefines its RDAs as ''recommended daily intake for the prevention of degenerative diseases,'' such as some types of cancer and heart disease, but suggests consultation with physicians.
- New guidelines established for vitamin and mineral supplementation.

2001 to 2010
- Immunologists accept vitamin C as acceptable treatment for impaired immune systems.
- Nutritional therapy proven to halt, and in some cases reverse, the devastating effects of Alzheimer's disease.
- Pharmacists fill increasing numbers of personalized vitamin prescriptions.
- The number of heart-related deaths under age 65 declines to an all-time low, due in large part to change in dietary habits and vitamin supplementation.
- Most major employers have nutrition education and dietary counseling programs.
- Biochemical laboratories available to the public in all 51 states (assuming that Puerto Rico will have become the 51st state).

2011 to 2020
- Vitamin E therapy accepted as beneficial in reversing cardiovascular damage.
- American Psychiatric Association validates nutritional therapy in the treatment of schizophrenia, childhood hyperactivity, and other disorders.
- The American Medical Association recognizes nutritional therapy as the first option in the prevention and treatment of many diseases.
- Culinary schools and most restaurants affiliated with medical or other health organizations.

2021 to 2030
- The number of incurable cases of schizophrenia dramatically declines through the use of nutritional therapy.
- Biochemical analyses mandated for all physical examinations.
- Reported cases of flu and colds decline significantly.
- Orthomolecular medicine becomes mainstream medicine.

=Access Guide=

Nutritional Medicine

The following organizations can provide the names of physicians who practice nutritional medicine and their specialties (general practice, pediatrics, gynecology, etc.) These organizations are currently working to expand their physican networks. Some, like the American Academy of Medical Preventives, have accreditation for their members, requiring examinations similar to the standard medical boards; others are working on developing such credentials. If they have no listing for a nutritional or preventive medicine physician in a requested area, they will make every effort to locate one. But in most cases, their referral services and membership directories are not recommendations.

Orthomolecular Medical Society
6151 West Century Boulevard, Suite 1114
Los Angeles, CA 90045

For information about the society and a directory of member orthomolecular physicians and psychiatrists, send $3.50 to the above address.

American Academy of Medical Preventics
6151 West Century Boulevard, Suite 1114
Los Angeles, CA 90045

For information about the Academy and a membership directory of doctors who practice preventive medicine, including those practicing nutritional medicine, send $3.50 to the above address.

American Academy of Environmental Medicine
P.O. Box 16106
Denver, CO 80216

(Formerly the Society for Clinical Ecology.)

International Academy of Preventive Medicine
P.O. Box 5832
Lincoln, NE 68505

The Academy offers a referral service with its expanding membership directory.

International College of Applied Nutrition
312 E. Las Tunas Drive
P. O. Box 1000
San Gabriel, CA 91776

The International College is an organization of qualified physicians, dentists, and Ph.D.'s with doctorate degrees engaged in practical application or research in applied nutrition. The group will supply a list of members in your area.

Colgan Institute of Nutritional Science
565 Pearl Street, Suite 301
La Jolla, CA 92037

The Institute provides individuals with nutrition and performance assessments based on more than 1,000 variables, and they need not be done at the institute itself. When laboratory tests and analysis are complete, the client receives a report including dietary and exercise programs, and vitamin, mineral, and amino acid supplements individually packed in daily packs. Re-assessments are recommended after six months and annually thereafter.

Princeton Brain Bio Center
862 Route 518
Skillman, NJ 08558
609-924-8607

The Center is an outpatient clinic and research center under the auspices of the Schizophrenia Foundation and the New Jersey Mental Health Research and Development Fund. It is actively engaged in the study of many disorders including hypoglycemia, childhood hyperactivity, epilepsy, arthritis, allergies and digestive disorders.

Health-Conscious Restaurants

The American Heart Association will provide a list of restaurant chains that participate in the Creative Cuisine program; for independent restaurants, contact the local chapter of the American Heart Association. For the names of restaurant chains write to:

Association National Center
7320 Greenville Avenue
Dallas, TX 75231
(214) 750-5300

Pritikin Longevity Center will also provide a list of its affiliate restaurants. Write:

"Pritikin Questions and Answers"
1910 Ocean Front Walk
Santa Monica, CA 90405

RESEARCH CENTERS FOR VOLUNTEERS

For food and nutrition studies, universities often recruit the schools' students because they are readily available, or they may advertise in local newspapers and on community bulletin boards. Studies run for specific lengths of time, and require participants with specific medical histories. Many universities and research centers do not have a central volunteer registry, and they do not always know their needs until a project is about to begin. But interested prospective volunteers can contact local universities that have a medical school, or a division of nutritional sciences, food science, biochemistry, or similar departments to inquire about their needs. University public relations or communications offices can also guide inquiries to the proper office or individual. The following are some research centers that seek volunteers.

Clayton Foundation Biochemical
  Institute
Nutrition Clinic
ESB 444
The University of Texas at Austin
Austin, TX 78712-1096

United States Department of
  Agriculture
Human Nutrition Research Center
  at Tufts University
711 Washington Street
Boston, MA 02111
(617) 956-0417

Kenneth L. Jordan Cardiac Center
Atherosclerosis Research Center
48 Plymouth Street
Montclair, NJ 07042
(201) 746-1268

University of Alabama in
  Birmingham
Department of Nutritional Sciences
University Station
Birmingham, AL 35294
(205) 934-4710

University of Miami School of
  Medicine
Nutrition Division
1550 Northwest 10th Avenue
Miami, FL 33136
(305) 547-6932

$$\underline{}13\underline{}$$

Immortality Made Easy:
A Short Guide to Longevity

When Durk Pearson and Sandy Shaw sit down for a meal, food is only a small part of the menu. They also ingest large quantities of other nutrients: calcium pantothenate, beta-carotene, selenium, vitamins C, E, B_b and A, choline, L-dopa, rutin, tryptophan, cysteine, the food preservative BHT, zinc, and RNA. No doctor prescribed these. Pearson and Shaw did it themselves. Although neither are physicians (Pearson has a degree in physics from MIT and Shaw graduated from UCLA with a degree in chemistry), they spent years culling the scientific literature looking for anything that might retard aging.

Like Ponce de Leon, who sailed the world in search of the fountain of youth, Pearson and Shaw seek the key to optimum health and, if not eternal, then extended, life. In their best-selling book, *Life Extension: A Practical Scientific Approach*, they explain how nutrients can slow aging. Having sold over 2 million copies of their book, Pearson and Shaw have become celebrities, appearing frequently on radio and television. But have they found a way to preserve youth, or at least, to push back the aging clock?

No one knows for sure, but Pearson and Shaw are convinced they will live forever—barring murder or accident—and have raised the hopes of thousands of others.

Their hypotheses, however, have also angered many scientists in the field of gerontology who think Pearson and Shaw are premature, if not reckless, in their assessments of current research. But many of the same scientists also realize that gerontology is in need of financial support, and the attention Pearson and Shaw have created may well mean an increase in public interest and government funding for research.

The quest for longevity is nothing new. For centuries, people have searched—sometimes desperately—for ways to prolong life. Not surprisingly, the history of this quest has been filled with quacks and secret potions. Even in the twentieth century, such unlikely items as novacaine, cells from unborn lambs, and ape testicles have been peddled as rejuvenators. The natives of Vilcabamba, Ecuador, and a group from the Caucasus mountains in Russia have their own way of extending life: exaggeration. Because respect comes with age in these societies, hundreds of people claim to be well into their one hundreds. One Russian from the Caucasus bragged of his 130 years, but investigators discovered that he was actually using his father's documents to verify his age. In reality, he was 78 years old. According to one Russian gerontologist, there are thousands of similar cases.

In the scientific examination of aging, the progress has been slow, but steady. Although few breakthroughs have been made, a growing number of studies have convinced scientists that it may indeed be possible to lengthen the average life span. Endocrinologists are exploring the role of hormones, and cancer specialists are probing the genetic code to see how genes might be involved in aging. Immunologists are studying why the body's immune system breaks down over time, producing a host of medical problems from arthritis to Parkinson's disease. Understanding the processes that age us is the first step toward learning how to prolong life. The most promising areas of study sweep the spectrum from genetic and hormonal manipulation to low-calorie diets and brain transplants.

Before researchers can understand why we age, we must examine why we live as long as we do. The time a person can expect to live in the United States today is 71 years for males and 78 years for females. Our natural, genetically potential life span, however, is much higher—110 years. The goal of all life extension studies is to enable people to live out their lives in good health and mind. Then, as physician and author Lewis Thomas wrote, we will be able to "zip from tennis court to deathbed at age 120." Prolonging youth as well as life is at the heart of the new science of aging.

How Old Are You Really?

When he was 70 years old, Noel Johnson's son threatened to put him in a nursing home. Noel refused. Instead he changed his diet and began exercising. Today at age 85 he runs the length of a marathon once every month. What gives Johnson the ability to run long distances while there are any number of 35-year-olds who, even with training, cannot? That's what William Regelson, a professor of medicine at the Medical College of Richmond, Virginia, wants to find out. "How can we study aging," he wrote in his book *Interventions in the Aging Process*, "unless we develop a way to measure it?"

Keeping track of a person's chronological age is easy, but determining his or her biological age (how old the person is physiologically) is not. The major problem is establishing reliable biomarkers, the physiological functions that change over time in a steady, irreversible fashion. Simply charting changes in blood pressure or cholesterol levels is not sufficient; both rise and fall throughout life.

But a few years ago, one researcher, Richard Hochschild, designed a machine that may have solved the problem. Called the *H-Scan*, the device tests 14 age-dependent physiological processes including hearing, lung function, motor reflexes, memory, and decision-making time. Once individuals have been evaluated, they can see how they measure up to others their age. More importantly, though, H-scan can be used repeatedly so a person can see how he or she has aged over time, say, a 2-year period, and whether a new diet, exercise program, or other youth-promoting regimen is working.

The H-Scan is already used by at least one major life insurance company—that company offers discounts to clients whose biological age undercuts their chronological age. The machine has also been purchased by a pharmaceutical firm for testing the effect that certain drugs have on aging.

The doctor's office of the future will make the H-Scan and machines like it the first order of business, using them to chart a patient's progress from one visit to the next. A still more sophisticated age monitor is being developed by Richard Cutler at the National Institute of Aging (NIA). He is working on a method of measuring the amount of biological damage experienced on a molecular level. Once the damage is identified, proper therapies can be administered to repair it. Using this technique, future checkups could be used to improve health, rather than just look for disease.

But learning to identify a person's biological age is only the first step in the quest for youth. The secret lies elsewhere, perhaps in our most basic selves—our genes.

Expressive Genes

Inside each one of us is a unique genetic code that remains constant throughout our lives. That code, the double helix of our DNA, constantly regenerates itself, a process that depends on the ability of the DNA to patch weak links along its strands so its messages are passed through the cells correctly. In young people, DNA efficiently repairs damage to itself caused by pollution, stress, or poor diet. But as we age, our DNA loses some of its vigor and often becomes distorted or scrambled; this means that we have some abnormal or less efficient cells. Such malfunctions can lead to cancer and other disease. Some researchers think that it is simply wear and tear over time that distorts DNA, but others disagree. They believe that certain genes actually initiate the process. Set like a time bomb, our genes may be programmed to make us grow old.

"The entire process of aging seems to be governed by only a few genes," says Richard Cutler, a foremost expert on aging. "And that means that if we can identify those genes, we may be able to manipulate them and correct a whole number of diseases."

Among the researchers looking for the "supergenes" that control aging is Roy Walford. His work at the University of California at Los Angeles has unveiled one likely contender: a cluster of genes known as the *major histocompatibility complex (MHC)*. In several controlled experiments, Walford showed that mice bred without the complex died before control mice, suggesting that DNA was unable to repair itself without MHC. Walford also suspects that MHC may play a crucial role in fighting off the effects of free radicals, which are highly unstable molecules that cruise through the body, searching for other, more stable, molecules with which to merge. One process initiated by free radicals (called cross-linking), turns healthy molecules into dangerous ones or prevents them from functioning. Some cross-linking occurs normally, but radiation, pollution, and stress can also create these unholy alliances. Cross-linking can make blood clot abnormally and may contribute to arthritis and lung ailments. In addition, free radicals linked to certain molecules can kill brain cells by cutting off their oxygen supply.

Although the body can defend itself to some degree against free radicals, researchers don't understand why. One possible explanation comes from Kenneth Munkres, a molecular biologist at the University of Wisconsin. He suggests that certain genes release an enzyme that reacts with free radicals, rendering them harmless. Munkres is now investigating ways of instructing the genes to release this enzyme, called *superoxide dismutase (SOD)*, when free radicals begin to proliferate. This would enable the body to destroy free radicals before they had a chance to damage cells.

SOD is not the only way to fight free radicals; similar compounds may also stave off these internal enemies. Called antioxidants, they are ingested every day by Dirk Pearson and Sandy Shaw. Antioxidant therapy is the heart of their life-extension plan.

Antioxidants are enzymes that curb the cross-linking activity of free radicals. Vitamins A, C, E, B_1, B_5, B_6, beta-carotene, the food preservative BHT, selenium, some sulfur-containing amino acids, and a number of brain-reactive drugs all help fight free radicals.

Antioxidant therapy consists of consuming these compounds, a practice that antioxidant adherents believe restores youth. After 10 years of megadosing antioxidants, Pearson and Shaw, both 42, had their biological ages estimated. Each was shown to be 10 years younger biologically than chronologically. But Pearson and Shaw pay a high price (about $64 a day each for the supplements) and perhaps an even steeper toll in terms of their health. "The actual nutrients Durk and Sandy recommend have to be considered as drugs when taken as self-prescribed supplements and in excessive doses," wrote one doctor in the *Journal of the American Medical Association*.

Indeed, megadosing antioxidants may lead to a number of maladies, including liver disease, and may cause the body to shed unneeded antioxidants, which would allow free-radicals levels to rise. Other research suggests that megadosing antioxidants can actually suppress the body's ability to produce them.

Even so, longevity researchers hope antioxdiants can allow us to control aging without gene manipulation. "We'd just have to replace the body's reserve of antioxidants as they become depleted with age," says Cutler. By keeping the body's supply of antioxidants high, cells will function at their peak, even in the elderly.

Maybe aging is caused by poorly functioning DNA, but for many researchers, the idea that genes carry the key to longevity seems suspect. They are convinced that the search should be focused on hormones and the glands that secrete them.

The Master Gland

Because a flu vaccine doesn't always keep people from getting the flu, doctors at the University of Wisconsin are trying a new tactic to defeat the virus. They inoculate some people with *thymosins*—a group of hormones produced by the thymus, which is a small gland located beneath the breastbone. The thymus is the master gland of the immune system, and doctors hope that a shot of thymosins will strengthen immunity, giving the elderly a better chance of fighting off viruses. Gerontologists also believe that thymosins may protect us from the diseases of old age.

Since he first isolated the hormone group 20 years ago, Allan Goldstein, who chairs the department of biochemistry at George Washington University, has believed thymosins could fight against cancer and other diseases. Already, clinical studies have shown thymosins can help in the treatment of rheumatoid arthritis, lupus, multiple sclerosis, and a wide range of allergies and infectious diseases. Thymosin supplements have also been used with some success to bolster the immune system in patients who have the early symptoms of AIDS. The thymus is particularly interesting to gerontologists because it shrinks to about one-tenth of its original size by late adulthood. Production of its hormones declines, which may be one reason we become progressively more susceptible to disease as we age. Goldstein believes that the gland's decreased efficiency, which begins at the onset of puberty, marks the start of aging.

He has developed a test to measure the level of thymosins in the blood and hopes it will become a routine part of physical examinations in the future. By charting the decreasing levels of thymosin production as we age, doctors in the twenty-first century will know when to begin replacing the hormones, thus delaying aging. As a first step toward this therapy, Goldstein has set up a company, Alpha-I Biomedical, based in Washington, D.C., to develop synthetic thymosins.

Some researchers question the thymus's status as the premier gland of aging. W. Donner Denckla, whose research into the cause of death has made him famous, believes that humans die because one of two major body systems—the cardiovascular or the immune system—fail. In other words, people do not really die of kidney failure or liver malfunction. We die because the immune system fails to protect us from disease, or because our blood vessels fail to deliver oxygen and nutrients. Denckla traces this failure to a marble-sized gland in the brain and its "death hormone," DECO.

The Death Hormone

An adult who loses his or her pituitary gland will die within a day. As the gland that controls growth and sexual maturity, the pituitary is not only essential to continued survival, it may also trigger the aging process.

The pituitary controls the thyroid gland, which regulates our metabolism, the rate at which we burn calories. As we age, Denckla discovered, the pituitary produces a substance that slows our metabolic rate. Dubbed DECO, (Decreasing Oxygen Consumption Hormone), the substance prevents cells from properly using thyroxine, a major pituitary hormone. Denckla found that when he removed the pituitary in rats and gave the rats injections of all the pituitary's hormones—except DECO, the efficiency with which the animals' systems processed thyroxine did not decrease. More startling, however, was the rats' sudden return to youth. In the absence of the pituitary, the rats' aortas (the main blood vessel in the heart) regained their flexibility, which normally declines with age. Their lung capacity improved, and white blood cell count increased, indicating a rejuvenated immune system.

Despite these improvements, Denckla's rats live only slightly longer than average. Alert and well one morning, they might be dead by night. Apparently, removing the pituitary extends youth, not life.

But why does the body produce a substance that eventually undermines its strength and resilience? Denckla suggests that the answer is related to the way the body regulates temperature. Most of the heat our bodies generate is released through the skin. As we grow older, our skin loses some of its ability to dissipate heat. If the body's thermostat did not help us continue to cool ourselves, we might literally cook to death. DECO apparently is produced to slow the rate at which we produce heat, by slowing down our metabolism. In this way, it actually protects us.

Nevertheless, researchers feel that it may be possible one day to block DECO's dangerous side effects without disrupting its beneficial action. Once DECO is isolated, a pill could be developed to block harmful action of the chemical without affecting DECO's cooling function. Denckla once believed that a DECO blocker would be available in pill form, at about the price of aspirin. But its development needed far more funding than he could find. Disheartened, he gave up his research to build sailboats.

But his work has continued. Two scientists, who want to remain anonymous until they complete their studies, believe they have identified the death hormone and predict that within the next 10 years, it will be possible to control this "neuroendocrine clock."

Steroid Link

When Vernon Reilly, an endocrinologist who died in 1980, placed mice with tumors onto a rotating turntable, he discovered something remarkable. The stress of riding a spinning wheel shrank their thymus glands and their tumors grew faster. In his next experiment Reilly administered the steroid *dehydroepianderosterone* (*DHEA*) to half of the mice and placed them on the turntable. (The control group was not given DHEA before being placed on the table.) The control group exhibited the usual shrinkage of the thymus; but the mice who had been given DHEA had no decrease in thymus size and no increase in the size of their tumors. DHEA apparently protected them from the ravages of stress.

Since then numerous studies have reaffirmed DHEA's role in fighting disease. At the Jackson Laboratories in Bar Harbor, Maine, researcher Doug Coleman found that DHEA can be used to treat diabetes in animals. Other animal research indicates that the hormone may also sensitize brain cells to cholines, chemicals that become depleted in victims of Alzheimer's disease. Because DHEA levels decrease dramatically in humans as they age, scientists believe there may be a link between a drop in the level of this hormone and the rise of certain age-related diseases.

This research is still preliminary. No clinical trials on humans have been conducted, and it is too soon to know if DHEA has positive effects on humans. Nevertheless, Progenics, a bioresearch firm in New York, has synthesized the hormone, and a DHEA compound is expected to be marketed within 2 years.

Diet, Exercise, and Body Temperature

Sixty-year-old Roy Walford is known for his brightly colored Indian shirts and his huge walrus mustache. He also heads the research laboratory for the study of immunology at the University of California at Los Angeles. In his book *Maximum Lifespan*, Walford presents his diet for a long life. It is a diet big eaters won't like.

Walford recommends total abstinence from food 2 successive days each week and a healthy, but sparse, diet the other 5 days. A typical breakfast might include scant quantities of brewer's yeast, rye cereal, wheat germ, wheat bran, strawberries, and milk, followed by a lunch of sweet potatoes, spinach, pears, and buttermilk. For dinner he recommends chicken, lima bean salad, green beans, and grapefruit.

His tip to dieters who might stray when invited to the home of a gourmet cook: "Let it be understood," he wrote, "that you're a fanatic or eccentric on this point, or that intermittent fasting makes you 'high,' as indeed it does . . . then turn noneating into a slightly risqué vice and your host will be charmed and alarmed at your wickedness."

Walford's diet stems from many studies. As far back as 1920, Cornell University researcher Clive McKay prolonged the lives of rats by placing them on a low-calorie diet. Other researchers, including Walford and his colleague Richard Weindruch, have gotten similar results with other animals. Eating little, but well, may slow the aging clock by reducing body temperature and improving DNA repair. It also appears to guard against autoimmune diseases. (Autoimmune diseases, such as rheumatoid arthritis and lupus, occur when the body perceives its own white blood cells as foreign bodies and begins destroying them.)

Although no one knows exactly why reducing food intake appears to prolong life, some researchers feel the apparent result may be linked to the lowering of body temperature. In 1917, researchers at the Rockefeller Institute in New York City discovered that they could significantly increase the life spans of fruit flies by keeping the temperature of their habitats 6 degrees lower than normal. Similarly, Walford doubled the life span of the South American fish *Cynolebias belotti* by cooling the water in which it lived. Even in warm-blooded animals, the aging rate seems to slow when body temperature is lowered. Researchers found that by injecting neuropeptides into the brains of chimpanzees, they could lower the chimps' body temperature, and they found that the chimps with lowered body temperatures lived longer.

After looking at this research, Walford wanted to examine people who lived beyond their life expectancy and had lower body temperatures than average. He traveled to India to study yogis, who, it had been reported, could raise or lower their body temperatures at will. He found a group of the holy men who agreed to take part in his experiments in the Jhilmil caves of northern India. The yogis could indeed control their body temperatures. While they were meditating, temperatures dropped from the normal 98.6 to 95 or 94 degrees. Unfortunately, Walford could not substantiate some yogis' claims to extremely long lives because no records proved their birth dates.

So the question remains: Does turning the human thermostat

down prolong life? Much more research is needed. Scientists have found that by placing heat-controlled rods in the hypothalamus of a rodent, they could lower the animal's body temperature. And certain drugs, including THC (the active ingredient in marijuana) and chlorpromazine (a tranquilizer) have been used to reduce body temperature in animals. "If humans are like animals," says gerontologist Bernard Strehler of the University of Southern California, "then a few degrees drop in body temperature could add something like 15 to 25 years to human life. And that could account for practically all the difference that one sees in human life span."

And the question remains about the value of limited diets.

Animal studies indicate that reduced food intake increases the number of years an animal lives, but little hard evidence exists for its effect on humans. Nor do researchers understand why eating lightly extends an animal's life. Besides the theory that limited food intake lowers body temperature, which in turn increases life span, other ideas are circulating. Donald Ingram, at the National Institute of Aging, hypothesizes that the answer involves an animal's hunt for food. "Part of living longer may have to do with having a commitment to life, a will to live," he says. "These rats are looking for food, it's something to do." To test his theory, Ingram built MouseWorld, a huge cage stocked with toys and food—everything, presumably, that a mouse could want. Although the mice in these cages grew fatter and bigger than normal mice, they also grew prematurely gray. The good life does not seem particularly conducive to longer life.

Although it is not as promising an avenue as limited diet, researchers are also exploring the effect of exercise on longevity. Research at NIA has shown that vigorous exercise prolongs the life of lab animals, and a continuing study of Harvard alumni indicates that moderate physical activity throughout adult life substantially increases life expectancy. "If exercise could be packed into a pill," says Robert Butler, former head of NIA, "it would be the single most widely prescribed and beneficial medicine in the nation."

Many fit 60-year-olds have better aerobic capacity (the ability of the body to use oxygen) than their younger, but inactive, counterparts. Exercise also guards against diabetes by shrinking fat cells, thus making the cells more sensitive to insulin and better able to break down glucose. Aerobic exercise keeps cholesterol levels low. Studies done at the University of Texas have also found that physically fit older men and women have better motor reflexes and mental skills than their sedentary peers.

But some people need far less exercise than others to push their systems to maximum capacity. Excessive exercise carries its own risks, from heat exhaustion to heart attacks. In the future, those who want to extend their lives will be given personal exercise regimens.

Aging and the Brain

Many investigators believe aging begins in the brain. As the master controlling organ of the body, the brain relays messages to and from the endocrine (hormonal), involuntary nervous, and muscular systems. Any deterioration of or damage to the brain can have widespread effects on other parts of the body. "The final common pathway as we age is the viability of the brain," says Vernon Marks of Boston University Medical School. "Everything else is a supporting organ."

One group of natural chemicals in the body might protect the brain against the deterioration that comes with age. Known as *neuropeptides*, these hormones appear to make brain cells more sensitive to other hormones. They may also stimulate memory and learning ability. Philip Landfield, a neurobiologist at the Bowman Gray School of Medicine in Winston-Salem, North Carolina, was one of the first researchers to test neuropeptide drugs. When he administered the drugs to middle-aged rats, the rate at which their brains aged seemed to slow. The test rats learned mazes as well as their younger counterparts, and better than control rats of the same age. In addition, analysis of the brains of those rats that had been given the peptides revealed far less cell deterioration than normal. "In other words," says Dr. Landfield, "these peptide drugs may have a cumulative effect not only on the function of the brain, but on its structure. They may be able to prevent deterioration."

Landfield's laboratory developed a neuropeptide-based drug that he hopes to market as a memory enhancer. It is being evaluated by the Food and Drug Administration, and, if approved, it will be available in a few years.

Perhaps the most radical life extension experiments underway, however, are those in which brain tissue is transplanted. By learning how to inject fetal brain cells into inactive or damaged portions of the brain, doctors may one day cure diseases that today seem hopeless. Transplants may eventually be used in cases of stroke, brain trauma, Alzheimer's disease, Parkinson's disease, and any other malady that is caused by the death of brain cells. "For millions of people," says Vernon Marks, "this is the only game in town."

Already animal research has paved the way. Carl Cotman of the University of California has successfully treated rats suffering from Alzheimer's disease by replacing disease-ridden cells with healthy ones from other animals, and William Freed of St. Elizabeth's Hospital in Washington, D.C., has demonstrated similar success with rats who have Parkinson's.

Researchers at Rochester University discovered the reason why brain transplants seem to work. After cutting away sections of rats' brains, they injected fetal cells into the area. The fetal cells fused with the remaining brain, actually filling in the space where the original cells had been. It's the cells' ability to reconnect successfully that makes brain cell transplants so promising.

Doctors in Stockholm attempted a brain transplant on a 45-year-old woman suffering from advanced Parkinson's disease. The woman's condition improved only slightly after adrenal gland cells taken from an embryo had been implanted in her brain. Even so, doctors were encouraged and believe someday they will use the technique to cure disease.

Despite the ethical problems connected with use of human fetal cell transplants that come from aborted embryos, the future of cell transplants seems secure. At least one laboratory is trying to synthesize fetal cells, and many researchers believe it will be only a matter of time before cells can be manufactured and obtained as easily as prescription drugs.

The day will also come, researchers believe, when they completely rejuvenate the brain. By removing 10 percent of the brain each year and replacing it with embryonic material, doctors will one day transform the brain into an ageless master of human life.

Timeline

1987 to 1990
- *Patients can find out their true biological age and learn their optimal exercise and nutrition program.*
- *Preventive health therapy becomes more effective as more potent antioxidants are produced.*
- *Victims of cancer and rheumatoid arthritis get a boost from thymosin supplements which strengthen the immune system response. Thymosin is used as a preventive by those susceptible to AIDS and the flu.*
- *DNA scanning ascertains the strength of patients' health and tags those who need extra protection from potential environmental threats.*

1991 to 2000
- *The "death hormone" is identified and neutralized by pill blockers.*
- *DHEA treats cancer, obesity, diabetes, and Alzheimer's disease.*
- *Senescense becomes rare as memory drugs sharpen cognitive thought and powers of recall.*
- *Supergenes that control the rate of aging are identified.*

2001 to 2010
- *Genetic engineers learn to retool supergenes and slow the rate of aging.*
- *Fetal brain cell transplants revive victims of paralysis, stroke, and Alzheimer's disease.*
- *The entire brain can be replaced, section by section, and made new.*

=Access Guide=

Life Extension Foundation
2835 Hollywood Boulevard
Hollywood, FL 33020
(800) 327-6110

Publishes *Life Extension Report*, sells life extension drugs and literature, and offers information on doctors practicing life extension medicine.

Harry Demopoulos
Health Maintenance Program
14 Madison Avenue
Valhalla, NY 10595
(914) 592-3155
1 (800) DOCTORD (out of state)

Antioxidant distributor.

Duke Center for the Study of Aging
Box 3003
Durham, NC 27710
(919) 684-2248 or 684-3654

Carrying on several clinical studies ranging from depression to the effects of neuropeptides on Alzheimer's disease. Will accept patients and exceptional subjects. Has a good public information office.

Waneen Spirduso
Department of Physicial and Health Education
University of Texas at Austin
Austin, TX 78712
(512) 471-1273

Conducting systematic clinical studies on the effects of exercise on aging and the brain.

John Holloszy
Director of Applied Physiology in Dept. of Medicine
Washington University Medical School
St. Louis, Missouri 63110
(314) 362-2344

Conducts frequent clinical studies on the effects of exercise on aging.

Arnold Lippa
Natrix Research
North Academic Complex 7-232
City College of New York
New York, NY 10031
(212) 368-7474

Produces active lipids to refluidize cell membrane and provides information on clinical research.

Norman Applezweig
Progenics
442 West 44th Street
New York, NY 10036
(212) 265-0653

Developing DHEA compounds and conducting clinical tests in Europe.

George Washington University School of Medicine
Department of Biochemistry
2300 I Street Northwest
Washington, D.C. 20037
(202) 676-3171

Conducts frequent clinical studies on effects of thymosin on cancer, rheumatoid arthritis, and AIDS.

William Hazzard
Blalock 1007
The Johns Hopkins Hospital
600 North Wolfe Street
Baltimore, MD 21205
(301) 955-8131

Experimenting with new forms of estrogen therapy in an effort to narrow the longevity gap between men and women. Receptive to questioning on estrogen therapy. Will help those interested in clinical participation.

American Paralysis Association
7655 Old Springline Road, No. 104
McLean, VA 22102
(703) 556-7782

Keeps an eye on latest developments in the field of fetal cell transplant.

American Longevity Association
1000 West Carson Street
Torance, CA 90509
(213) 533-2233

Scientists and lay persons interested in the acceleration of research programs which study the mechanisms of aging.

American Foundation for Aging Research
117 Tucker Hall
University of Missouri
Columbia, MO 65211
(314) 882-6426

Funds basic research and education opportunities for the study of age-related diseases and biology of aging. Awards scholarships and grants in aging research.

Denham Harmon American Aging Association
College of Medicine
University of Nebraska
Omaha, NE 68105
(402) 559-4416

Dedicated to "helping people live better, longer" by promoting biomedical studies directed toward slowing the aging process.

National Cancer Institute
9000 Rockville Pike
Bethesda, MD (301) 496-4000

Conducts frequent clinical studies, particularly on effects of antioxidants on cancer.

Gerontological Research Center
National Institute on Aging
National Institute of Health
4940 Eastern Avenue
Baltimore, MD 21224
(301) 955-1707

Federal agency that oversees research on aging.

Richard Hochschild
Hoch Company
2915 Pebble Drive
Corona Del Mar, CA 92625
(714) 759-8066

Sells the H-Scan, a machine that can help ascertain one's "true," or biological, age.

Longevity
OMNI Publications
1965 Broadway
New York, NY 10023
(212) 496-6100

A monthly newsletter designed to be a practical guide to staying young.

14

The Last
Whole Body Catalog

As we assembled this almanac, we constantly came across medical breakthroughs—or research in progress—that didn't fit neatly under any of the previous chapter heads. This research raised some interesting questions. For example, will ant venom one day be accepted as the best treatment for lupus and rheumatoid arthritis? Will tryptophan, an amino acid found in milk, replace synthetic painkillers? Will the application of sugar or honey to a wound be the preferred treatment for burns? Rather than discard such potentially valuable medical news items because they defy conventional classification, we include them here in a final Last Whole Body Catalog. We cannot promise that the following therapies, medicines, or procedures will become standard practice in the future, but they are worth your scrutiny.

Breathing Easier

Emphysema sufferers often look forward to nothing better than a slow and tortured death by long-term asphyxiation. But at West Hollywood Hospital in Los Angeles, a surgical procedure called *bilateral carotid body resection* makes patients breathe easier. By removing two small glands—the carotid bodies—from the neck, the surgeon frees good lung tissue that had previously been blocked.

This procedure is considered so controversial that West Hollywood's Benjamin Winter is the only surgeon in the country who performs the operation. Many lung specialists contend that the carotid bodies are responsible for monitoring blood levels of oxygen and carbon dioxide. The removal of these glands can make the patient unaware that he or she is short of oxygen. Winter, who has successfully performed 1,600 of these operations, counters by citing research that shows that oxygen- and carbon dioxide-monitoring functions are carried on primarily in the brain, so that the removal of the carotid bodies presents no danger to the patient.

"The real reason other doctors won't do it," says Dr. Winter, "is that Medicare and the insurance companies won't cover the cost of this operation." Winter has filed suit against the insurance establishment to force them to pay, and the suit is now being heard in California. "If we win, surgeons all over the country will be performing this operation," he adds.

Bucktoothed Kids

Most people with buckteeth owe their overbites to underdeveloped jawbones—not the position of the teeth themselves. As a result, efforts to correct the problem with standard braces often prove unsatisfactory. Now, bucktoothed children are finding that a simple device developed in Germany some 30 years ago can actually change the shape of their jaws. Named after its inventor, Dr. Rolf Frankel, the *Frankel appliance* is made of stainless steel wire and acrylic. The appliance, worn most of the day, reminds the child to hold the jaw in a forward position. This effort strengthens the jaw muscles, and when the muscles are working well, the bone grows normally. If the Frankel appliance is used for 18 to 24 months, conventional braces need be worn for less than a year to adjust the position of the teeth. The device is available from the Foundation for Craniofacial Research, 555 Peachtree Dunubody Road, Suite 301, Atlanta, Georgia 33342 (contact Dr. Michael Dierkes).

Knifeless Face-Lifts

People who want a face-lift but would prefer to avoid a surgeon's scalpel now may have a tooth lift. New York City dentist Irwin Smigel invented the procedure he calls "plastic surgery without a scalpel" and teaches it nationwide. Smigel "plumps" the back tooth on each side of a patient's mouth or inserts a similarly raised denture. This technique, Smigel explains, "raises the cheekbones, softens radial lines that run from the corner of the nose to the edge of the lips, and gives the face a balanced appearance."

The procedure takes about an hour to perform on each tooth. Smigel developed the procedure after finding he could eliminate "denture look" by building out the plastic base of the denture to compensate for bone sinking. Although Smigel cautions that the procedure, for various reasons, is not for everyone, the dental face-lifts are available in most major cities.

Pollen Cure

Hay fever sufferers are finding relief from spring-summer allergy problems by using *local nasal immunotherapy (LNIT)*. LNIT patients inhale gradually increasing doses of pollen extracts, starting 8 weeks before the onset of the hay fever season. In trials since 1979, extracted pollen in various forms and strengths has proved effective in desensitizing patients, according to a research team at the State University of New York at Buffalo. "We are now working out appropriate dosing, but the treatment provides a convenient, effective, relatively inexpensive alternative to the conventional series of injections now used," says immunologist Robert Reisman.

Pain Free, Naturally

Tryptophan, an amino acid found in milk, is nature's sleep inducer. Now, research indicates that tryptophan is a painkiller as well. Dr. Samuel Seltzer and his colleagues at Temple University's Maxillofacial Pain Control Center have been experimenting with tryptophan to see if it can raise pain resistance. The Temple team concentrated on 30 patients who were troubled by head and neck pain, including migraine, arthritis, and several types of neuralgia. Test results show that tryptophan, when combined with a low-protein, low-fat, high-carbohydrate diet is effective as a pain reliever. It stimulates the brain's production of serotonin, a neurotransmitter thought to be involved in regulation of sleep, antidepressant activity, and now analgesia.

Short-Circuiting Migraines

Medical science may be on the verge of a breakthrough in the treatment of migraine headaches. Using a class of drugs known as *calcium channel blockers*, John Meyer and Jeffrey Hardenburg, of Baylor University in Waco, Texas, and the Veterans Administration Medical Center in Houston, have been able to "significantly reduce" migraines in up to 90 percent of their patients.

Calcium channel blockers stop the movement of calcium ions across the cell membranes of smooth muscle tissue in the blood vessels. Because calcium ions are at least partially responsible for constricting blood vessels, cutting those ions off at the pass, as it were, allows the blood vessels to open again. That's where migraine comes in. The headache itself is preceded by constriction of blood vessels in the head. The pain begins when those vessels open again and fill rapidly with blood. The researchers reasoned that if the constriction phase could be short-circuited with calcium channel blockers, the migraine itself could be stopped before it started.

Tests with hundreds of sufferers showed that Meyer and Hardenburg were right. Of the four calcium channel blockers used in double blind experiments, "the best is nimodipine (Nimotop), because it's designed specifically for blood vessels in the head," Meyer says. Side effects of nimodipine are minor: slight constipation in some patients or mild muscle cramping in women. Nimodipine is undergoing final approval by the Food and Drug Administration and will be distributed by Miles Laboratory. Scientists in the United States and Europe have been testing calcium channel blockers and have confirmed the effectiveness of several of them.

Dry Mouth

Thousands of people are unable to salivate because they suffer from xerostomia (dry mouth), a condition that makes eating and speaking difficult and can also lead to oral health problems.

Now there's relief in the form of an artificial saliva called *MOI-STIR*, which works by creating a lubricating film in the mouth. The film holds water against the tissue in the mouth and lasts 1 to 2 hours. Designed for patients with radiation-damaged salivary glands, it can also relieve dry mouth caused by surgery near the salivary glands, certain medications, and Sjogren-Larsson syndrome, which dries up a person's saliva, tears, and (sometimes) gastrointestinal juices.

MOI-STIR is approved by the Council on Dental Therapeutics of the American Dental Association and is available at local pharmacies. Two other products, MOI-STIR 10 Throat Spray and MOI-STIR Oral Swabsticks, have been developed recently. MOI-STIR 10 protects the mucous membranes in the throat and acts as a voice lubricant. It was specifically designed for professional singers, entertainers, and speakers. By protecting the larynx from dryness, esophagitis, and other conditions, it allows these people to use their voices without risk from damaging stresses. Inquiries may be directed to Kingswood Laboratories, Inc., P.O. Box 744, Carmel, Indiana 46032; (317) 846-7452.

Innovative Hearing

There are approximately 12 million Americans who suffer from mild to moderate hearing loss due to a variety of causes: aging, environmental exposure to noise, heredity, congenital abnormalities, physical damage, and disease. Many of these persons have great difficulty hearing clearly in the presence of background noise, particularly at restaurants, parties, or meetings.

Innovaid 600 is a clear plastic bubble—the size of the end of a man's thumb—with a pencil-thin hole in it. The bubble, designed by Richard L. Goode, professor of surgery at Stanford University, outperforms electronic hearing aids for people who have partial hearing loss. This is because it boosts frequencies in the range of the voice—1000 to 2500 cycles per second (cps)—without amplifying background noise.

The 10- to 15-decibel improvement is about the same as the effect produced by a hand cupped against the head. It occurs because the device, which is individually fitted to—and nestles inside—the helix of the ear, changes the opening size and volume of the cavity, shifting its resonant frequency downward from the 4000-cps range to the 2800-cps range. This minimizes perceptions of the higher-frequency background sounds. The device works better than more powerful electronic aids because it "selects" vocal sounds and "ignores" noise.

The Innovaid 600, manufactured by Innovative Hearing Corporation, San Francisco, California (415) 863-1111, is available through professional dispensing practices around the country.

Sweet Treatment

Putting sugar or honey on a wound is an old folk remedy. After 10 years of research, Dr. Richard Knutson's slightly revised version of the folk treatment has proved effective on 3,000 patients, including 800 burn patients. Initially, Knutson, who works out of the Delta Medical Center in Greenville, Mississippi, tried the remedy on an elderly patient's bedsore at the suggestion of a nurse. "The ulcer went clear to the bone and wouldn't respond to conventional treatment," Knutson recalls. "I knew I couldn't make it any worse; so I tried sugar, and a day and a half later we had clean tissue and no infection. This primitive medicine beat the hell out of everything we knew to use."

Knutson's experiments show that ordinary granulated table sugar combined with providone iodine works best. In addition to helping sugar adhere to the wound, providone iodine has antibacterial and antifungal properties that speed the pace of healing. Powdered and brown sugars contain starches that neutralize the effect of the iodine against the bacteria and fungi. Note: Plain iodine is an extremely harsh substance on exposed tissue; it truly destroys certain cells.

The treatment provides low-cost healing for deep wounds, burns, and bedsores. It has an enormous impact on the cost of treating wounds, and it allows skin to cover even large wounds, such as those made by a shotgun blast. "Since we've discovered the sugar treatment," Knutson says, "our use of antibiotics is 10 percent of normal." Knutson suspects the sugar treatment works because it provides nutrients to surface cells, promoting rapid tissue growth in the wounds.

Development of a stable medication is being pursued; one will be introduced in Western Europe and Scandinavia within the next 2 years.

Anti-inflammatory Drug

Tests at the University of Miami in Florida have shown that a Bolivian ant's venom can cause a 2- to 3-year remission of rheumatoid arthritis. Bolivian Indians have been using the venom of this ant, a member of the genus *Pseudomyrmexm*, to treat arthritis for generations.

During the first phase of research, the Miami doctors injected the natural venom into volunteers at the rate of a milliliter a day for 14 days. "It's very impressive," researcher Duane Schultz comments. "The medicine is taken for 2 weeks, and 6 months later most of the patients are doing well." The researchers have developed a purified extract of the natural venom and have successfully treated patients with chronic active hepatitis. "It's our feeling now," Schultz says, "that this material is a general anti-inflammatory drug. We are going to be testing more diseases, such as lupus, in which inflammation is the characteristic symptom."

Male Infertility

Elevated testicular temperature often plays a crucial role in male infertility. A jockstrap called the *testicular hypothermia device* (*THD*), may help thousands of infertile couples to conceive by cooling overheated testicles.

The sperm-producing cells in the testicles require temperatures lower than the overall normal body temperature to multiply properly—which is why testicles hang outside the body. The blood entering the genitals in the arteries is normally cooled by an exchange of heat with chillier blood returning in the nearby veins.

In perhaps as many as 75 percent of men with fertility problems, this exchange doesn't take place because the blood in the veins flows the wrong way. Some of these men have a condition called a varicocele, an enlarged vein that twists around the testicles. In others, no varicocele can be identified, but the temperature of the blood is elevated anyway, adversely affecting the number, motility, and shape of the sperm.

Physically the THD consists of a cotton pouch fitted around the genitals and kept cool by the controlled evaporation of distilled water via a constant pressure pump with a metering device. As evaporation occurs, scrotal temperature decreases by about 2 degrees Celsius—producing a more suitable temperature for sperm maturation.

The device is available by prescription and marketed by Repro-Med Systems, Inc., 713 North Street, Middletown, New York 10940; 1 (800) 637-9990.

Allergy Consult

The uncomfortable and often costly scratch test for allergies, which may require 45 to 90 needles, in many cases can now be replaced by a simple blood test called *Arest*. A modification of the *Radio-AllergoSorption Test* (*RAST*), the Arest program uses radioisotopes and gamma-ray counters to measure extremely low levels of antibodies in a patient's blood.

Arest screens for a variety of common allergens: pollens, grasses, danders, dust, and several food groups. The Arest Patient Management System provides diagnostic and toll free scientific consultation and individually formulated therapeutics for the allergy patient. Call 1 (800) ALLERGY. Consultation for asthma patients on theophylline is also available: 1 (800) 4-CONSULT.

Healing Bubbles

Manufacturers in the United States and abroad are now producing surgical dressings made from polyurethane that not only lack the adhesive strip's shortcomings but actually promote healing and cost less, too. The adhesive bandage has many drawbacks: It keeps healing oxygen and moisture away from the wound, it kills all skin under the adhesive, and it rips out hair when it's removed.

The new bandages have the stretch and consistency of plastic food wrap, although they are opaque, and come in all sizes from 1-inch squares to large sheets of several feet. A protective paper backing peels off to expose an underside completely coated with adhesive material that does not stick to injured skin. When applied over a wound, the dressing forms a bubble that looks like a blister.

The reason for the dramatic difference between the new dressing and the adhesive bandage is that the bubble breathes. Because oxygen is allowed to reach the wound, a greater number of bacteria-eating white blood cells are attracted to defend the wound site against infection. And because there is no gauze covering to clog the blood, clots are smaller and can be broken down more rapidly as new skin grows. But the nonadhesive characteristic of the new bandages is the biggest advantage. When removed, adhesive materials reinjure the wound.

While the new bandages are now only marketed for hospitals, they will be available for consumers in the near future. Johnson and Johnson makes *Bioclusive*; 3-M makes *Tegaderm*; Smith and Nephew, in England, produces *Op-Site*.

Titanium Teeth

When most people lose their teeth, their gums and jawbones begin to shrink, and many of them can no longer chew properly or speak clearly with conventionally replaced dentures. These problems now can be corrected by a new implantation technique—which is good news for 30 million Americans who are totally or partially toothless.

"In the past, efforts to replace teeth with dental implants—devices that attached replacement teeth to gums or bones in the mouth—met with limited success," says New York City periodontist Stuart J. Froum. In fact the risk of bone deterioration and infection was so great that most dentists abandoned the notion of implantation and relied chiefly on the conventional denture.

That is no longer necessary due to refinements in the *osseointegrated technique*, which involves the surgical implantation of small, pure titanium screws into the jawbone while the patient is under local anesthesia. The titanium molecules actually bond with the bone cells in the jaw, anchoring the screws—five for a full denture, two for a partial bridge—and providing a solid foundation for the patient's artificial teeth.

Because the titanium is compatible with body tissue, there is far less chance of infection than with other implants. After a 3- to 6-month healing period is completed, the titanium screws are topped with cylinders to which the artificial teeth are attached, and then the patient is fitted with a semipermanent bone-anchored bridge.

The procedure is currently available at five dental facilities around the country, including the Mayo Clinic, as well as from such trained practitioners as Froum. For further information, contact Nobelpharma USA, Inc., P.O. Box 9051, Waltham, Massachusetts 02254–9051.

Heart Patches

For those who suffer from angina pectoris, climbing stairs, running, even a brisk walk, can keep oxygen from the heart and inflict stabbing chest pain. But now angina sufferers can step up their physical activities without suffering, thanks to an adhesive patch called *Transderm-Nitro*. The patch, worn on the chest, allows continuous absorption of nitroglycerin through the skin.

Nitroglycerin has long been used to expand the coronary arteries and relieve angina pain. A standard pill under the tongue provides a blast of nitroglycerin into the bloodstream within a minute, but the effect is short-lived—15 to 20 minutes. Transderm-Nitro, however, delivers a steady, low dose that minimizes the side effect of the standard medication—splitting headaches. Nitroglycerin goes through the mucous membranes directly to the bloodstream, providing immediate relief to the angina patient. The patch is convenient, and it improves patients' quality of life. They can pursue daily activities without having to carry or take medication.

Two other patches are available from Ciba-Geigy. *Transderm Scop*, which is worn behind the ear for 3 days, relieves motion sickness. The *Estraderm* patch relieves menopausal symptoms. The patches are available by prescription.

Bioptic Lenses

Electrical engineer David Green voluntarily gave up driving due to a serious eye condition that had severely limited his vision. He no longer felt safe behind the wheel. His visual loss also cost him his job, which required enormous precision and dexterity. But now corrective glasses and an attached telescopic lens allow Green to see clearly enough to reconsider driving and to enroll in vocational rehabilitation classes.

The new device, called the *bioptic telescope*, offers improved vision through two sources—the telescope, which contains 14 magnifying lenses, and the corrective glasses themselves. When wearers need to magnify an object just a bit, they look through the glasses; when more magnification is required, they simply dip their heads and look through the telescope.

According to Randall Jose of the University of Houston College of Optometry, bioptic lenses are appropriate for individuals with good peripheral vision who have trouble with details like newspaper type. Approximately 1500 people nationwide were fitted with bioptic lenses last year, and many have been able to drive safely again. Twenty-four states currently issue driver's licenses to low-vision individuals wearing bioptic lenses. The lenses are manufactured by Designs for Vision, in New York City. "We are making two improvements on the lenses right now," says Jose. "We have a prototype that is cosmetically more acceptable. Instead of attaching the telescope to the front of the glasses, we have miniaturized the lenses to fit behind the glasses. The device is better looking. And, a new focusing system allows the wearer to adjust for distance or for close work by turning a screw on the lenses."

Healing Toxin

The toxin that causes botulism is one of the deadliest poisons known. Every so often the toxin, botulin, turns up in canned foods. When ingested, the substance heads straight for the nervous system. There it inhibits release of the chemical acetylcholine, which in turn prevents the muscles from contracting.

So when San Francisco ophthalmologist Alan Scott began looking for a way to end the muscle spasms that cause crossed eyes, he naturally thought of botulin. He thought it might be just the substance to help the skewed eye muscles to relax. Working at the Smith-Kettlewell Eye Research Foundation in conjunction with Dr. Edward Schantz, an authority on the toxin, Scott and other investigators injected minute amounts of botulin into the eye muscles of over 3000 strabismic (cross-eyed) patients, many of whom had undergone unsuccessful eye surgery. The results, he says, were overwhelmingly positive.

"In most cases," Scott says, "it took several weeks and two or three injections to realign the eyes, but the procedure was less traumatic than surgery and essentially painless."

Scott also has successfully treated 1,800 patients suffering from blepharospasm, a disorder characterized by an involuntary closure of the eyelid, and other conditions, including spasmatic torticollis of the neck, cerebral palsy, and other disorders characterized by spastic or contracted muscles.

The drug is safe and will be widely available in the next few months.

Blood-Clotting Aid

Thromb-Aid is a bandage that dramatically accelerates blood clotting and stops capillary bleeding within 30 seconds. Developed by hematologist John Altshuler of the University of Colorado, Thromb-Aid is a gauze pad saturated with beef thrombin, a blood-clotting protein similar to one produced by humans. The thrombin converts a blood protein called fibrinogen to a jellylike substance known as fibrin. Fibrin is the meshwork that constitutes the structure of a normal blood clot.

The new bandage will be important for hemophiliacs, whose bodies do not produce normal levels of thrombin near the surface of a cut. In case of an accident in which a major artery has been severed, however, the bandage will be ineffective, because the very high pressure in these larger vessels prevents clot formation.

Thrombin has long been recognized as a clotting agent, but its shelf life of 48 hours prevented widespread use. Altshuler, however, discovered that if he added a glycerin-based solution to thrombin, it could be stored for 1 year under refrigeration.

The FDA has approved Thromb-Aid for prescription use, and it will be available in the near future.

Index